Oncology Nursing in Practice

Edited by
JANICE GABRIEL

MPhil, PgD, BSc(Hons), RGN, FETC, ONC, Cert.MHS
Lead Nurse, Cancer Services
Portsmouth Hospitals NHS Trust

W
WHURR PUBLISHERS
LONDON AND PHILADELPHIA

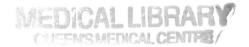
© 2001 Whurr Publishers
First published 2001 by
Whurr Publishers Ltd
19b Compton Terrace, London N1 2UN, England and
325 Chestnut Street, Philadelphia PA 1906, USA

British Library Cataloguing in Publication Data
A catalogue record for this book is available from the British
Library.

ISBN: 1 8615 6 165 2   1002116240

Printed and bound in the UK by Athenaeum Press Ltd,
Gateshead, Tyne & Wear

Contents

Contributors   viii

Preface   x

Introduction   xi

PART 1

Chapter 1   1

Cancer: health promotion, early detection and staging
Janice Gabriel

PART 2

Chapter 2   11

Understanding radiotherapy and its applications
Antony Palmer

Chapter 3   30

Understanding cytotoxic chemotherapy
Janice Gabriel

PART 3

Chapter 4   51

Breast cancer
Carmel Sheppard

Chapter 5   71

Colorectal cancer
Janie Whittaker

Chapter 6   **91**

Lung cancer
Christine Fehrenbach

Chapter 7   **102**

Gynaecological cancers
Tracey Wilson

Chapter 8   **122**

Skin cancers
Janice Gabriel

Chapter 9   **138**

Haematological malignancies
Joanne Todd

Chapter 10   **169**

Urological cancers
Audrey Hayward

Chapter 11   **193**

Head and neck malignancies
Kay Howard

Chapter 12   **212**

Childhood cancers
Ruth Sadik

PART 4

Chapter 13   **231**

Fungating tumours
Sylvia Hampton

Chapter 14   **246**

Nutritional support
Jo Hunt

Chapter 15   **265**

Infection control issues
Sarah Balchin

Chapter 16   **296**

Body image and sexuality
Janie Whittaker
Carmel Sheppard

PART 5

Chapter 17   **308**

Complementary therapies
Derek John Ace

Chapter 18   **311**

Pain control in palliative care
Wendy Young

Chapter 19   **328**

Breaking bad news
Wendy Young

References   **333**
Useful addresses/support groups   **350**
Index   **355**

Contributors

Derek John Ace, BEd, MIFA, Cert Ed, RCNT, RMN, RGN
Senior Lecturer, School of Health Studies, University of Portsmouth

Sarah Balchin, BA (Hons), RN
Associate Nurse Director, Portsmouth Hospitals NHS Trust

Christine Fehrenbach, RGN
Respiratory Nurse Specialist, Portsmouth Hospitals NHS Trust

Sylvia Hampton, BSc (Hons), Dip SN, RGN
Tissue Viability Nurse Specialist, Eastbourne Hospitals NHS Trust

Audrey Hayward, BSc (Hons), RGN, Dipl Nursing (London), FEATC
Continence Nurse Advisor (formerly Urology Course Teacher),
Urology Department, St Mary's Hospital, Portsmouth

Kay Howard, BA (Hons), RGN, Diploma Professional Studies in
Nursing
formerly Macmillan Head and Neck Specialist Nurse, University
Hospital, Queens Medical Centre, Nottingham

Jo Hunt, RGN, BSc (Hons)
Sister, Intestinal Failure Unit, St. Mark's Hospital, Middx

Antony Palmer, BSc, MSc, DipIPEM, MIPEM
Clinical Scientist, Radiotherapy Physics, Medical Physics Department, Portsmouth Hospitals NHS Trust

Ruth Sadik, MSc, BA (Hons), RSCN, RGN, RNT, Cert Ed (FE)
Child Branch Co-ordinator, School of Health Studies, University of Portsmouth

Carmel Sheppard, BSc (Hons), MSc, RGN
Breast Care Nurse Specialist, Portsmouth Hospitals NHS Trust

Joanne Todd, BSc, RGN
Senior Lead Nurse/Service Manager, Suffolk Cancer Centre, Ipswich Hospital NHS Trust

Janie Whittaker, BSc (Hons), RGN
Clinical Nurse Specialist, Stoma Care, Portsmouth Hospitals NHS Trust

Tracey Wilson, DPSN, RGN, ENG
Staff Nurse, Lincoln County Hospital

Wendy Young, MSc, RGN, Cert Ed, RNT, PG DipEd
Hospice Tutor, Earl Mountbatten Hospice, Newport, Isle of Wight

Preface

Although the speciality of oncology nursing is covered by an array of books, many are very specialized and fail to address the needs of the student or newly qualified nurse caring for patients with cancer. This book addresses the main areas of cancer nursing, taking into account recent Department of Health publications and recommendations, and drawing upon the knowledge and experience of specialist cancer nurses.

It is primarily intended to be an informative text for students and newly qualified nurses. However, it will also be a useful reference book for nurses already working in the speciality to update their knowledge, and for students undertaking oncology or palliative care courses such as ENB 237, ENB 931, etc.

The aims and objectives of this book are:

- To describe what cancer is, its disease process and predisposing factors for developing certain types of malignant conditions
- To define how radiotherapy and cytotoxic chemotherapy work to combat this group of diseases
- To focus on caring for patients with site-specific malignancies, taking into account the range of problems an individual with a diagnosis of cancer could face, e.g. psychosocial, altered body image, etc.
- To enable nurses working in the speciality of oncology to keep abreast of developments that can influence their patients' care.

Introduction

This book is written for nurses by nurses. It will focus not on the medical models of managing a patient with cancer, but on meeting the needs of cancer patients and their families by helping nurses to understand the disease process, and the impact the disease and its treatment can have on individuals.

This book is not designed to overwhelm the reader with excessive information on the disease process, but to illustrate how the needs of individual patients with site-specific cancers can be met. Each site-specific chapter addresses the pathology, investigation and management of each malignancy, but emphasis is placed upon how potential problems can be prevented, alleviated or solved by the nurse. Each chapter concludes with some case histories of how patients with specific problems were managed. It is intended that these examples will illustrate the theoretical points addressed by the authors of the chapter on site-specific cancers, with particular emphasis on nursing care.

No attempt has been made to cover every oncological condition, as some conditions are rare. While patients may be diagnosed at their local hospital, further investigations and management may well be undertaken at a specialist centre. Some of the patients with these types of rare malignant conditions may well be part of a clinical trial, and not receiving 'standard' treatment. Consequently their inclusion in this text could cause confusion for those nurses not familiar with the current care of such groups of patients. This book will concentrate on the patients who present with cancer at their local cancer unit or cancer centre.

The text is divided into five main sections. Section one provides the reader with a definition of cancer and explains how a malignant lesion differs from a benign one. It also discusses the epidemiology of cancer, taking into account the results of recent epidemiological studies, including the effects of genetic susceptibility, lifestyle, diet, occupational exposure, etc. This section concludes by discussing what staging of a patient's cancer involves and why it is important in relation to treatment options.

The second part of the text looks at the main treatment options for patients with cancer. It discusses what radiotherapy is and the types of radiotherapy that can be used to treat different types of malignancies, including curative and palliative regimens. This section also looks at cytotoxic chemotherapy, its clinical indications, methods of administration, etc.

The third section consists of nine chapters dealing with site-specific malignancies. It is intended that each of these chapters will not only address the treatment for the specific stage of the patient's disease, but address the potential problems associated with the disease and its treatment, e.g. lymphoma, psychosocial problems, etc. Each of these chapters concludes with case histories to help identify to the nurse the holistic care available to individual patients.

The fourth section looks at specific problems that can be encountered by the cancer patient, e.g. management of fungating wounds, nutritional problems, infection susceptibility, altered body image and sexuality problems.

The final section deals with complementary therapies and their integration into the main framework of cancer treatments. Pain control, the spiritual/cultural aspects of cancer, and the complex issue of breaking bad news are also addressed in this section.

It is not intended that this text will be read through in its entirety at one sitting, but that it will be used by students as a basic oncology nursing textbook to support them throughout their training. It is also intended to support the newly qualified nurse caring for a patient with a specific cancer or cancer-related problem.

The philosophy of this book is to provide clear, up-to-date practical support and information for students and newly qualified nurses. It is hoped that it will encourage discussion on the rapidly developing and changing area of cancer nursing, thereby influencing the care of the patient with a diagnosis of cancer.

Chapter 1
Cancer: health promotion, early detection and staging

Janice Gabriel

Introduction

It is estimated that one in three people in the United Kingdom (UK) will develop a malignancy by the age of 70. This equates to approximately 270,000 individuals receiving a cancer diagnosis each year (Cornwell, 1997). The UK incidence of cancer is expected to increase, affecting one in two of the population in the next 25 years (Cornwell, 1997).

This chapter will look at the definition of cancer and discuss how this group of diseases differs from benign growths. It will also address the predisposing risk factors for the development of some malignant conditions and the steps that can be taken to eliminate, or minimize, the risk to individuals and specific groups of people. It will also consider the importance of 'staging' an individual's cancer in order to ensure that he or she is offered the most appropriate treatment.

The definition of cancer

Cancer is a generic term, encompassing a group of diseases characterized by the unregulated growth and spread of cells. That is, a mass of tumour cells will not only grow uncontrollably locally, but cells can spread to other parts of the body via the lymphatic system and bloodstream, creating secondary deposits known as 'metastases' (BMA, 1997). The overgrowth of these cells is controlled by mutated genes, which cause subsequent generations of cells to become malignant (BMA, 1997). Every cell in our body requires a 'blueprint' in order to replicate itself. This 'blueprint' is known as a gene. Genes are a collection of *codons* which can be found in deoxyribonucleic acid (DNA) and ribonucleic acid (RNA). If the gene becomes damaged, mutation can occur (Davies, 1978).

Possible causes of cancer

As a society becomes more affluent, so the incidence of cancer increases. There could be a number of reasons for this, including the fact that increased wealth and improved healthcare enable individuals to live longer. People are also surviving previously life-threatening illnesses, such as infectious diseases, major accidents, etc., only to live longer and develop cancer. We also know that more affluent societies consume higher amounts of convenience foods, alcohol and tobacco, and are exposed to higher levels of chemicals and pollutants compared with people living in some third world countries. All of these factors can contribute to an individual developing a malignancy (Venitt ,1978; Cartmel and Reid, 1993). Other factors include past exposure to radiation, viruses and a genetic predisposition (Cartmel and Reid, 1993).

Diet

Cartmel and Reid (1993) discuss how modifying an individual's diet can greatly contribute to reducing the incidence of colorectal cancer. In Europe it is estimated that a third of all cancers are directly linked to diet. So what are the causal links believed to be?

In 1990, Trock et al. highlighted a possible link between a diet that was low in fibre and an increased risk of developing colon cancer. It is now widely accepted that a diet high in animal fats can also be a contributing factor to this particular type of cancer (Cartmel and Reid, 1993). Gillis, writing as long ago as 1978, highlighted that the commonest predisposing factor for developing carcinoma of the large bowel is a low fibre, high animal fat diet. Diet is linked not only to colorectal cancer, but also to breast cancer (Armstrong and Doll, 1975).

Alcohol

A number of cancers are believed to be linked directly to an individual's alcohol consumption (Gillis, 1978; Cartmel and Reid, 1993). These can include carcinomas of the:

- oral cavity
- larynx
- oesophagus
- liver
- stomach
- colon and rectum

With the exception of colorectal cancer, the other malignancies listed above are strongly linked to the consumption of large amounts of alcoholic spirits (Gillis, 1978). Colorectal cancer can be linked to excessive consumption of beer in some individuals (Cartmel and Reid, 1993).

Tobacco

While smoking unquestionably contributes significantly to the development of a range of malignant conditions, it must not be forgotten that tobacco can be consumed in a variety of ways (Cartmel and Reid, 1993). These can include chewing, sniffing and inhalation from passive smoking, as well as inhalation from active smoking. The malignant conditions linked to the use of/exposure to tobacco can include:

- small cell carcinoma of the lung
- oropharyngeal cancer
- bladder cancer
- cervical cancer
- gastric cancer
- lip cancer

Lung cancer is the commonest cancer affecting men and women in the UK. Although its prevalence is declining in men, it is still rising in the female population (Gillis, 1978). This is not a pattern solely confined to the UK, as the incidence of smoking-related lung cancers is not expected to peak among American women until 2010 (Cartmel and Reid, 1993). Studies in both the

United States of America (USA) and the UK indicate that, despite the publicity linked to cigarette smoking and cancer, the incidence of smoking is still rising among females from lower socioeconomic groups (Gillis, 1978; Cartmel and Reid, 1993).

Passive smoking is also linked to the development of cancer among non-smokers. There have been a number of litigation cases in the USA for compensation from individuals diagnosed with smoking-related cancers, who have had to share offices with smokers for many years (Fielding and Phenow, 1988).

In some parts of the world, notably India, cancer of the oral cavity accounts for a high percentage of all cancers registered annually. This high incidence is linked to the social habit of chewing quids of betel, lime and tobacco. The constant irritation to the tissues of the cheek and gum predispose the individual to developing a malignancy in this area (Gillis, 1978).

Bladder cancer, especially in the UK, is also closely linked to an individual's smoking habits (Gillis, 1978).

Viruses

Hausen (1991) suggested that up to 15% of cancers were linked to past viral exposure. These viruses and their possible resulting malignancies are listed in Table 1.1.

Table 1.1 Viruses linked to specific cancers

Virus	Cancer
Human papilloma virus	Cervical cancer
Hepatitis B & C	Hepatic cancer
Epstein-Barr virus	Burkitt's lymphoma
Human T-lymphotropic virus (HTLV 1)	T-Cell leukaemia/lymphoma
Human immunodeficiency virus (HIV)	Kaposi's sarcoma

Radiation

Today it is well recognized that exposure to ionizing radiation can have a carcinogenic effect on living cells, but this has not always been the case. Sadly, previous exposure to ionizing radiation, whether in small repeated doses or in one isolated incident, can predispose an individual to developing a cancer in later life (Walter, 1977). Individuals exposed to ionizing radiation can go on to develop a range of cancers, including haematological malignancies, thyroid cancer and squamous cell carcinoma of the skin (Venitt, 1978; Cartmel and Reid, 1993).

Radiation is naturally occurring, as it is found all around us in our everyday life. Consequently, the commonest cause of carcinomas of the skin is ultraviolet radiation (Cartmel and Reid, 1993) (see Chapter 8).

Chemicals / other agents

As long ago as 1775, Percival Pot, a London surgeon, described the link between cancer of the scrotum and chimney sweeps' boys. This was probably one of the first occupational malignant diseases reported (Walter, 1977).

Today it is well recognized that exposure to a number of chemicals, many of which are used in industry, are linked to developing or giving a predisposition to certain malignant conditions (these are summarized in Table 1.2). For individuals who do encounter occupational exposure to agents such as asbestos, aniline dyes, etc., there is legislation to ensure that their exposure is minimized and their health is regularly monitored (Cartmel and Reid, 1993).

Table 1.2 Past exposure to chemicals/agents linked to specific cancers

Chemical/agent	Cancer
Asbestos	Mesothelioma
Pitch, soot, coal tar, oil	Squamous cell carcinoma of the skin, scrotum
Vinyl chloride	Liver
Arsenic	Sinuses, lung
Benzidine	Bladder
Wood/leather dust	Nasal sinuses
Aniline dyes	Bladder

Pollution

As our society becomes more developed, so we consume more and generate more waste products which can lead to pollution. One example of pollution is the destruction of the ozone layer by chlorofluorocarbons (CFCs). The destruction of the ozone layer has led to an increase in ultraviolet light reaching the earth. Consequently, this is a contributing factor to the increase in the number of skin cancers (Cartmel and Reid, 1993) (see Chapter 8).

Genetics

While there are unquestionably a number of predisposing factors linked to an individual developing cancer, it is clear that some people are more susceptible than others. Many, if not all, healthcare professionals involved in caring for cancer patients over a prolonged period of time can recall families where a number of members have been treated for cancer. Medicine has now reached a stage where it can identify some gene defects that predispose family members to developing specific cancers. One example of a genetic predisposition to colorectal cancer is *familial adenomatous polyposis* (Walter, 1977). Another is retinoblastoma, a malignant condition where a child inherits a defective gene from one of its parents.

While medicine is making great advances in identifying defective genes that could give rise to cancer, the presence of one of these defects does not mean that an individual will inevitably develop the associated cancer. For this reason, it is important that any individual contemplating genetic testing receives adequate counselling before such a test is carried out. The repercussions of a positive test could affect an individual's eligibility for life insurance, health insurance, etc. It could also influence the individual's decision about starting a family, etc.

Health promotion

Health promotion needs to start at an early age, in order to have a maximum impact in reducing an individual's risk of developing cancer in later life. The overriding problem behind the success of any health promotion campaign is bringing about a change in an individual's lifestyle. As the majority of cancers take many years to develop, the targeted recipients of such campaigns fail to recognize, or indeed ignore, the message. An example of a difficult health promotion campaign is persuading teenagers/young adults of the associated risks of cigarette smoking. Teenagers often feel immortal, and what might happen to them 30 years down the road seems too far away to influence their lifestyle at the present time.

One example of a high-profile and effective health promotion campaign is that of raising the public's awareness of the associated risks of developing skin cancer. Today, many individuals are aware of the potential for developing skin cancer from exposure to the sun's ultraviolet radiation.

Cancer screening

It is important to be aware of the differences between the terms 'screening' and 'testing'. Screening is intended to look at large numbers of asymptomatic individuals in an attempt to identify a small number of positive cases. 'Testing' is a specific intention to eliminate or prove the cause of an individual's symptoms. Individuals included in a screening programme tend to have very generalized characteristics; for example, they fall into a specific age band, or are of the same sex. An example of one such programme is 'breast screening', i.e. women between the ages of 50 and 64 are regularly screened for signs of breast cancer in the UK.

The other important differences between screening and testing are the potential risk factors linked to the investigations, and their costs. A 'screening' investigation should be minimally invasive and not too uncomfortable, in order to ensure maximum 'take-up' by the target population. If the associated risk(s) linked to a screening programme were too high, it would not be practical, or indeed ethical, to offer it to large numbers of individuals where the incidence of cancer would be low. If an individual has a 'positive' screening result, it would not necessarily mean that a cancer had been identified. Individuals with 'positive' results would then go on to have a 'diagnostic' test. As they would then have an 'abnormality' to be investigated, the diagnostic test might cause them more discomfort or inconvenience when compared with the screening investigation (Chamberlain, 1978; Frank-Stromborg and Cohen, 1993). The purpose of the diagnostic test would be to confirm or eliminate the diagnosis of cancer.

As long ago as 1978, Chamberlain addressed the dilemma of the cost-effectiveness of cancer screening. Can society actually afford to offer expensive screening programmes for specific cancers, especially if there is no proven financial gain in treating that individual's cancer at an earlier stage?

There is also the psychological impact on the individual of

having a 'positive' screening result. Would the anxiety potentially generated by such a result be justified, only to be confirmed as a 'false-positive' some days or weeks later? Would a positive test result influence the long-term survival of the asymptomatic patient?

As cancer can develop over a period of years, and commonly present with increasing age, any screening programme has to be ongoing. Individuals do not have a 'one-off' investigation to provide them with a negative test for life (Chamberlain, 1978). Screening needs to be undertaken on a regular basis. The frequency with which individuals in a screening population need to be investigated depends upon the specific cancer being looked for, the sensitivity of the screening test, the compliance of the screening population, the potential number of treatable cancers identified and the costs involved.

Chamberlain (1978) emphasizes that a screening programme must not be viewed in isolation. She states that such programmes cannot meet their objectives unless they are supported by the services necessary to promptly investigate and act upon positive results.

Staging of disease

Once a patient has received a diagnosis of cancer, the treatment that he or she is offered will depend very much upon the histological features of the tumour, together with the extent of its spread. Other factors are also considered, such as the patient's general health and age (O'Mary, 1993).

The majority of solid tumours are 'staged' using the internationally recognized TNM classification system (UICC, 1978). The TNM classification system was introduced into clinical practice in the 1950s. It aims to ensure each individual patient is offered the most appropriate treatment for his or her cancer, depending upon its exact extent. It also aims to give an indication of the individual's prognosis, by ensuring that clinicians have standardized information when discussing specific patients' cases and their anticipated responses to treatment (UICC, 1978; O'Mary, 1993).

The TNM classification works by assessing the extent of the primary tumour, the involvement of the lymph glands and the presence of metastases (see Table 1.3) (UICC, 1978). A patient classified with a stage TIV disease commonly has a less favourable prognosis than a patient with a tumour classified as TI.

Table 1.3 TNM Classification System

T = Tumour size

e.g.

T0 – No evidence of primary tumour

TI, II, III & IV – number allocated to size of primary tumour.
I represents smallest size, ranging up to stage IV.

TX – minimum requirements to assess primary tumour unable to be met.

N = Regional lymph node involvement

e.g.

N0 – No evidence of regional lymph node involvement

NI, II, III & IV – number allocated to involvement of regional lymph nodes ranging
from I, confined to 1 group, up to IV, involving several groups.

NX – minimum requirements to assess regional lymph nodes unable to be met.

M = Distant metastases

e.g.

M0 – no evidence of distant metastatic spread.

MI – evidence of distant metastatic spread.

MX – minimum requirement to assess metastatic spread unable to be met.

NB: Example only. Not all stages applicable to some cancers.

The staging process will inevitably follow on from the initial diagnostic procedure. This can be a very frustrating time for patients. After all, they have been given a diagnosis of cancer and, unless the rationale for further investigations is explained, will often become anxious regarding the delay in the commencement of treatment. If a woman with a diagnosis of breast cancer is identified from the staging investigations as having liver metastases, it would not be appropriate to advise her to undergo mastectomy. The rationale is that the disease is no longer confined to the breast. On the other hand, if staging investigations demonstrate that a patient has a small carcinoma confined solely to his larynx, he may well be successfully treated with radiotherapy, and not have to undergo laryngectomy.

While the TNM classification system is commonly used throughout the world for solid tumours, other classification systems do exist. These include the 'Dukes' staging system for colorectal cancer and 'Clark's' classification for malignant melanomas.

For haematological malignancies the TNM classification system is not applicable because of the systemic nature of the diseases involved (O'Mary 1993). O'Mary (1993) lists a variety of classification systems for haematological malignancies, including:

- Hodgkin's and non-Hodgkin's – Ann Arbor classification
- Myeloblastic leukaemia – French–American–British classification
- Chronic lymphocytic leukaemia – Rai classification

Conclusions

Nurses can play an important role in reducing the numbers of individuals diagnosed with cancer. Through health education, our knowledge about diet, the dangers of tobacco and alcohol consumption, ultraviolet radiation, occupational exposure to hazardous substances, etc., we can help to bring about a change in people's lifestyles to minimize their risk of developing cancer in later life.

The one thing that those diagnosed with cancer have in common is fear and uncertainty about the future. Whatever the cause of an individual's cancer, the nurse will have a key role. Not only does he or she have the opportunity to participate actively in the treatment of the patient, but the nurse can provide psychological support, often over many years.

Chapter 2
Understanding radiotherapy and its applications

ANTONY PALMER

Introduction

An understanding of the basic principles of radiotherapy is of great benefit to those involved with the care and support of patients undergoing cancer treatment. This chapter will provide the necessary background knowledge in the therapeutic use of ionizing radiation.

A basic description of the physics of radiotherapy is presented in a manner that does not require a deep knowledge of mathematics, then a short history of radiotherapy is given. This is followed by a description of the biological effects of ionizing radiation, and a summary of radiotherapy treatment doses and regimes. Examples of the use of radiation for palliative and curative intent and the different types of radiotherapy are then described, followed by an explanation of how radiotherapy treatments are planned. The fundamentals of radiation protection to enable safe working in a radiotherapy department are also discussed. The chapter concludes with several case histories of patients who have undergone a variety of radiotherapy treatments.

The basics

To understand the procedures involved in radiotherapy, it is useful to have an appreciation of basic radiation physics. A little perseverance will provide an insight into many aspects of radiotherapy, from the fundamental principles of patient treatments to techniques of radiation safety. This section answers some commonly asked questions about radiation and gives uncomplicated explanations of terms that are frequently used in an oncology department, such as: *radiation, radioactivity, decay, half-life* and *inverse square law*.

What is radiation ?

Radiation is simply the means by which energy is transferred from a source to a location some distance away. This energy transfer may be in the form of waves or particles, neither of which can be directly seen or felt.

The waves, called electromagnetic radiation, travel in straight lines and are categorized in terms of their wavelength (the distance between crests of the wave). Examples include familiar waves such as radio waves, infrared (heat radiation), visible light, ultraviolet light, X-rays and γ (gamma) rays. These are listed in order of reducing wavelength and increasing energy. The electromagnetic radiations used in radiotherapy are X-rays and gamma-rays, which have very short wavelengths and high energies. In fact, these two types of radiation are exactly the same, with their names indicating only a differing origin. If the radiation comes from radioactive substances (see below) it is called gamma-ray, but if produced by electrical machines the waves are called X-ray. High energy X-rays are produced by machines with large generating voltages, megavoltage (MV) radiation, while lower energy X-rays come from kilovoltage (kV) equipment (Walter, 1977a).

Particulate radiation involves alpha (α) particles, beta (β) particles, electrons, neutrons or protons (Walter, 1977a). It is necessary to consider briefly the structure of matter to understand what these particles are. The atom is the basic building-block from which all solids, liquids and gases are composed, including our own bodies. The atom is extremely small, much too small to be seen by the eye, and so small that 100 million atoms side by side would occupy a length of 1 cm. Atoms consist of a small central nucleus containing protons and neutrons, with electrons moving around the nucleus in a similar way to planets moving around the sun. Beta particles are fast-moving electrons emitted by radioactive materials. Electrons produced in treatment machines are physically indistinguishable from beta particles but have higher energies. Alpha particles, which are the nuclei of helium atoms, are emitted from radioactive substances, but are of limited use in radiotherapy. Neutrons and protons require prohibitively expensive machinery for their production; such machines are available only in a very small number of institutions, mainly those involved in research.

What is ionizing radiation?

Some types of radiation have the ability to dislodge electrons from atoms. This process is called ionization. X-rays, gamma-rays and each of the particle radiations considered above are ionizing radiations. The nucleus of an atom has a positive electrical charge, balanced by an equal negative charge of the orbiting electrons. When ionizing radiation is absorbed, electrons are ejected from the atoms, leaving an unbalanced positive charge. The electron is caught by a neighbouring atom, which then becomes negatively charged. The positive and negative atoms are called ions. This ionization causes physical and chemical changes in living cells, which results in the biological effects (Stryker, 1992).

What is radioactivity and which materials are radioactive?

Matter can be broken down into roughly 100 different substances, called elements, such as oxygen, copper and lead. The chemical element of an atom is determined by the number of protons it contains. Atoms of a particular element with differing numbers of neutrons are called isotopes of the element. The total number of protons and neutrons in an atom is used to designate the isotope. For example, the element iodine always has 53 protons in each atom, and the particular isotope with 78 neutrons is iodine-131 (I^{131}). The majority of naturally occurring isotopes remain permanently unchanged; they are stable. Some elements, such as radium, have large numbers of protons and neutrons and are unstable, undergoing spontaneous re-adjustments of the atoms (transformations) to attain a stable state. It is possible to artificially produce unstable isotopes of any element in a nuclear reactor. All unstable materials are termed *radioactive*. This means the atoms will spontaneously and randomly disintegrate. When they undergo these transformations they emit ionizing radiation, either alpha, beta or gamma, in a process called radioactivity (Wehr et al., 1984).

Radioactive decay and half-life

When radioactive isotopes undergo transformations they are said to decay. The rate of decay is described by the half-life, which is the time taken for half of the radioactive atoms in a material to decay. If the half-life of a particular isotope was one day, then after one day only half of the radioactivity would remain. After two days there would be one-quarter of the original activity, and after three days only one-eighth. Each isotope has a different half-life, which is constant and a characteristic of the isotope. The half-life may vary considerably between isotopes, as shown in Table 2.1.

Table 2.1 Half-lives of radioactive substances commonly used in medicine

Radioactive isotope	Half-life
Caesium-137	30 years
Cobalt-60	5.3 years
Gold-198	2.7 days
Iodine-131	8 days
Iridium-192	74 days
Radium-226	1,622 years
Technetium-99	6 hours

The penetration of radiation

An understanding of the penetration of radiation is essential. How far into the tissue will penetration, and ionization, take place? What thickness of materials is needed to safely absorb the radiation? The answers can be found by considering the penetration of the radiation, which depends on the type and energy. Alpha particles are relatively heavy and slow moving, interacting easily and travelling only a fraction of a millimetre in tissue. Beta particles are much smaller, lighter, travel faster and interact less easily, travelling several millimetres in tissue. High energy electrons can travel several centimetres in tissue. X-rays are the most penetrating, travelling tens of centimetres in tissue, with high energy X-rays travelling large distances in dense materials.

Inverse square law

The inverse square law describes how the intensity of radiation falls as the distance from the source of radiation is increased. Doubling the distance from a source reduces the radiation intensity to one-quarter of the original value, and trebling the distance reduces the intensity to one-ninth. Figure 2.1 demonstrates this reduction in intensity.

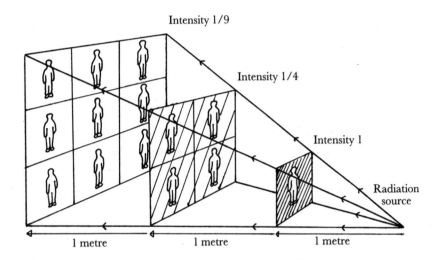

Figure 2.1 Example of the inverse square law. The radiation intensity is reduced to 1/4 as the distance from the source is doubled, and to 1/9 as the distance is trebled.

What is radiotherapy?

Radiotherapy is the use of ionizing radiation to treat disease. The radiation may be in the form of electromagnetic waves or subatomic particles, which cause ionization in cells leading to biological effects. The radiation damage will occur in normal tissues as well as tumours. Therefore, the therapeutic usefulness of radiotherapy depends on careful treatment planning and dose prescription to minimize damage to normal tissues, and on the relative sensitivity of tumours to radiation. Radiotherapy is usually given as a series of daily treatments, called fractions, over a period of weeks. The radiation dose is prescribed in terms of a unit called the Gray (Gy). Tissues have received 1 Gy when 1 joule of radiation energy is absorbed per kilogram (Greening, 1985).

Historical background

Wilhelm Roentgen discovered X-rays in 1895. In 1896 Henri Becquerel discovered radioactivity, and in 1898 Marie and Pierre Curie discovered radium. Within months of their discovery, the medical applications of X-rays were realized, in terms of both diagnosis and treatment. It took much longer to appreciate the harmful effects of the radiation, however. Several years after the first use of radiation, many people had reported problems with their eyes, hair loss and reddening of the skin after irradiation. Few heeded the warnings of these early effects of radiation. In fact, the perception of radiation in the early twentieth century was very different from today. Radium had been shown useful in certain treatments, but it became fashionable as a 'cure-all', with several commercially available products, such as a radioactive water generator available in 1913 intended for a number of benign conditions. The hazard of radiation was still not fully understood as recently as the 1950s when X-ray pedoscopes were used in shoe shops, exposing customers to significant radiation doses. In the early years, the limit at which radiation was dangerous was not even approximately known. With time, an increasing awareness of the dangers of radiation was obtained. Guidelines and legislation for the use of radiation have since been published, and the recommended exposure limits are becoming increasingly restrictive with time, having reduced by around a factor of ten in the last 60 years (Mould, 1993).

Cancers were treated with X-rays as early as 1903 but the kilovoltage beams had poor penetration, allowing only skin treatments. Radiotherapists required higher X-ray energies for greater penetration. Between 1920 and 1940, the energies slowly increased towards megavoltage. During their early use, the intensity of X-rays would often be assessed using the 'erythema dose', measuring the reddening of the hand when irradiated! In the 1930s, instruments were developed to measure the radiation dose, permitting reproducible treatments. After the Second World War, the first linear accelerators (linacs) were designed, making use of microwave technology developed during the war. 1950 saw the first installation of linacs providing X-rays of several megavolts (MV). By the mid-1960s, the indications for MV treatments were established and many linacs were installed worldwide. By 1980, linacs were widely available for delivering X-rays up to 25 MV and electrons of variable energies.

Radiotherapy by the local application of radium was introduced in 1901. Clinicians would often instruct patients to hold the radioactive sources on their skin, with little understanding of dose quantification or dosimetry and no concept of radiation protection. In 1930, the first comprehensive system of dosimetry for the use of radium was put forward, describing the required strength and positioning of sources. Today, radium is considered a dangerous source and its medical use has been abandoned in most countries. It has been replaced by artificially produced radioactive materials, such as caesium-137 and iridium-192, which were available by the 1950s. During the 1960s, the safe use of radioactive sources was improved by the development of afterloading techniques (see below).

How does radiotherapy work? The biological effects of ionizing radiation

When ionizing radiation is absorbed by human tissue, electrons are ejected from atoms causing ionization within cells and the production of ions. This leads to chemical changes resulting in biological damage. Radiation damage to DNA, which may result in single or double strand breaks, is considered most significant. Partial damage may cause chromosomal abnormalities leading to cell mutations, with severe damage resulting in reproductive death of the cell. Mammalian cells reproduce by the process of mitosis. Their sensitivity to radiation varies through the cell cycle, with radiation injury most likely during the mitotic phase. It follows that tissues most easily damaged by radiation are those whose cells are rapidly dividing. Cell survival curves describe the relationship between radiation dose and the proportion of cells which survive with the ability to form colonies. These curves have been important in understanding the radiobiology of tissue (Stryker, 1992).

The success of radiotherapy depends not only on delivering a higher radiation dose to the tumour than to the normal tissue, but also on the differing response to radiation. Tumour cells in general divide more rapidly than normal tissue, and have a greater degree of radiosensitivity. After irradiation, some cells will die and a proportion will be repaired, retaining their viability. Normal cells have a greater capacity for repair than malignant cells. This is relied upon in a course of fractionated radiotherapy treatment, where normal cells are allowed to recover more than malignant cells between fractions, increasing the differential cell kill between tumour and normal tissue. Tissues with a decreased oxygen supply are considered relatively radioresistant. The centre of a tumour mass may contain hypoxic tissues with limited blood supply. Fractionation of the radiotherapy allows reoxygenation to occur between treatments as the tumour shrinks and blood flow improves. Cells that survive a first dose of radiation will tend to be in a resistant phase of the cell cycle. Redistribution of cells into resistant phases of the cell cycle could occur during a fractionated course of radiotherapy. At the next fraction of radiation, these cells may have progressed into a more sensitive phase. This is known as reassortment, or redistribution in the cell cycle. During a course of radiotherapy, tumour cells that survive irradiation may proliferate, increasing the number of cells to be killed. This repopulation may be significant if there are inappropriate gaps between treatment fractions. The biological factors of radiosensitivity, repair, reoxygenation, redistribution and repopulation are termed the five Rs of radiotherapy (Bomford et al., 1993).

The level of success of radiotherapy depends on the type of tumour and on the stage of disease; some tumours are highly curable and others not. Tumours can vary considerably in their radiosensitivity, with the dose of radiation for tumour control larger in those with a lower sensitivity to radiation.

It is unavoidable that normal tissues will be irradiated when giving an adequate treatment to the tumour. The tolerance to radiation varies considerably with tissue type, and the treatment dose is limited by the level of normal tissue damage the patient can tolerate. The effect of radiation on normal tissue can be divided into early effects, occurring a few hours to a few weeks after exposure, and late effects, after months or years (Sweetenham et al., 1989). Tables 2.2 and 2.3 provide examples and onset doses of acute and delayed effects of radiation, for typical fractionated radiotherapy treatments.

Radical and palliative radiotherapy and treatment regimes

The clinician will decide whether a radical or palliative treatment is appropriate on the basis of the general condition of the patient and the extent of his or her disease.

Table 2.2 Examples of early effects of radiation damage to normal tissue, with typical occurrence dose during a conventional course of fractionated radiotherapy

Tissue	Early effect of radiation	Dose (Gy)
Bladder	Frequency and dysuria	40–50
Bone marrow	Suppression	10–20
GI tract	Nausea and vomiting	Any dose
	Diarrhoea	30–40
Hair	Alopecia	30–40
Lung	Pneumonitis, cough, dyspnoea	35–50
Mucous membranes	Mucositis	30–40
Skin	Erythema	10–20
	Dry desquamation	40–50
	Moist desquamation	45–55

Table 2.3 Examples of late effects of radiation damage to normal tissue, with typical occurrence dose, during a conventional course of fractionated radiotherapy

Tissue	Late effect of radiation	Dose (Gy)
Bowel	Stricture or fistula	45–60
Brain	Necrosis	55–60
Eye	Progressive cataract	8–10
	Retinal damage	50–60
Kidney	Nephritis	15–20
Liver	Fibrosis	30–50
Lung	Fibrosis	40–50
Skin	Fibrosis	50–60
	Necrosis	60
Spinal cord	Necrosis	40–50

Radical treatment aims to produce a permanent cure, destroying all malignant cells present in the primary tumour growth and in surrounding tissues that may be involved (e.g. lymph nodes). Radical radiotherapy is usually indicated in early stages of disease. The treatment generally produces some acute toxicity with a finite risk of longer term damage. Radical radiotherapy requires high doses of radiation to eliminate the tumour, divided into smaller fractions to improve the effectiveness of the treatment while minimizing side effects and remaining within the tolerance of normal tissue. A typical treatment regime is a total dose of 60 Gy delivered in 30 fractions

(2 Gy per fraction), with 1 fraction each weekday over 6 weeks.

Palliative treatment is used in the management of advanced malignant disease, where radical treatment is impractical. The intention is not to effect a cure but to improve the quality of the patient's life, relieving symptoms (e.g. pain, bleeding, cough) and improving ulceration or fungation. Examples of palliative treatment include relief of symptoms of lung cancer, control of haematuria in patients with bladder cancer, and the relief of pain for those with bone metastases. Treatment is often given as a single dose, or fractionated over one or two weeks, with minimal acute reactions to the radiation, and little concern for late effects. Typical treatment regimes are 10 Gy in a single dose, or 20 Gy in 5 daily fractions.

The different types of radiotherapy

There are a variety of techniques available for delivering radiotherapy treatments. The methods are grouped into 'external beam', 'brachytherapy' and 'unsealed source' therapy. The clinician will decide on the most appropriate treatment based on many factors including the location, type and size of the individual patient's tumour and whether the treatment intention is radical or palliative.

External beam therapy

The most common form of radiotherapy treatment is external beam therapy (or teletherapy). In this method radiation beams are applied from outside the body. Low energy X-ray beams (kV), penetrating between 1 and 3 cm below the skin surface, are produced by 'superficial' or 'orthovoltage' treatment machines. High energy X-rays (MV), with much greater penetration, are produced by linacs. These are used for the vast majority (about 90%) of radiotherapy treatments. Electron beams, for the treatment of superficial tumours, can also be produced by many modern linacs.

Radiation from a linac emerges from the 'head' of the machine. The head is mounted on a gantry that may be rotated around the patient to deliver treatment fields from any direction. Radiographers will 'set up' the patient in the correct position for treatment using predefined marks on the surface of the patient's body and a light beam from the linac head which mimics the shape of the radiation beam. The radiation beam size can be adjusted to match the size of the tumour. The radiographers will then leave the treatment room and switch on the radiation from outside. Linacs only produce radiation while they are switched on, usually for short periods (e.g. 60 seconds), unlike radioactive sources that continuously emit radiation. Radiographers must leave the room during treatments, even though the radiation beam is accurately directed at the tumour, to avoid exposure from radiation scattered off the patient and surroundings. Warning signs and interlocked doors prevent people from entering the treatment room during a radiation treatment (Tschudin, 1988).

Brachytherapy

Brachytherapy is the use of sealed radioactive sources placed within or on the site of a patient's tumour. A very localized dose of radiation is given with minimal effect on surrounding normal tissues, due to a rapid reduction of dose only short distances from the source (inverse square law, Figure 2.1). Brachytherapy is used for small localized tumours that are accessible for the application of sources, which are then removed after the required dose has been delivered. There are three types of brachytherapy: interstitial, intracavitary and surface applicator (or mould) treatments.

Interstitial treatments involve the implantation of radioactive sources, in the form of needles, pins, hairpins or seeds, directly into the tumour. Rigid guide tubes may be first inserted into the tissue and after verifying their position is correct, the radioactive source is introduced, such as flexible iridium-192 wire. This approach is termed 'afterloading' and reduces the radiation exposure to staff as well as increasing the accuracy of source placement. Caesium-137 needles may be used as an alternative to iridium wire. Sites most commonly treated by interstitial brachytherapy are the tongue, breast, vulva and anus. Figure 2.2 shows an interstitial treatment to the breast. From the time of insertion of the radioactive sources to their removal, which could be several days, the patient is effectively a source of radiation. Patients must therefore remain in their own private rooms with appropriate radiation shielding. There are limits to visiting times and the time that staff can spend caring for the patient. Once the sources have been removed, the patient is no longer a source of radiation. Recently, equipment has been developed to provide high dose rate

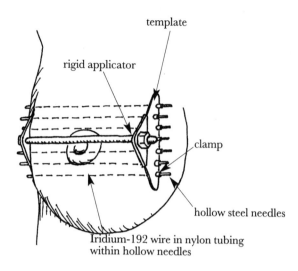

Figure 2.2 Interstitial brachytherapy treatment to the breast with iridium-192 wire sources in a rigid applicator.

brachytherapy, enabling some treatments to be performed much more rapidly (typically between 5 and 25 minutes per treatment), without the need for patients to remain isolated on the ward (e.g. Nucletron's MicroSelectron-HDR unit). Less accessible sites such as the prostate may be treated with radioactive gold or iodine seeds.

Intracavitary brachytherapy involves placing sealed radioactive sources (usually caesium-137), within natural body cavities. The most common application of the technique is for gynaecological tumours of the cervix, uterus and vagina. Standard applicator systems have been developed to fit within the cavity to be treated, consisting of rubber or plastic tubes, ovoids or spacers. The applicators can be loaded with varying amounts of sources depending on the volume to be treated. Figure 2.3 shows an intracavitary treatment of the cervix. It is now common for afterloading systems to be used, in which inactive applicators are placed within the patient, their correct position is verified, and only then are the radioactive sources introduced. Intraluminal brachytherapy is possible for the treatment of tumours of the bronchus or oesophagus. Catheters are positioned into which a small high activity source is later introduced.

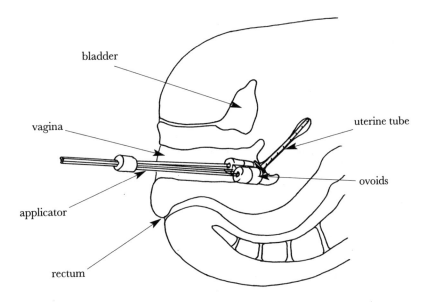

Figure 2.3 Intracavitary brachytherapy treatment to the cervix using caesium-137 manual afterloading sources in a plastic applicator (with two vaginal ovoids and intra-uterine tube).

The source may be remotely controlled, termed remote afterloading, which significantly reduces radiation exposure to staff. Again, special arrangements are required for the care of a patient while radioactive sources are in situ (Tiffany, 1979).

Surface applicators or moulds are used to treat superficial tumours. The plastic moulds are designed individually for each patient and contain a distribution of sealed radioactive sources. They are worn externally continuously or intermittently for an accurately prescribed time while the patient is isolated in hospital. Sites suitable for treatment with moulds include the hand, the pinna and the lip. Surface applicators are also used for ocular tumours. With the increasing availability of electron treatment units the usefulness of this form of brachytherapy is diminishing.

Unsealed source therapy

Unsealed source therapy involves the administration (orally or intra-venously) of radioactive liquids. There is preferential uptake and prolonged retention of the agent by the tumour, resulting in a higher radiation dose to the tumour than to normal tissue. The procedure is non-invasive and can deliver large radiation doses to the malignant tissue more selectively than external beam treatments. An example is Iodine-131, which, when given orally, is taken up selectively in thyroid tissue and associated tumours. This results in localized irradiation for thyrotoxicosis, thyroid carcinoma and associated metastases. In general, the patient must be admitted and isolated until the administered radioactivity has diminished through decay and excretion. Phosphorus-32 is given for the treatment of polycythaemia rubra vera, resulting in 'whole body' bone marrow suppression. Strontium-89 is given for the relief of bone pain associated with bone metastases.

Planning radiotherapy treatments

Radiotherapy treatment planning is the process by which a set of treatment instructions is decided upon to realize the delivery of the radiation dose prescribed by the clinician. The aim is to deliver a homogeneous dose of radiation to an accurately localized target volume whilst minimizing the dose to the surrounding normal tissue, especially radiosensitive organs. The target volume contains the gross tumour volume as well as a margin for spread and geometrical variations and inaccuracies. The clinician will have determined the type of tumour and extent of malignancy before deciding on the most appropriate treatment technique and the volume to be irradiated (Bleehen et al., 1983).

The level of complexity of treatment planning for external beam radiotherapy depends on the site of the tumour and on the treatment intent: radical or palliative. Superficial tumours require little planning, with often a single low energy X-ray beam or electron beam directed at the visible lesion. A simple calculation will determine the exposure time required to deliver the prescribed radiation dose. For external beam treatments of deep-seated tumours the situation is more complex and patients will first attend a planning session on a treatment simulator. This machine has a similar appearance and the same movements as a linac but takes diagnostic X-ray images instead of delivering treatment. The clinician uses the X-ray images to localize the tumour in the patient and to decide on the size and

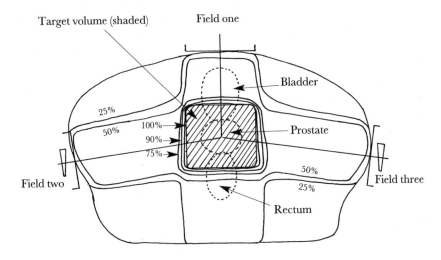

Figure 2.4 External beam radiotherapy treatment plan for carcinoma of the prostate. Isodoses (numbered lines) indicate regions of equal radiation dose.

location of the target volume. A radiographer will then mark the patient's skin at the level of the tumour, enabling accurate and reproducible location of the field at each treatment fraction. An outline of the patient's body, through the centre of the treatment volume, is obtained. It is increasingly common for CT images to be used to locate the target volume and provide the patient outline. This information is then used on a treatment planning computer. The computer calculates the effect of delivering X-ray beams from several directions, generating a plan showing the resultant distribution of radiation dose within the patient (isodose distribution). The arrangement of radiation fields can then be optimized to give a uniform dose in the target and minimal dose elsewhere. Figure 2.4 is an isodose distribution generated by the computer for the treatment of carcinoma of the prostate using three radiation fields. Single fields are inadequate for deep tumours because the dose delivered reaches a maximum just below the surface and gradually diminishes with depth. However, if several fields are positioned to overlap at the target volume, the tumour will receive a higher dose than surrounding tissue.

The planning of brachytherapy treatments (interstitial, intra-cavitary and surface application), is often accomplished using one of a number of published 'dosimetry systems'. These provide reference points for dose prescription, rules for the distribution of radioactive sources to deliver a uniform dose to the target volume, and precal-culated tables to derive treatment times. The most commonly used dosimetry systems are the Manchester system (Paterson and Parker, 1938; Meredith, 1967) developed in the 1930s for the use of radium and later caesium, and the Paris system (Pierquin et al., 1978) from the 1960s for iridium wire treatments. The Manchester system for gynaecological treatments defines a dose prescription point 'A', 20 mm lateral to the uterine canal and 20 mm above the level of the vaginal fornices. The Paris system for interstitial implants defines a prescription dose-rate as 85% of the minimum between sources (the basal dose-rate). Because of practical difficulties of implantation, the sources are rarely positioned exactly as prescribed. It is there-fore often necessary to make retrospective calculations of dose-rate from the actual implant geometry rather than the idealized posi-tions of the dosimetry system. X-ray images are taken to determine the precise positions of the sources. Dose-rates can then be calcu-lated and, using the prescribed dose, the source removal times determined.

The planning of unsealed source treatments is straightforward compared with other radiotherapy techniques. The oral or intra-venous delivery of radiation is the same for all patients, and the dose of radiation is decided by the clinician. For example, the dose of radioactive iodine required for treatment of thyrotoxicosis is calcu-lated from the size of the gland and the uptake of iodine (measured in a tracer test). Pre-treatment dosimetry calculations are rarely performed for unsealed source therapy and although dosimetry systems exist (Loevinger et al., 1989), it is difficult to achieve precise estimates of the magnitude and distribution of internal radiation doses from unsealed sources.

Radiation safety

Staff, patients and visitors must be protected from the harmful effects of unintentional exposure to ionizing radiation. There are strict guidelines governing the use of radiation (IRR 1999; IR(ME)R

2000), and staff working with radiation or caring for patients with radioactive sources in situ must understand the dangers and their own responsibility for safe practice. There are three fundamental techniques to reduce exposure of personnel: **time**, **distance**, and **shielding**. It is intuitive that less time in the vicinity of a source of radiation means less radiation exposure. Increasing the distance from a source of radiation reduces the dose rate, in accordance with the inverse square law (see Figure 2.1). The radiation intensity can be reduced significantly if appropriate shielding equipment is used to screen the source of radiation.

Each radiotherapy treatment technique (brachytherapy, unsealed source and external beam) has unique radiation protection aspects that should be noted. A brachytherapy treatment with sealed radioactive sources lends itself to the direct application of the three principles of radiation safety (above). For example, the implantation of sources should be done as quickly as possible, with long-handled forceps, directly from the lead shielded transfer container. Once the sources are in place, the patient must be isolated with lead shields placed at the sides of the bed. Essential nursing procedures should be carried out as quickly as possible and visiting times minimized. The distance from the patient must be maximized whenever possible. The use of unsealed sources has additional radiation safety implications. Bodily fluids can carry radioactivity which can in turn contaminate bedding, equipment and the room. Patients must be totally isolated with their own toilet and washing facilities, with nursing interventions minimized. All waste from the room must be bagged, labelled 'radioactive waste' and destroyed in a controlled manner according to the regulations, or stored until the activity has decayed. Radiation safety for external beam radiotherapy treatments is relatively straightforward. The linacs are surrounded by thick concrete walls, adequate to absorb all but a negligible intensity of radiation. It is necessary for staff to leave the room during the actual irradiations to benefit from this shielding. External beam radiotherapy treatments impart no radioactivity to the patient, so there is no risk of contaminating staff. All staff involved with the care of patients undergoing radiotherapy wear film badges. It is a surprisingly common misconception that these badges convey some magic protection to the wearer! In fact they measure the amount of radiation to which the wearer has been exposed.

Case histories

Mr James

Mr James was 75 when he presented with urinary outflow symptoms and an episode of urinary retention. After ultrasound scans and a prostatic biopsy had been carried out, a localized well differentiated carcinoma of the prostate was diagnosed. There was no evidence of metastases on a nuclear medicine bone scan. Mr James was referred for radical external beam radiotherapy to the prostate. The side effects of the treatment and the risk of inducing impotence were explained. An abdominal CT scan was requested, from which the radiotherapy planning was carried out. The clinical oncologist prescribed 64 Gy tumour dose in 32 fractions over 6 weeks and 2 days. The external beam treatment plan consisted of three radiation fields, overlapping at the tumour volume. Mr James can expect a reasonable five-year survival probability. He will be followed up by his urologist and clinical oncologist.

Mrs Barry

Mrs Barry was 65 when she went to her GP with a brief history of post-menopausal bleeding. He suspected cervical cancer from his examination and referred her to a gynaecologist. A biopsy was performed which confirmed a moderately differentiated invasive squamous cell carcinoma of the cervix. The patient was then seen by the clinical oncologist, who decided to give radical external beam radiotherapy. The external beam treatment delivered 45 Gy in 25 fractions over 5 weeks, with four radiation fields converging on the cervix. She was also admitted for brachytherapy, which consisted of caesium insertions to the uterus and vagina, delivering an additional 20 Gy (to point 'A' of the Manchester dosimetry system) during a 39-hour treatment time. The tolerance dose of the rectum and bladder were considered when prescribing the treatment doses. Mrs Barry was followed up by her gynaecologist and clinical oncologist, initially at three-monthly intervals.

Mrs Evans

Mrs Evans was 59 when she discovered a lump in her left breast. She had no previous breast problems and no family history of note.

Mammography revealed an ill-defined dense 2 cm mass in the left breast, consistent with carcinoma. She underwent wedge resection of the mass and axillary dissection. X-ray, ultrasound and isotope bone scan showed no evidence of metastases. The clinician decided to give radical external beam irradiation followed by an interstitial iridium wire implant as a localized boost. The external beam radiotherapy consisted of two tangential fields delivering 50 Gy in 25 fractions over 5 weeks. This was followed by the brachytherapy treatment, as an inpatient, consisting of a breast implant of seven iridium wires, 6 cm in length. The prescribed dose of 16 Gy (to 85% basal dose on the Paris dosimetry system) was delivered in 47 hours, after which the sources were removed and she was discharged. Mrs Evans had an excellent cosmetic result from the local excision and radiotherapy, which she tolerated well, and has remained free of recurrence for five years. She was followed up by her surgeon and oncologist.

Conclusions

This chapter has presented an introduction to radiation physics, radiobiology, and the principles of radiotherapy treatments. The field of radiotherapy is continually advancing with developments in dosimetry and treatment planning techniques, the introduction of sophisticated new treatment equipment, and the application of advanced imaging technology, making it possible to direct radiation ever more accurately at lesions, whilst sparing normal tissues and minimizing complications.

Chapter 3
Understanding cytotoxic chemotherapy

JANICE GABRIEL

Introduction

The term 'cytotoxic chemotherapy' conjures up impressions of exhausted bald-headed patients racked by uncontrolled nausea and vomiting. This is not the case. Yet many patients dread the prospect of having to undergo chemotherapy because of this popular misconception.

This chapter will look at the development of cytotoxic drugs, how they work and how they can be administered. It will also address the safety aspects of handling and disposal of these agents. The chapter will conclude with some case histories of patients who have undergone chemotherapy. It will explain how some potential problems have been prevented or minimized, to offer patients effective treatment with the minimum of side effects.

The history of cytotoxic drugs

Calvert and McElwain (1978) discuss how the medical profession identified that soldiers who died after exposure to mustard gas during the First World War had severely depleted bone marrows. For those soldiers who did survive the initial exposure and returned to England, it was noticed that they succumbed readily to infections and died prematurely. This led to research into the effects of mustard gas on bone marrow, with a view to developing a therapeutic agent for treating haematological malignancies. The drug that was eventually developed was nitrogen mustard, which was introduced into clinical practice in the 1940s (Calvert and McElwain, 1978).

Since the 1940s we have seen the development of an increasing range of cytotoxic drugs, especially during the last 20 years (Calvert and McElwain, 1978; Allwood and Wright, 1993). The 1940s saw the development of methotrexate, a drug still widely used today. Chemists noticed that children affected by leukaemia had low levels of folic acid. Yet, when they were given a folic acid supplement, their disease process appeared to advance rapidly. Consequently, methotrexate was developed with a view to acting as an antagonist of folic acid (Calvert and McElwain, 1978).

In the late 1950s extracts of the periwinkle plant were being investigated for their potential as a treatment for diabetes. However, it was noticed that the extracts caused bone marrow suppression in mice, and tissue necrosis if they were injected. As a result of this research extracts of the periwinkle plant did not prove fruitful as a treatment for diabetes, but two cytotoxic agents, i.e., vincristine and vinblastine, were developed. Both of these drugs are still widely used today (Calvert and McElwain, 1978). More recent extracts from plants have led to the development of such drugs as paclitaxel, in the 1990s.

How do cytotoxic drugs work?

Regardless of where the cell is situated in the body, every cell has four essential features, i.e.

- It requires oxygen and produces carbon dioxide
- It contains enzymes
- It has selective permeability
- It contains ribonucleic acid (RNA) and deoxyribonucleic acid (DNA), which are essential for cell replication.

All cells have to go through five key stages in order to replicate (Figure 3.1). Each cell is capable of replication. Every cell contains genetic information within its DNA, which will be passed on to the next generation of cells (Calvert and McElwain, 1978). The five stages the cell undergoes in order to replicate are summarized in Table 3.1 (Knobf and Durivage, 1993).

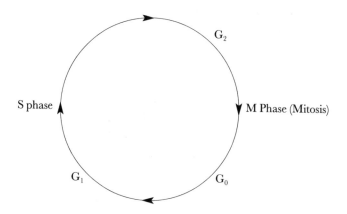

Figure 3.1 The cell cycle.

Table 3.1 Five phases of cell replication

Phase	Activity
G_1	RNA and protein synthesis
G_2	Cells complete DNA synthesis and prepare to enter mitosis phase
G_0	Dormant phase
S	DNA synthesis takes place
M	During the M phase, mitosis (cell division) takes place

Different groups of cells require different lengths of time to complete their cycle of replication. In the treatment of malignant disease, knowledge of the cell cycle is one of the key factors in planning effective treatment for an individual's specific cancer (Knobf and Durivage, 1993).

There are four main groups of cytotoxic agents. These are **antimetabolites, alkylating agents, vinca alkaloids** and **cytotoxic antibiotics**. Each group of drugs affects the cell at a specific phase during its cycle (Calvert and McElwain, 1978).

Antimetabolites

Antimetabolites work by preventing the cell from manufacturing the extra DNA that is necessary for replication. This leads ultimately to the death of the cell (Walter, 1977b).

Examples of drugs within this group are:

- Methotrexate
- 5-Fluorouracil (5FU)
- Fludarabine
- Gemcitabine
- Thioguanine

Alkylating agents

Alkylating agents are chemically related to the first known cytotoxic drug, i.e. mustine. They work by damaging the DNA and preventing it from separating into two distinct strands in order to replicate (Walter, 1977b; Calvert and McElwain, 1978).

Examples of drugs within this group are:

- Cyclophosphamide
- Mustine
- Ifosfamide
- Melphalan
- Chlorambucil

Vinca alkaloids

Vinca alkaloids work on the final stage of the cell cycle by preventing the cell from dividing.

Examples of drugs within this group are:

- Vinblastine
- Vincristine
- Vindesine
- Etoposide
- Vinorelbine

Cytotoxic antibiotics

Cytotoxic antibiotics work on the G_2 phase of the cell's cycle. The drug binds to the DNA, so preventing it from completing its synthesis.

Drugs within this group include:

- Doxorubicin
- Epirubicin
- Daunorubicin
- Mitozantrone
- Bleomycin
- Mitomycin

Treatment with cytotoxic drugs

Not all malignant cells are sensitive to cytotoxic chemotherapy, e.g. some types of head and neck cancers. For this reason, it is important that an individual diagnosed with cancer is referred to a clinician who is experienced in the management of patients with malignant disease. Treatment will depend upon exactly what type of cancer the patient has, and how localized or widespread it is. Other factors to be taken into consideration are any other underlying medical conditions. For example, if the patient has an underlying cardiac condition, the use of doxorubicin may be contraindicated, as it can lead to cardiomyopathy (Table 3.2 overleaf).

The overall objective of treating patients with cytotoxic chemotherapy is to achieve a response, i.e. to see a disappearance of all or part of the disease and its associated symptoms (Calvert and McElwain, 1978). Calvert and McElwain (1978) define five levels of response to cytotoxic drugs. These are summarized in Table 3.3.

Table 3.3 Five levels of response to cytotoxic drugs

Complete response	disappearance of all detectable signs of disease
Partial response	reduction of 50% in signs of the disease
Minor response	a slight improvement in the detectable signs of disease
Static response	no improvement/disease stable
Progressive disease	the disease process has continued despite the treatment

Cytotoxic chemotherapy is a systemic treatment, that is all the body's cells with the exception of the central nervous system are exposed to the drug(s) as they circulate via the bloodstream. Many cytotoxic agents are incapable of crossing the blood/brain barrier, unless they are injected directly into the cerebrospinal fluid (CSF) by means of a lumbar puncture (intrathecally).

Curative chemotherapy

Chemotherapy can be prescribed as the main or sole treatment for some cancers, e.g. haematological malignancies. This is because haematological malignancies are usually disseminated throughout the body and the chemotherapy will exert a systemic effect (Calvert and McElwain, 1978).

Neoadjuvant chemotherapy

Cytotoxic chemotherapy can also be used prior to surgery and/or radiotherapy, in an attempt to reduce the size of the tumour. This is known as neoadjuvant chemotherapy. Neoadjuvant chemotherapy can be used with the aim of improving the 'cure rate' for any subsequent treatment with radiotherapy and/or surgery (Calvert and McElwain, 1978).

Adjuvant chemotherapy

Adjuvant chemotherapy is a term used to describe the treatment with cytotoxic chemotherapy following surgery and/or radiotherapy. It is aimed at eliminating any remaining malignant cells and so minimizing the possibility of future disease recurrence (Calvert and McElwain, 1978). It is widely used in the management of breast and bowel cancers.

Salvage chemotherapy

Salvage chemotherapy can be used to actively treat a patient who has relapsed following earlier treatment. It is not the same as 'palliative chemotherapy'.

Palliative ch2emotherapy

Palliative chemotherapy is prescribed with the specific intention of improving symptoms, and hopefully improving the quality of life, for patients with advanced disease (Calvert and McElwain, 1978).

Effect of cytotoxic chemotherapy on the cell cycle

As a tumour is composed of many millions of cells, it is inevitable that they will be at different stages of the cell cycle when the cytotoxic drug(s) is/are administered. Consequently, the majority of patients diagnosed with a malignant disease are treated by a combination of drugs (Walter, 1977b; Calvert and McElwain, 1978; Allwood and Wright, 1993; Knobf and Durivage, 1993). By administering drugs from more than one group of cytotoxic agents, it is hoped that as many of the malignant cells as possible will be 'killed' by the actions of these drugs on the different phases of the cells' cycle

Table 3.2 Examples of cytotoxic drugs and their common side effects

Group	Drug	Method of administration	Vesicant	Degree of nausea	Degree of alopecia	Other common side effects
Cytotoxic antibiotics	Doxorubicin	IV or IVI bladder instillation	yes	+++	+++	cardiotoxic, myelosuppression, mucositis
	Epirubicin	IV or IVI bladder instillation	yes	+++	++	cardiotoxic, myelosuppression, mucositis
	Daunorubicin	IV or IVI	yes	+++	+++	cardiotoxic, myelosuppression, mucositis
	Mitozantrone	IV or IVI	yes	+	++	myelosuppression, mucositis
	Bleomycin	IV, IVI, IM or intracavity	no	-	-	mucositis, hypersensitivity reactions, pulmonary fibrosis, increased pigmentation
	Mitomycin	IV, bladder instillation	yes	-	-	pulmonary fibrosis, renal damage
Alkylating agents	Cyclophosphamide	IV, PO, IVI	No	++	+	haemorrhagic cystitis can occur

	Route	Vesicant			Side-effects
Ifosfamide	IV or IVI	No	++	+	with high doses or in dehydrated patients; haemorrhagic cystitis can occur with high doses or in dehydrated patients
Antimetabolites					
Chlorambucil	PO	N/A	-	-	
Melphalan	PO, IV or IVI	No	+	+	
Mustine	IV or IVI	Yes	+++	+++	
Methotrexate	PO, IV, IVI, IM	No	+	+	mucositis, myelosuppression
Fludarabine	IV or IVI	No	+	+	myelosuppression
Gemcitabine	IVI	No	+	+	rash, GI disturbances, flu-like symptoms, renal impairment
Fluorouracil	PO, IV, IVI or topically	No	+	+	mucositis
Vinca alkaloids					
Vincristine	IV	Yes	+	+	peripheral neuropathy
Vinblastine	IV	Yes	+	+	peripheral neuropathy, mucositis
Vindesine	IV	Yes	+	+	peripheral neuropathy
Etoposide	PO or IVI	No	++	++	myelosuppression

(Figure 3.1). However, as healthy cells are also susceptible to the toxic effects of these drugs, careful prescribing and monitoring of the patient needs to take place (Knobf and Durivage, 1993).

Prescribing cytotoxic chemotherapy

Each individual patient will have a dosage of drugs specifically worked out for them. This takes into account their height and weight, from which their surface area is calculated. All cytotoxic drug regimens are prescribed 'per metre squared', e.g.

Cyclophosphamide 1 g per m^2
Doxorubicin 50 mg per m^2

So if a patient's surface area is 1.5 m^2, the drug dosages they will receive will be as follows:

Cyclophosphamide 1.5 g
Doxorubicin 75 mg

As the cells composing the tumour will be at different stages of their cell cycle when the cytotoxic chemotherapy is administered, it would be impossible to rid the patient of the disease with one treatment. Knowledge of the disease allows the clinician to deliver the treatment in divided doses, known as pulses, at daily, weekly, three-weekly intervals, etc. Knowledge of the specific disease, and how it generally responds to treatment with cytotoxic agents, allows for a maximum 'kill rate' to the malignant cells, but at the same time minimizes the toxic effects on healthy cells. Prior to each pulse of chemotherapy, it is common practice for the patient to have a blood sample analysed to check the following: haemoglobin; platelets; and white blood cells, especially neutrophils

The levels of these cells within the blood will give an indication of how toxic the previous pulse of cytotoxic agents was on the patient's bone marrow. If the clinician is concerned that the levels of these cells are 'too low', he or she may either reduce the individual doses of the drugs to be administered, or delay the patient's treatment. Either scenario should allow the patient's bone marrow time to recover from its previous exposure to the cytotoxic agents.

Common side effects

As cytotoxic drugs have been developed with the specific intention of curbing the activity of malignant cell growth and replication, it is inevitable that they will exert some effect on 'normal' cell growth and replication (Walter, 1977b).

Bone marrow suppression

Virtually all cytotoxic drugs have an adverse effect on the patient's bone marrow. How long this will take to manifest will very much depend on the specific drug(s) used as part of the individual patient's treatment regimen. The time span can commonly range from 7 to 28 days. For this reason it is important that patients have their blood count monitored before each pulse of chemotherapy (Walter, 1977b; Knobf and Durivage, 1993).

As the patient's white blood count may be reduced, he or she could be at increased risk of infection. There could also be an increased risk of haemorrhage if the platelets are also reduced (Walter, 1977b). It is important that patients receiving their treatment on an outpatient basis or in the home care setting are made aware of these potential risks and who to contact if they experience any of the following symptoms:

- sore throat/mouth
- productive cough
- shivering
- raised temperature
- frequency of micturition
- diarrhoea
- excessive bruising
- bleeding, e.g. nose bleed

Nausea and vomiting

Probably two of the most widely known side effects of cytotoxic chemotherapy are alopecia and nausea/vomiting. However, not all drugs used in the treatment of malignant disease result in these side effects (Table 3.2) (Calvert and McElwain, 1978; Allwood and Wright, 1993). Some cytotoxic drugs, such as vincristine, chlorambucil and 5-fluourouracil have very little emetogenic effect on the individual, while others, such as doxorubicin, epirubicin and mustine, can be highly emetogenic (Table 3.2) (Calvert and McElwain, 1978; Allwood and Wright, 1993). The emetogenic effect of cytotoxic drugs is believed to be coordinated by the vomiting centre, close to the fourth ventricle in the brain. Once the vomiting centre has been stimulated, it initiates the vomiting process. It is therefore vitally important that the emetogenic potential of cytotoxic drugs is known to the individual who will be administering/prescribing them. In the majority of cases this will be the patient's chemotherapy nurse. The nurse should ensure that if a drug with emetogenic potential is to be administered to the patient, it is accompanied by an appropriately prescribed anti-emetic on a prophylactic basis (Allwood and Wright, 1993).

Drugs such as metoclopramide, domperidone and prochlorperazine can be effective in eliminating or minimizing nausea/vomiting associated with cytotoxic drugs which have a low emetogenic potential (Table 3.2) (McLaughlin and Thompson, 1995; Abdulla and Daneshmend, 1995). For drugs which are highly emetogenic, the prophylactic administration of one of the $5HT_3$ receptor antagonists can prove highly effective in preventing nausea/vomiting. Damage to the gastrointestinal mucosa stimulates the release of 5HT. The 5HT then binds to $5HT_3$ receptors of the vagus nerve. These then convey emetogenic impulses to the vomiting centre of the patient's brain. By administering a $5HT_3$ receptor antagonist, these messages are blocked. Drugs within the $5HT_3$ receptor antagonist group include granisetron, ondansetron and tropisetron. The addition of dexamethasone at the time of administering the $5HT_3$ receptor antagonist has been demonstrated to enhance its efficiency (Abdulla and Daneshmend, 1995).

Alopecia

Hair loss with cytotoxic chemotherapy, like nausea and vomiting, is very much dependent upon *which* drugs are used. Some drugs, such as chlorambucil and bleomycin, have little effect on the patient's hair, while others, such as daunorubicin, will probably render the patient bald within 2–3 weeks of their first treatment (Goodman et al., 1993).

It is important to remember that although any hair loss a patient does experience, as a result of the cytotoxic chemotherapy, is only going to be temporary, its psychological impact should not be underestimated. Alopecia associated with cytotoxic chemotherapy is rapid. Sadly its regrowth is not. Regrowth of hair will be visible approximately 4–6 weeks after the last pulse of treatment. In some cases visible hair regrowth will commence prior to the last treatment (Goodman et al., 1993).

Loss of head hair is often more noticeable to the patient than loss of hair elsewhere on the body. This is because about 85% of head hair is in its active stage of replication at any given time, compared to a much lower percentage of other body hair, e.g. pubic hair, eyebrows, etc. (Goodman et al., 1993).

There have been attempts to minimize the degree of alopecia associated with cytotoxic chemotherapy. These have included the use of a scalp tourniquet and hypothermia cap. Both techniques involve reducing the blood supply to the scalp immediately prior to the administration of the cytotoxic drugs, and for a short period afterwards. Scalp hypothermia is the more widely used of the two techniques. It not only restricts the blood flow to the hair follicles, but also reduces the metabolic rate of the scalp cells (Goodman et al., 1993). The technique involves the patient wearing an ice-pack, or commercially available hypothermia cap, for approximately 15–30 minutes prior to the administration of the cytotoxic drug(s), during the administration and for about 30 minutes following the administration.

The use of hair preservation techniques is less successful in patients receiving combination cytotoxic chemotherapy, especially if intravenous agents are followed by several days of oral treatment. It is also not recommended for patients with haematological malignancies, as the technique prevents or hinders the drugs from reaching the cells of the scalp (Goodman et al., 1993).

Mucositis

Mucosal epithelial cells are found throughout the gastrointestinal tract and vagina, and are particularly sensitive to effects of cytotoxic chemotherapy. Painful ulceration, known as mucositis, can occur. This can result in bleeding, infection, indigestion and diarrhoea (Goodman et al., 1993).

The nurse can play an important role in ensuring the patient does not neglect mouth care, which will minimize the risks of oral mucosal problems.

Nails

Changes can often be seen in the nails of both the patient's hands and feet when undergoing a course of cytotoxic chemotherapy.

Occasionally separation of the nail plate can occur, but more commonly a condition known as *Beau's lines* can develop. This is when the nail ceases to grow, as a response to cytotoxic drugs, and white lines develop across the nail. Each line corresponds to a pulse of treatment.

Fertility

No automatic assumption should be made that after receiving a course of cytotoxic chemotherapy the patient will become infertile, or should refrain from having children.

Krebs (1993) discusses how infertility and sterility have been reported in both men and women after receiving cytotoxic chemotherapy. However, this depends very much upon the drugs used and the age of the individual.

It has been known for some time that long-term exposure to alkylating agents can be responsible for infertility, but other drugs can also be responsible. These can include:

- Vinblastine
- Vincristine
- Cisplatin
- Procarbazine
- 5-Fluourouracil

In women, exposure to cytotoxic agents can lead to an early menopause, especially if they are in their late thirties or their forties when treatment is initiated. In men, exposure to cytotoxic drugs can cause a depletion in their testicular volume, which can result in infertility (Krebs, 1993). It is important that potential fertility problems are discussed with the patient before the commencement of cytotoxic chemotherapy treatment. For men who are to be exposed to chemotherapy regimes believed to be linked to a potentially high risk of causing infertility, 'sperm banking' can be considered. This procedure should be undertaken *prior* to commencing treatment.

While individuals are undergoing cytotoxic chemotherapy it is important that they are given contraceptive advice, so that pregnancy is avoided. This advice should be given to both men and women.

Methods of administration

The majority of cytotoxic drugs are administered orally or by injection (IV, IVI, continuous IV infusion and occasionally IM and S/C). Consequently their effects on the individual are systemic, i.e. the whole body is exposed to the effects of the treatment (Walter, 1977b). The exceptions to this are drugs administered by the following routes:

Intrathecally

Drugs administered directly into the cerebrospinal fluid (CSF), e.g. methotrexate, for the treatment of haematological malignancies.

Into serous cavities

Drugs administered directly into the pleural or peritoneal cavities, e.g. bleomycin, for use in malignant effusions.

Into the bladder

Drugs instilled into the bladder, by means of a urinary catheter, for localized treatment of bladder cancers.

Limb perfusion

By isolating the main artery and vein to a limb, then placing a tourniquet around the limb, a cytotoxic drug is administered via a catheter with the intention of delivering a high dose of the drug to the tumour. This minimizes the systemic side effects of the treatment for the patient. After a period of time, e.g. 20 minutes, the drug is pumped out via the vein. This treatment is used for management of malignant melanoma. The patient is anaesthetized for the procedure.

Topically

A topical application of some drugs, e.g. 5-fluourouracil, can be used for basal cell carcinomas.

Types of vascular access devices

As many cytotoxic drugs are vesicant, or require to be administered intravenously over a period of time, it is important that the most appropriate intravenous access device is selected. Today we have a range of vascular access devices available to meet the individual patient's clinical needs and, where appropriate, lifestyle away from the hospital environment. These devices are listed in Table 3.4.

Centrally placed devices, that is devices with their tips terminating in the superior vena cava, are more appropriate for the administration of vesicant cytotoxic drugs. This is because the location of the catheter's tip will ensure that the drugs are delivered into the central venous system, therefore minimizing the risk of chemical phlebitis and extravasation (Gabriel, 1999). Centrally placed devices are also used for patients prescribed 'continuous ambulatory infusion'. This is a method of continuously administering parenteral chemotherapy by means of an intermediate to long-term central venous access device, e.g. a PICC or a skin-tunnelled line.

Cytotoxic extravasation

Cytotoxic extravasation occurs when a vesicant drug has leaked out of the vein and infiltrated the surrounding tissues. Its resulting tissue damage can range from erythema to severe necrosis which will require surgical intervention. As it is virtually impossible to reverse the effects of cytotoxic extravasation, prevention is obviously going to be more effective than any subsequent remedial action. Each hospital will have its own policy and procedures relating to the prevention and management of extravasation (Goodman et al., 1993). The general principles in preventing cytotoxic drug extravasation are:

- Use the most appropriate IV access device for the drug(s) to be administered (see Table 3.4)
- Ensure you select a venepuncture site where the vein can easily be observed for early signs of swelling (the ante-cubital fossa veins and veins overlying a joint should be avoided. If they are used, they should only be considered as a last resort, as extravasation in these areas can lead to tendon and nerve damage)
- Ensure that there is adequate blood return from the IV access device

Table 3. 4 Vascular access devices

Type of device	Placement setting	Centrally placed?	Suitable for long-term use	Number of lumens	Long-term maintenance
Winged needle	Ward, clinic or home	No	No – unless resited for each pulse of chemotherapy	1	N/A
Peripheral cannula	Ward, clinic or home	No	No – unless resited for each pulse of chemotherapy	1	N/A
Midline Catheter	Ward, clinic or home	No	Will last for a number of days	1	Regular flushing with 0.9% sodium chloride/heparin
Peripherally Inserted central catheter (PICC)	Ward, clinic or X-ray dept	Yes	Yes	1 or 2	Weekly flush for valved PICCs. More frequent flushing for open-ended PICCs
Skin-tunnelled catheters	Ward, X-ray dept or operating dept	Yes	Yes	1, 2 or 3	Weekly flush for valved catheters More frequent flushing for open-ended catheters
Implantable injection ports	X-ray dept or operating dept	Yes	Yes	1 or 2	Monthly flush

- Always test the IV access device for patency with 0.9% sodium chloride before administering/infusing the cytotoxic drug(s)
- Observe the infusion site for signs of swelling during the administration of the drug(s).Constantly check that your patient is not experiencing any pain/discomfort during the administration of the drug(s).Flush the IV device well with 0.9% sodium chloride after the administration of the drug(s) (Allwood and Wright, 1993).

If extravasation of a cytotoxic drug occurs, or is suspected, you should follow the procedures recommended by your own hospital.

The general advice for managing cytotoxic extravasation is as follows:

- Stop administration of the drug immediately and attempt to aspirate back from the IV access device
- Remove the IV access device
- Inject 100 mg of hydrocortisone S/C around the area of extravasation
- Apply an ice-pack periodically to the affected area for up to 24 hours
- Apply 1X hydrocortisone cream on and around the affected area for 2–3 days, or until the redness and discomfort subside
- Record the incident.

Although extravasation is more likely to occur with peripheral venous access devices, it can be a rare occurrence of centrally placed devices due to the formation of fibrin sheaths enveloping the catheter, resulting in backtracking of the drug as it is injected/infused (Gabriel, 1999).

Safe handling and disposal of cytotoxic agents

As cytotoxic drugs have mutagenic, teratogenic and carcinogenic potential, healthcare professionals handling these agents must be aware of these hazards, and receive adequate training to minimize the risks to themselves, colleagues and the environment (Allwood and Wright, 1993; Reyman, 1993). Cumulative exposure to these agents can occur during reconstitution/preparation, handling, administration and disposal. As a response to this growing body of knowledge relating to the potential risks to healthcare professionals, safety measures have been implemented and are closely monitored. These will ensure that the risks to staff involved with cytotoxic agents are minimized and the health of the staff involved regularly monitored (Allwood and Wright, 1993).

Each hospital and community trust should have its own guidelines for staff involved in the handling and disposal of cytotoxic materials.

Preparation and administration

All cytotoxic drugs should be prepared for administration in a suitable safety cabinet. These are usually situated within the hospital's pharmacy department or oncology department. On the rare occasion when it is not possible to undertake the preparation of these agents in a designated area, the following protective clothing should be worn when preparing an injection/infusion:

- disposable water repellent gown/apron
- disposable gauntlets (if the gown does not have long sleeves)
- disposable gloves
- face mask with visor

The only protective clothing required for the administration of an injection/infusion are disposable gloves. Tablets can be administered to a patient by using a 'non-touch' technique. On no account should cytotoxic tablets be crushed or broken.

Disposal

All cytotoxic waste should be disposed of safely to comply with national and local guidelines (Allwood and Wright, 1993). Sharps should be placed immediately into the correct container. Other waste materials, e.g. disposable protective clothing, IV tubing, etc., should be segregated from other waste materials and disposed of in the appropriate container to await collection for incineration (Allwood and Wright, 1993).

Spillage

Every clinical area using cytotoxic drugs should have access to a designated spillage kit. This will contain all the necessary materials to deal with the spillage of a cytotoxic drug, therefore minimizing the potential risks to staff, patients and the environment (Reyman, 1993).

No member of staff should undertake the preparation or administration of cytotoxic drugs until he or she has received adequate training. No member of staff who is pregnant should be involved in handling cytotoxic agents.

Support

The support available to individual patients and their families varies immensely throughout the UK. As it is now common practice for specially trained chemotherapy nurses to assume responsibility for the administration of cytotoxic drugs, they can prove invaluable in providing practical and psychological support. This small group of nurses will become familiar with the common fears, concerns and problems experienced by patients undergoing chemotherapy. Their specialist training, ongoing experience, and regular contact with the patient will help them to develop a close relationship with their patients. This can prove to be highly beneficial in identifying potential problems and addressing other issues sooner rather than later.

In addition to the support offered by the patient's chemotherapy nurse, Macmillan Cancer Relief sponsors a number of nursing, medical and professions allied to medicine posts. These individuals provide specialist support for many thousands of patients.

Case histories

Paul

Paul, a 26-year-old bus driver, has been diagnosed with Hodgkin's Disease and is to undergo a 12-week course of cytotoxic chemotherapy. He is married with three children under the age of six. He and his wife have recently purchased a house, for which he is relying on his overtime payments to meet his monthly outgoings. His wife does not work outside the home, as she is kept fully occupied looking after the children.

While Paul is obviously worried about his long-term outlook, he is reassured by his chemotherapy nurse and medical oncologist that there is a very good chance of him responding well to his treatment, and being able to resume his job.

During the administration of his second week of treatment Paul confides in his chemotherapy nurse that the treatment was not as bad as he expected it to be, but he was worried about 'other things'. After some gentle questioning Paul's nurse ascertains that although he is receiving 'sick pay' from his employer, it is only at the basic rate and far short of what he has been used to with the additional overtime. In an attempt to find a practical solution to what will only be a short-term problem, Paul's nurse suggests a referral to the hospital social worker and Macmillan Nurse. The intention of these referrals is to find out if there are any benefits which Paul is unaware he is entitled to.

Jean

Jean, a 52-year-old with a two-year history of metastatic breast cancer, is just about to embark upon a course of palliative cytotoxic chemotherapy. However, the regimen prescribed includes doxorubicin, which will result in alopecia. Jean confesses to the nurse that although she knows the intention of the chemotherapy is to make her feel better, she is devastated at the thought of losing her hair.

Jean's nurse explains that a wig will be provided before she experiences any hair loss, and that the alopecia will not be permanent. However, Jean still has reservations about commencing the treatment. As her treatment is for palliation the nurse discusses the feasibility of scalp cooling with Jean's consultant. The consultant is quite happy for this suggestion to be put to Jean. Although there is no absolute guarantee that scalp cooling will totally prevent alopecia, Jean is very happy to try it, even though it will prolong her outpatient visits on the days she is to receive chemotherapy.

Anne

Anne, a 44-year-old secretary, is receiving chemotherapy each Tuesday morning for cancer of the colon. She is married with two grown-up children living away from home. Several weeks into her treatment Anne states that she is becoming very depressed as she feels quite nauseated on the day of her chemotherapy. Although a change in anti-emetics has improved the situation, she is really worried that she is letting her employer down by her lack of concentration.

After discussions with Anne's consultant it is suggested that her treatment day is moved from Tuesday to Friday. The intention of this is to allow Anne time to recover from her treatment on Saturday and Sunday. Anne was very amenable to this suggestion and after a couple of weeks was feeling much better psychologically.

Conclusions

Cytotoxic chemotherapy is undoubtedly a rapidly developing area of cancer care, both as a primary treatment and for palliation. Sadly, as more individuals are diagnosed with cancer, so the number of recipients of cytotoxic chemotherapy is set to rise.

Nurses can play a key role in dispelling some of the outdated myths surrounding chemotherapy, and provide practical and psychological support for this growing patient population.

Chapter 4
Breast cancer

CARMEL SHEPPARD

Introduction

This chapter looks at the current situation in the UK, the role of breast screening for early detection, and risk factors associated with breast cancer. It also explains the process of diagnosis, and possible treatment options available, as well as highlighting the psychological outcomes associated with the diagnosis of breast cancer. Finally, two case histories describe a variation of patient processes, treatments, and outcomes.

The current situation

In 1991 approximately 34,5000 women were diagnosed with breast cancer (CRC, 1996a). It is by far the most common cancer in women, and accounts for one in five female cancers within the UK.

The mortality rate in the UK remains high in comparison to other European countries with only an average of 64% of women alive five years following diagnosis (CRC, 1996b). During the past 15 years or so there has been much pressure on the government to tackle this problem. In 1988 the National Breast Screening Programme was set up following the recommendations of the Forrest Report (1986). Evidence in other countries had shown that a 30% reduction in mortality could be achieved with breast screening.

In 1992 the Health of the Nation document was published, which set a target to reduce deaths in the UK by 25% by the year 2000. More recently, the Calman-Hine Report (1995) recommended the introduction of specialized treatment centres. Traditionally, most patients with breast cancer were treated by a general surgeon; however, recent papers have indicated that women have a better prognosis if treated in a specialized centre (Gillis and Holes, 1996), where the surgeon has a specialized interest in breast cancer, treats over 100 new cases per year, and is part of a multidisciplinary team.

Survival of breast cancer does depend on a number of different prognostic factors, such as size and grade of tumour, tumour type, lymph node involvement and metastasis (Miller et al., 1994). Recent statistics have shown evidence of a sudden fall in mortality rates, with 15,180 deaths in 1990, compared with 14,080 in 1995 (CRC, 1996c). It was initially thought that this fall in mortality was influenced by the introduction of the national screening programme. However, many have disputed the likelihood of screening having such an early impact, claiming that it is far more likely that the fall is attributable to the widespread use of the drug tamoxifen since the early 1980s (Baum, 1995).

Breast screening

Britain's National Breast Screening Programme aims to screen all women between the ages of 50 and 64 years at three-yearly intervals (Forrest, 1986). Each screening unit throughout the country identifies women via the Family Health Authority (FHA) and duly sends a list of all women in this age group to each GP practice. Ideally this list is checked by the GP, and any women unsuitable for screening (i.e. patients with a prior diagnosis of breast cancer) are removed from the list. Following this, all eligible women in this age group are invited to attend for screening.

There are many reasons why women decline their screening invitation (Fallowfield, 1991). These include:

- Fear of what might be found, and fear of possible subsequent treatment
- Fear that the mammogram might be painful
- A personal belief that breast cancer will not affect them
- Other personal priorities, e.g. lack of time, work commitments, family commitments, other illnesses, etc.
- A lack of understanding of the process of breast screening
- Embarrassment – an invasion of privacy

Nurses working in health promotion roles should be aware of these reasons for non-attendance and optimize opportunities during patient contact to promote and encourage breast awareness. Approximately 90% of breast cancers are found by women themselves (Department of Health, 1991). However, there is little evidence that breast examination alone is effective in reducing mortality. The concept of breast awareness does not follow a ritualistic pattern of examination, but is aimed to educate women to become more aware of what is normal for them, and to both look at and feel their breasts during normal daily activities, e.g. during a bath or shower (Department of Health, 1998).

Nurses should equally be aware of the recommendations and guidance on breast examination issued by both the Royal College of Nursing and the Department of Health. This recommends that nurses (excepting breast care nurses with specialist training in breast palpation) should not undertake the role of breast palpation (Royal College of Nursing, 1995).

Assessment phase of screening

Following the initial screening procedure approximately one in ten patients will be recalled for further assessment. Patients may be recalled for a variety of reasons, e.g. poor film quality, normal asymmetry or aggregation of the breast tissue, and benign breast disease such as cysts or fibroadenomas. The majority of patients recalled will not have cancer.

During the assessment phase, the patient may undergo further investigations as required. This may include further mammography, ultrasound, clinical examination, cytology and/or core biopsy to confirm the diagnosis. Patients found to have abnormalities will be referred to a surgeon.

Patients with breast symptoms will usually have been sent by their GP to a symptomatic breast clinic for assessment. Symptoms that would require further investigation include any palpable lump, bloodstained nipple discharge, sudden nipple inversion, skin dimpling, itchiness and flaky skin around the nipple area, or unilateral pain.

Classification of cytology

C1 = Inadequate sample/insufficient cells for diagnosis
C2 = Benign cells present
C3 = Atypical cells
C4 = Suspicious of malignancy
C5 = Carcinoma cells present

Benefits of breast screening

- Reassurance for women with a negative result
- Detection of early breast disease – has been demonstrated to reduce mortality
- Less aggressive treatments, i.e. more conservative surgical treatment is possible if disease detected early
- Improved national standards of care both within the screening and symptomatic breast care services
- Increase in breast awareness within the general population
- Increased profile of breast cancer – leading to an increase in charitable funds
- The introduction of clinical trials to investigate the treatment of early breast cancer and thus more knowledge of the disease

Criticisms of breast screening

Many critics of the breast screening programme bemoan the fact that it is not accessible to women over 64 and under 50.

Why not screen the over 64s? It must be made clear that being over 64 does not prohibit women attending for screening. On the contrary, women over this age are welcome to telephone their nearest screening unit to make an appointment. However, evidence from other countries has shown that the acceptance rate for women over 64 years declines, consequently not justifying a heavy investment in administrative costs in organizing sent appointments (Forrest, 1986). It is also thought that some women over this age may already be suffering from other illnesses, and therefore may not regard breast screening as a priority.

Why not screen women under 50? There is insufficient evidence from studies in other countries that screening women under 50 reduces mortality (Forrest, 1986). Generally, mammography in this age group is less reliable as a screening tool because of the dense glandular tissue in a premenopausal breast. In addition, a three-yearly programme may be far from adequate, due to the often aggressive nature of breast cancers in some younger women.

Initially, many of the critics of screening suggested that breast screening causes unnecessary anxiety in women found to have benign breast disease. In recent studies there is little evidence to support this. To the contrary, many studies suggest little evidence of prolonged anxiety (Farmer et al., 1995).

The most significant point raised amongst the critics is in relation to the benefits of screening in terms of long-term survival. Many claim that whilst breast screening appears to reduce mortality, it may in fact be simply detecting a cancer earlier. Whilst survival appears to be prolonged, in reality, the time scale between diagnosis and death is extended rather than overall survival (Rodgers, 1990):

> in effect we are asking people whether they want to find out if they have cancer earlier than they would have … this action, without adequate counselling of women before the screen to inform them of the implications and risks of screening, is ethically unjustifiable.

In conclusion, it will be many years before one can truly reflect on the evidence, experience, and real benefits of breast screening in relation to overall survival.

Risk factors

HRT

The influence of HRT on breast cancer has recently attracted much publicity. A study by Beral (cited in Wise, 1997) suggests that the relative risk was 1 in 35 in those women who had taken HRT for five years.

Family history

The risk of breast cancer caused by a genetic link accounts for less than 5% of all breast cancers. A moderate risk includes women who have a first degree relative diagnosed with breast cancer under 50 years of age, or two first or second degree relatives under the age of 60 years (White and Mackay, 1997). Women with a moderate to high risk might consider having annual mammography, although this is not currently widely offered within the NHS.

Some hospitals have a genetic clinic through which women can be referred via their GP. Women can now be screened for two of the genes associated with breast cancer (BRCA1 and BRCA2). However, all women considering genetic testing should be offered appropriate counselling to explore the issues associated with a positive result, e.g. does the patient then have a prophylactic mastectomy? How does the patient cope with this knowledge? One of the genes mentioned above is also associated with an increase risk of ovarian cancer.

Presently, some hospitals are participating in the tamoxifen prevention trial. This national trial recruits women willing to participate in a research trial who have a moderate to high risk of breast cancer, to assess the value of tamoxifen as a preventative drug.

Table 4.1 Risk factors for breast cancer

Known risks	Age – incidence increases with age
	Early menarche
	Nulliparity or first pregnancy after 30
	History of benign breast disease
	Family history
	Prior history of breast cancer
	Ionizing radiation
Possible risks	HRT/oral contraceptive pill. Lifestyles, e.g. high fat diet, and alcohol intake exceeding 14 units per week.

Classifications of breast cancer

Ductal carcinoma in situ (DCIS)

This is a pre-invasive stage of the disease, whereby the cancer is confined to within the duct (Figure 4.1).

Invasive tumours

The classification of tumour relates to overall prognosis. Specific types of breast cancers often hold a better overall prognosis; however, all tumours are usually graded I–III. The grades represent the extent to which the cells are differentiated, i.e. represent normal breast tissue, and also the mitotic activity of the cells; e.g. a grade III tumour would be a poorly differentiated tumour cell unrecognizable as a normal breast cell, with a high mitotic rate, and thus be considered to be more aggressive. Grade I cancers generally have a better overall prognosis.

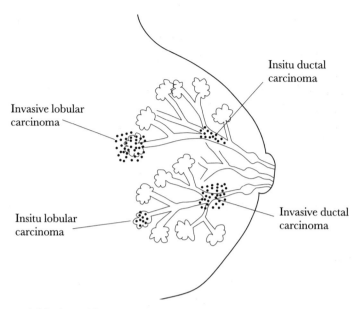

Figure 4.1 Insitu and invasive carcinoma.

Prognosis is also related to the extent to which the lymph glands are involved (Table 4.2).

Table 4.2 Survival of patients with breast cancer according to involvement of axillary lymph nodes

	Survival at 10 years
Negative axillary lymph nodes	64.9%
Positive axillary lymph nodes	24.9%
1–3 nodes involved	37.5%
>4 nodes involved	13.4%

(CRC, 1996c)

Spread of disease

Breast cancer may spread via the lymphatic or vascular channels. The most common sites of metastatic disease are bone, liver and brain.

Treatments

Ideally, each patient will be seen by both a breast surgeon and oncologist, who will provide an overview of the treatment options available. It is important at this stage that the breast care nurse is involved as she may provide an opportunity for further discussion of treatment options, as well as providing information to the patient regarding what to expect.

Surgery still remains the primary treatment, although in some cases (for example large or aggressive tumours), radiotherapy or chemotherapy may be more appropriate in order to downstage or gain control of the disease.

Surgery

Surgical treatment usually involves either mastectomy or wide local excision.

Mastectomy

This involves removal of the breast, and remains the treatment of choice in some circumstances. These include:

- Patients presenting with a large lump >4 cm
- Patient choice
- Multifocal tumours
- Patients who may be unsuitable for radiotherapy, which is usually given following wide local excision

Wide local excision

This is the removal of the tumour plus a circumference of normal breast tissue surrounding it. The patient should be informed that this might bring about some distortion of the normal breast architecture, causing some indentation of the breast.

It is important to remember that the overall survival outcome for both types of surgery is the same. The risk for local recurrence following mastectomy is approximately 10%. The risk of local recurrence after wide local excision followed by radiotherapy is also 10%. Wide local excision alone may have a 30% risk of local recurrence (Fisher et. al, 1989).

It would be wrong to assume that the psychological morbidity would be less for those undergoing wide local excision than for mastectomy. To the contrary, studies have suggested an equal scoring for psychological morbidity amongst both groups of women (Fallow-field et al., 1990). The woman who keeps her breast may fear recurrence, have a constant reminder of the cancer when she looks at her scar, not be able to touch her breast due to its association with cancer, and may envy those whom have undergone mastectomy.

Axillary surgery

It is usual for some axillary surgery to be done at the time of surgery. This may range from a sampling of glands from the axilla to gain a random picture of axillary node status, or complete axillary clearance. There is some debate nationally as to what is the most effective; however, there is an increased incidence in lymphoedema in patients following complete axillary clearance (Bundred et al., 1994).

Sentinel node biopsy

This is one of the most recent innovations in breast cancer treatment. There is evidence that 30% of node negative patients relapse within five years, possibly due to micrometastasis in the lymph nodes being missed, or the relevant affected nodes not being included in random axillary sampling. If the relevant lymph node responsible for drainage of the cancer could be identified, then appropriate treatment could be offered. The technique of sentinel node biopsy enables the identification of the primary node draining the tumour through the injection of a radioactive label into the tumour, which is then traced to the actual specific lymph node(s) responsible for draining the tumour (Veronesi et al., 1997). Further research will continue to evaluate the reliability of this technique.

Breast reconstruction

Both immediate and delayed breast reconstruction is available to all patients on the NHS following mastectomy. There has been much controversy recently regarding the use of silicone implants. A recent report to the department of health (Independent Review Group, 1998) reported no significant harm or dangers from silicone gel implants.

Breast reconstruction can be achieved in a number of different ways:

Tissue expanders

Following mastectomy an expandable implant is inserted under the chest wall muscle and pectoralis major. The implant is usually part silicone with a sac through which saline can be injected over time via a subcutaneous port. The implants are usually expanded during an outpatient visit over several weeks. Whilst this is quite a simple method, cosmetically it tends to be the least favourable. This method is also not suitable for patients who may require radiotherapy post-surgery.

Latisimus dorsi flap

Following mastectomy, the latisimus dorsi muscle, overlying skin, and its blood supply are rotated from the back and then tunnelled under the arm on to the anterior chest wall. A silicone implant is then placed underneath the transposed muscle. This method of reconstruction tends to be the most favourable.

Rectus abdominis myocutaneous flap

This abdominal muscle along with its superficial skin and blood supply is rotated, and tunnelled up on to the chest wall. Mesh is usually placed over the abdominal wall to minimize the risk of hernia. Due to the large amount of tissue that can be transposed, this method may avoid the need for a silicone implant. This method tends overall to be less favourable due to the increased risk (up to 10%) of possible flap necrosis (Watson et al., 1995).

Nipple reconstruction

This can be done as a day case, or overnight stay. It is not completed until the reconstructed breast has healed and thus may be done several months after the initial operation. The most frequent method is to utilize the skin of the reconstructed breast to create the nipple or use part of the contralateral nipple (nipple sharing), and then to create the areola by taking a graft of the skin from the inner thigh. Tattooing has also been used.

Many patients choose not to undergo reconstruction and are happy to continue wearing a external silicone breast prosthesis. This is usually fitted around 4–6 weeks post-surgery by either the breast care nurse or the hospital appliance officer. There is a variety of shapes and sizes of prostheses, including partial prosthesis for women who are left with a size difference following wide local excision. The silicone prosthesis will usually last several years and is replaced if the woman gains or loses weight, or when it perishes.

Endocrine therapy, radiotherapy, chemotherapy

Endocrine therapy

It is thought that many breast cancers are dependent on oestrogens. Consequently, treatments for breast cancer often include some form of hormone manipulation. Patients are usually advised not to take the combined contraceptive pill or to become pregnant for a least two years post-treatment. Patients on HRT are usually advised to discontinue.

Tamoxifen (20 mg daily) remains the most popular choice of adjuvant therapy post-surgery, and has been found to reduce the risk of contralateral breast cancer by up to 40% (Richards et al., 1994). The side effects include weight gain, hot flushes, altered libido, vaginal dryness and gastrointestinal disturbance; some patients may experience some menstrual disturbances if still menstruating. These side effects can be quite distressing in terms of quality of life, for example, not being able to wear their normal clothes and facing a further alteration of body image, as well as sleepless nights due to hot sweats – in this situation a progesterone, e.g. megestrol, may be of some value in controlling hot flushes. Visual disturbances can be a rare complication of tamoxifen, and patients should be advised to discontinue its use if reported. Another reported side effect is the slightly increased risk of blood clots; therefore tamoxifen is not usually prescribed concurrently with chemotherapy. More recently the risk of developing cancer of the uterus has been identified. Because this risk affects only one in 10,000 women, the benefits outweigh the risks; nevertheless patients who report any abnormal vaginal bleeding should be referred for investigation (Assikis et al., 1996).

For the future, the benefits of Arimidex versus tamoxifen are currently under evaluation. Trials have already shown a significantly improved survival benefit with Arimidex versus megestrol in post-menopausal advanced breast cancer (Buzdar et al., 1996).

Cessation of the ovaries can be achieved either by laparascopic oophorectomy, which will bring about an immediate reduction in oestrogen levels, or by radiotherapy to the ovaries which is a more gradual process, or through the use of drugs such as Zoladex.

Radiotherapy

After wide local excision of their tumour, all patients are offered adjuvant radiotherapy to the remainder of the breast. Patients post-mastectomy are also offered radiotherapy to the chest wall if the original tumour extends to the chest wall, and to the axilla if lymph nodes were involved. Radiotherapy may also be offered as a primary treatment to patients with particularly large or inflammatory tumours to downstage the disease prior to surgery.

Some women may choose to avoid any surgery to their breast and consequently opt for radiotherapy as a primary treatment. Radiotherapy may also be given as a palliative treatment to improve quality of life, e.g. to a fungating breast to control the extent of ulceration, fungation, and haemorrhage. Radiotherapy is also useful in the relief of symptoms caused by metastatic disease, e.g. to the bone to control pain and reduce the possibility of pathological fracture, and to control symptoms in other metastatic sites such as the brain and liver.

Patients often find their first visit to the radiotherapy department quite daunting, and it is important to explore their fears with them. Providing information regarding expectations and side effects may help to ameliorate the patient's anxiety. Treatment is usually given for a few minutes each day over a period of 4–6 weeks, hence practical issues such as transport, taking time off work, childcare, etc., may be of concern to the patient.

Side effects can include erythema and irritation of the skin. Patients are usually given instruction with regard to skin care, e.g. to avoid the use of perfumed soaps, deodorants, moisturizing creams, etc., on the specific treated area, and to avoid shaving under the affected arm during treatment. Other side effects may include tiredness, lethargy and depression.

The combination of both surgery and radiotherapy to the axilla increases the risk of lymphoedema. Approximately 5% of patients will develop a frozen shoulder (Bundred et al., 1994). Rare complications include brachial plexopathy, cardiac damage and pneumonitis.

Chemotherapy

Chemotherapy may be used:

- As an adjuvant treatment (in addition/as a backup to the primary treatment). It is most commonly offered to patients with node positive histology and to those with a grade III histology. The benefits of adjuvant chemotherapy are greatest in patients under the age of 50. However, a small benefit is also seen in women over 50.
- As a primary treatment or neoadjuvant treatment prior to other treatment in an attempt to downstage the cancer. This may be offered in the case of a particularly large or inflammatory cancer, or to gain control of the disease when lymph nodes are palpable at the patient's initial presentation. The use of neoadjuvant chemotherapy has increased in recent years, with about 70% of patients showing a partial response, and a possible 10–15% a complete response (Richards et al., 1994).
- For treatment of metastatic disease as a palliative measure. However, the benefits versus the side effects in terms of quality of life must be considered.

Treatment usually lasts approximately six months. The length of the cycles will vary according to the regimen.

Side effects will depend on the types of drugs used (see Chapter 3).

The nursing care of a patient undergoing chemotherapy should include psychological care in offering support. The patient might have to cope not only with her diagnosis and possible disfigurement in relation to mastectomy, but also with further disfigurement from hair loss and other side effects. Information should be given with regard to the expectations and side effects, as well as help and advice in relation to anti-emetic therapy, adequate nutrition, the risk of infection, and what to do if they are concerned. Information regarding hair loss should include advice on wigs, turbans, scalp cooling, and avoiding any harsh chemicals or frequent washing of the hair to preserve it as much as possible. Some patients prefer to have their hair cut short so they do not have to contend with long lengths of hair falling out, which can be quite alarming.

It is essential that the patient is given a contact number for help and advice.

Finance may also be a great concern for many patients, especially if the side effects render them unable to work. Help can be sought from charitable bodies, e.g. Macmillan grants.

Social workers, health visitors and community nurses should be involved as required.

Psychological reactions to breast cancer

Studies have shown that approximately 20–40% of women develop anxiety and/or depression within the first two years of diagnosis (Maguire et al., 1978., Maguire, 1994). One-third of women will also suffer psychosexual problems (Maguire et al., 1978). These factors support the need for long-term follow-up by the breast care nurse, who can recognize those patients in need of further support and counselling. Patients who are in need of further psychological help should be referred via their GP to a psychologist or psychiatrist.

It is not surprising that these psychological reactions occur when the news of a life-threatening illness is combined with the side effects of treatments. Many people still view cancer as a death sentence associated with pain and a lack of dignity. This view is particularly influenced by their own past experiences and encounters with the disease, e.g. the death of a close relative. For some, cancer or 'the big C' represents the stigma of a disease that might be catching, making the patient feel quite isolated or dirty. Patients may experience feelings of guilt, which often arise during their search for reasons to explain 'why me?'

The diagnosis may also cause a total disruption of patients' family and social life. This may result in the need for time off work, guilt that the disease has caused emotional upset for the rest of her family, and feeling that perhaps she might be a future burden on the family, etc.

Treatments also add to the psychological morbidity through bodily mutilation, fear of rejection by partner, lowered self-esteem, alopecia, weight gain, induced menopause, hot flushes, skin irritation, lethargy, lowered libido, etc.

Patients may react to the news of their diagnosis in a variety of ways e.g. denial, fighting spirit, helplessness, anxiety/depression, stoic acceptance (Fallowfield, 1991).

As the reactions vary, so does the need for information. It is important that the nurse assesses the individual need for information and gives it accordingly. It would be wrong, for example, to overload a patient in denial with an exhaustive amount of information as this clearly does not allow the patient to utilize her own coping strategy. Equally, it would be wrong not to offer information to a patient who copes through active participation in her treatment.

Nurses may be faced with a variety of emotional responses from the patient. It is often very easy to avoid difficult situations because of feelings of inadequacy in dealing with such situations. There is evidence to suggest that sometimes health professionals block conversations with patients, avoid questions such as 'am I going to die?' or avoid tearful situations and uncomfortable topics like sexual problems (Wilkinson, 1991). This may be in the form of avoiding cues that the patient gives, or distancing themselves from the patient in an attempt to protect themselves from becoming too emotionally involved.

Giving inappropriate encouragement or reassurance may result in the patient either feeling silly because they are worrying unnecessarily, or believing that perhaps these feelings are not normal. Denying patients the opportunity to express their emotions can result in suppression of their feelings, which can lead to long-term psychological problems. Alternatively, it may make the patient quite angry that the health professional has not demonstrated empathy. Premature reassurance may lead to a lack of trust and frequently only serves to make the health professional feel better. It is never appropriate to say you understand, as even if you have suffered a similar occurrence no two people will necessarily feel the same.

Try to offer the opportunity to see the patient in private if at all possible. Use open questions to allow the conversation to become deeper, for example:

'I am wondering how you are really coping with your diagnosis?'
'How have you been feeling about losing your breast?'
'What impact has your treatment had on your relationship with your partner?'

Observe both the verbal and non-verbal cues the patient is giving. If the patient becomes tearful avoid rushing off to make a cup of tea; stay with the patient instead. Allow adequate time for silences as silence is often a valuable time for patients to reflect and express their true feelings. Acknowledging their distress, providing the opportunity to talk and giving the permission to cry may be all that the patient wants. It is not always appropriate to reach forward and put an arm round someone, as many people find this offputting and may suppress their feelings to avoid the physical contact. It might be helpful to ask the patient if there is anything you can do for her.

Equally, denial can be a coping strategy. It is important that the nurse does not attempt to destroy this strategy. When breaking bad news, give warning shots prior to breaking the news so that the patient is in control of what she wants to hear (Maguire, 1994). Ask the patient if there is anything that they want from you, and give opportunities for the patient to return at a later date for further information. It may be helpful to give a list of where and what information, help and advice is available in your area so that the patient is able to access this as she requires.

Some patients appear anxious, and tend to ask an exhaustive amount of questions regarding their diagnosis, prognosis, and treatments. Whilst it is important to provide the information that the patient has asked for, it is often helpful to check how she is coping with all the information. Although she has asked for information she may have difficulty in thinking rationally or assimilating all the information given. Checking this with the patient may help to slow her down and provide the opportunity to express how she is really feeling with regard to the diagnosis. Relaxation tapes, exercises, and deep breathing exercises can be helpful. Some patients find the telephone numbers of support groups useful.

Case histories

Kate

Kate was 27, lived alone, and had a partner whom she had been seeing for six months. Her parents and sister lived close by. Kate had a very active social life, and had already developed a highly successful career.

Kate was referred by her GP to the breast clinic with a lump in her left breast. On examination there was a 3 cm lump directly behind the nipple. A mammogram, ultrasound and cytology confirmed the presence of carcinoma cells. Both the surgeon and oncologist discussed the treatment options available to Kate, but because of the position of the lump a mastectomy was advised. Kate was quite devastated at the thought of losing her breast so she opted for a mastectomy and immediate reconstruction. Kate appeared quite shocked and distressed, and at this time did not ask any questions but described feeling quite numb. She was given the contact number of the breast care nurse, and arrangements were made for her admission to hospital.

Whilst Kate was awaiting admission she contacted the breast care nurse. Kate had spent several days collecting information regarding breast cancer and treatment and wanted to have a further discussion regarding her treatment. The breast care nurse gave her the opportunity to explore her fears and concerns. Kate felt it was unfair that this was happening; she was quite tearful at this time and expressed concerns regarding her relationship with her partner, her future, and her fears of possibly needing chemotherapy as this might affect her fertility. Kate also feared losing her job, and felt her dreams had been shattered.

As well as providing the opportunity for Kate to explore her fears, the breast care nurse was able to provide further information regarding breast reconstruction. Kate also agreed to meet a former patient who provided her with the opportunity to see the scars and final outcome of a reconstructed breast.

Kate was admitted to the ward. Naturally, on admission she was quite tense. The nurse explained what was happening and took a brief history prior to surgery.

Postoperatively, Kate appeared initially relieved and euphoric that the operation was over. By the third day she began to focus more on what the scars would look like, and how her partner might react. During a routine change of dressing the nurse offered the opportunity for Kate to look at her breast. Prior to this, the nurse had warned Kate that the wound would still appear quite bruised and bloody, and that initially the positioning of the breast might appear quite high on the chest wall, but that this would gain a more natural shape over time. Once Kate had seen the scar she felt relief and was quite pleased with the cosmetic outcome. A little while later the nurse returned to find out how Kate was feeling. Kate had spoken to her partner and now felt quite positive about her relationship.

The physiotherapist provided a programme of arm exercises and Kate was informed of the possible nerve twinges/shooting pains she might temporarily experience as a result of her surgery. Prior to discharge the nurse arranged for the district nurse to visit to check the wound.

Two weeks later Kate returned to the breast clinic for her histological results. These showed a grade 1 cancer, and all ten lymph glands were clear of cancer. This meant that Kate would not need chemotherapy, which was a tremendous relief to her. Kate was advised to take tamoxifen for a period of five years. She was also advised to avoid the use of hormonal contraceptives for the future, and ideally not to consider pregnancy for the first two years due to the uncertainty of hormonal effects on the breast. For the future, provided she remains disease-free Kate will be able to fulfil her dream of having children.

Four weeks later Kate was seen again by the breast care nurse. Kate was now back at work and seemed to be coping well. She and her partner had resumed their normal sexual relationship, and Kate was awaiting a nipple reconstruction.

Wendy

Wendy was a 53-year-old married housewife with 3 children aged 18, 20, and 22. Wendy had discovered a lump in her breast a year previously. At this time the effects of the menopause were causing some depression. She had seen her GP, who had prescribed HRT. Six months later Wendy felt less depressed but now felt guilty that she had not mentioned her breast lump. Although she had received an invitation to attend breast screening she declined this due to fear that perhaps it was now too late, and the cancer could have spread.

Two weeks earlier Wendy had been invited for a well woman check with her local practice nurse. The nurse had noted that Wendy had not attended screening and gently questioned her about this so as not to make her feel victimized. Eventually, Wendy became tearful and explained to the nurse the events during the last year. The nurse asked the doctor on duty to examine Wendy. The GP could feel a 2 cm lump in the upper outer quadrant of the right breast. The nurse sat with Wendy for some time to offer support and explained to her what would happen at the hospital.

Two weeks later at the breast clinic Wendy had several mammograms, and a cytology sample was taken from the lump. The tests confirmed breast cancer, and the surgeon and breast care nurse explained to Wendy the treatment options available. Due to the position and small size of the lump Wendy was suitable for a wide local excision. She agreed to this and was admitted a week later.

Wendy had been quite tearful during the admission process, and told the nurse that she had felt quite guilty for leaving the lump a year. The nurse was able to sit and hold Wendy's hand and allow her to tell her story.

Wendy recovered well from her operation and was discharged two days later. Prior to discharge she was seen by the breast care nurse, who would offer long-term support.

Two weeks later Wendy returned for her histological results. These showed a grade III tumour with four of the lymph glands sampled involved. The oncologist told Wendy that chemotherapy would be advisable, followed by radiotherapy and tamoxifen. Wendy was shocked and devastated. She sat quietly, not uttering a word while her husband held her. Although the treatments were explained, Wendy took little in.

Two days later the breast care nurse visited Wendy at home. She still felt very guilty about leaving her lump, and felt that she would not have needed further treatment if she had acted more quickly. The initial shock had subsided and although Wendy still felt very low she was able to ask more questions about her treatment. The breast care nurse explained the possible side effects of treatments and offered Wendy the opportunity to see her on a regular basis.

One month into chemotherapy Wendy had lost all her hair. She had not been sleeping well due to her worries about the cancer, and she was now beginning to think quite negatively about her future. Although her breast had healed she associated it with cancer and feared that the cancer might return. Wendy's GP prescribed a mild antidepressant and referred her to a qualified counsellor.

Six months later Wendy had finished her chemotherapy and had only one week of her radiotherapy left.

Wendy had initially been quite apprehensive regarding her

radiotherapy. The treatment lasted approximately ten minutes each day over a six-week period. Wendy had only experienced minimal side effects, i.e. minor burning of the skin, and recently some tiredness towards the end of her treatment. During her treatment she was advised to avoid the use of any perfumed soaps or deodorants on the treated area in case they might irritate the skin during the treatment.

Although Wendy was still seeing her counsellor she appeared to be coping well. She was relieved to have come to near the end of her treatment, and although she remained tired from the treatment she was now sleeping. She still thought about the possibility of recurrence, but appeared less negative and more able to enjoy a normal life style. She was looking forward to her hair growing back.

Conclusions

Despite a recent fall in mortality rates from breast cancer, the reality is that breast cancer still assumes the highest mortality rate among women in the UK, and it will be many years before one can truly reflect on the evidence and real benefits of breast screening on overall survival. Since the introduction of tamoxifen, little in terms of treatment has changed. However, it is encouraging that there appears to be a widespread commitment to both national and international breast cancer trials. Whilst we continue to wait for the answers, it is important that we do not forget the present sufferers. Caring for patients should not be solely disease-focused. The devastating psychological effects of coping with the knowledge of a life-threatening disease, the family and social disruption, as well as the financial implications and side effects of treatment, must all remain an integral part of care.

Chapter 5
Colorectal cancer

JANIE WHITTAKER

Introduction

Colorectal cancer is one of the least talked about and least publicized types of cancer, and yet it accounts for 12% of all cancer deaths (breast cancer, for example, accounts for 9% of cancer deaths) (Cancer Guidance subgroup, 1997). One of the possible reasons for this lack of public recognition or discussion may be the embarrassment and social stigma attached to bowel function within our society. Other cancers, such as breast cancer, are widely publicized within the media and are the subject of many television programmes and newspaper articles. Celebrities even openly discuss their diagnosis and treatments for such cancers. That is not the case at present with bowel cancer, and there is very little public declaration, although a public awareness campaign has been launched by television presenter Lynne Faulds-Wood. It is hoped that this will change soon with campaigns to raise public awareness.

This chapter will look at the predisposing factors contributing to bowel cancer, as well as investigations and management. It will also discuss how individuals may reduce their risks of developing bowel cancer, and touch on current research into a national screening programme.

Colorectal cancer (large bowel cancer) is the second most common cause of cancer death in England and Wales after lung cancer. It is the sixth most common cause of death overall. In 1996, 15,000 deaths were recorded in England and Wales (Office of National Statistics, 1997), 68% of which were colon and 32% rectal cancers. Some 25,000 new cases of colorectal cancer are recorded each year. One in 50 people will develop the disease (Harrocopus, 1996).

Colorectal cancer (large bowel cancer) is a disease that predominantly affects the elderly population. About 75% of cases present at 65 years and over, the median age being 70. At present, there appears to be a slightly higher incidence of colon cancer in women and rectal cancer in men. A report entitled 'Effective Health Care in the management of colorectal cancer' from the Office of National Statistics Monitor (1997) recorded the incidence per 100,000 of the population (all ages) as 15.35 for men and 36.7 for women.

The incidence in the UK is considered high, as it is in other highly developed regions such as the United States, Australia and Western Europe. Low incidence of the disease is recorded in Africa and Asia.

Incidence in the United Kingdom

- 4 per 100,000 among people under 50
- 100 per 100,000 among people 50–69
- 300 per 100,000 among people over 70

Aetiology

When exploring the possible aetiology of bowel cancer, the global variations were originally considered to be due to the dietary differences of the populations concerned. In other words, geographical dietary differences such as high animal fat and a low fibre diet in the Western world and a high fibre and low animal fat intake in underdeveloped countries were believed to have a causal effect on the incidence of bowel cancer.

Supporting the hypothesis that diet does play some part in its causation was evidence from the USA that Africans who adopt a Western diet do appear to develop a higher number of colonic tumours than their contemporaries who adhere to their ethnic dietary regimes.

However, contradictory evidence from the Eskimos would appear to discredit that belief, as their ethnic diet high in animal fat and low in fibre diet indicates a high incidence of colorectal disease. In fact, Eskimos have a low recorded incidence (Schofield and Jones, 1993).

Schofield and Jones (1993) also report that there are several research projects exploring whether environmental factors increase the incidence of colon cancer. Some of the hypotheses being researched include smoking, alcohol consumption, high intake of red meat and the transit time of stools influenced by intake of fibre.

Evidence from two trials in America positively linked the consumption of large amounts of red meat with colon cancer. The highest risk was in the group that consumed more than 130 g per day, approximately two portions of red meat a day. The lowest risk was in the group that ate only two portions a week (Cummings and Bingham, 1998).

Research undertaken by Gregory et al. (1995) suggests that a reduction in the intake of fats, increase in fibre and five portions of fruit and vegetables a day, together with an increase in exercise, could help to protect against bowel cancer. Presently there does not appear to be a consensus on any specific environmental or specific carcinogens that are causal in the development of colorectal cancer.

However, there is evidence that a small number of cases – perhaps 5% to 8% of all colorectal cases – have a genetic syndrome that is hereditary.

Familial adenomatous polyposis (FAP) is a hereditary syndrome known to cause bowel cancer. It affects 1:10,000 live births and is inherited in an autosomal dominant fashion (Jarvinen, 1992). About 50% of family members are affected and without treatment death from colorectal cancer is universal by the age of 50. The commonest place for polyps to grow is in the large bowel. They grow in large numbers; often thousands are present at diagnosis. Polyps may develop as early as 15 years, at which age screening is appropriate. The treatment is surgical; the patient will discuss the options with the surgeon. Presently there are three surgical options: colectomy and ileorectal anastomosis, ileo-anal reservoir or proctocolectomy and ileostomy.

Another group of patients that has been identified as having a higher than normal risk of developing colorectal cancer is the *hereditary non-polyposis colon cancer* (HNPCC) group. These patients also inherit their disease in an autsomal dominant pattern; they grow fewer polyps and seem to develop cancers in the right colon. The mean age of diagnosis of cancer in this group is the mid-50s and it accounts for about 5% of all large bowel cancers.

Polyps

A polyp is a descriptive term used for a pedunculated lesion that projects into the bowel lumen. Polyps can be benign or premalignant. There is significant evidence that most colon tumours evolve from a specific type of polyp.

Morson (cited in Myers, 1996, p.249) describes the sequence from benign polyp to malignant polyp to carcinoma. The rate of progression is considered to be variable. In some patients the polyps may grow slowly and can be asymptomatic for many years, while for others it may be more aggressive (Mountnay et al., 1994). These polyps can be removed by colonoscopy if they are small enough. However, if on histology an invasive carcinoma is found, colectomy (i.e. removal of a part of the large bowel) may be required.

It is therefore important for the patient that the bowel tumour be classified so that the appropriate treatment can be offered The most common approach to obtain classification is to obtain a small piece of the tumour for histology by flexible sigmoidoscopy or by colonoscopy. Once the histological report has been obtained the doctor can discuss a possible treatment plan with the patient.

The most common histology in the large bowel is adenocarcinoma, present in 90–94% of cases (Black, 1997).

The presenting clinical features of colorectal cancer can include one or more of the following:

- Persistent change in bowel habit
- Blood on or mixed with stools
- Anaemia
- Nausea and anorexia
- Unexplained weight loss
- Abdominal pain
- Tenesmus
- Frequent, sometimes painful wind

(Cancer Guidance subgroup, 1997)

As these symptoms are frequently found in the elderly population, problems with obtaining an early diagnosis and treatment can occur. A large number of the elderly believe rectal bleeding to be a symptom of haemorrhoids and ignore this symptom. A percentage of patients with these clinical features will have the more significant disease of colorectal cancer.

At present, research indicates that the survival rate of patients may be linked closely to the classification and staging at presentation and surgical intervention. Staging of the disease is performed at surgical intervention by removing the tumour and sending it to the histopathology department for their opinion. In some areas this can be obtained intra-operatively, whereas in other centres it takes approximately 10–14 days for a definitive classification. This is significant, as many patients will wish to know the extent of the tumour spread and whether further treatment such as radiotherapy or chemotherapy will be offered.

In the UK the most common mode of disease classification of bowel tumours is Dukes classification (Dukes, 1932), which was introduced in the 1930s. It is still widely used today (see Table 5.1).

Cancers of the large intestine include all cancers in the colon and rectum. The incidence of specific sites is illustrated in Figure 5.1.

Table 5.1 Dukes classification

Dukes A:	The tumour has not penetrated the bowel wall
Dukes B:	The bowel wall has been penetrated but the lymph nodes are not involved
Dukes C:	The bowel wall has been invaded and the lymph nodes have also been invaded
Dukes D:	The bowel wall and lymph nodes have been invaded and there are distal metastases, e.g. liver.

Staging of bowel cancer

Survival rates

Dukes A:	83%	5-year survival
Dukes B:	64%	5-year survival
Dukes C:	38%	5-year survival
Dukes D:	3%	5-year survival

Percent of classification at initial diagnosis (or presentation)

Dukes A:	11%
Dukes B:	35%
Dukes C:	26%
Dukes D:	29%

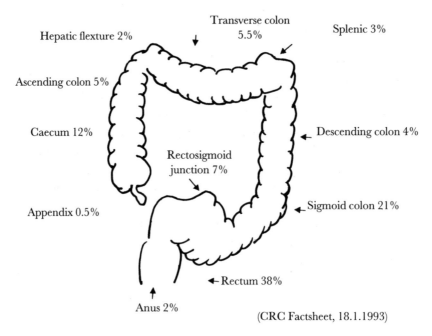

Figure 5:1 Site incidence of large bowel tumours.

Screening

As previously stated, survival is clearly linked to early diagnosis at Dukes A or B, so early detection offers the best chance. Various research projects are currently being undertaken to establish whether a bowel-screening programme would be a cost-effective method of reducing mortality and morbidity of colorectal cancer within the UK.

One method of screening for bowel cancer is to test the faeces for blood – the haemoccult test is a way of doing this. This involves using impregnated strips of paper that change colour in the presence of partially digested blood. Supporters of this method of screening insist that this is a simple non-invasive procedure. However, critics of this method suggest that due to its poor sensitivity many patients have tested positive and have shown minor colonic diseases but yielded very few colonic carcinomas (Schofield and Jones, 1993, Robinson et al, 1999).

Another research project being undertaken in centres around England is the Flexi-scope trial. This involves patients over the age of 50 who are asymptomatic (that is they have no previous history of colon disease or any symptoms) being examined by flexible sigmoi-doscopy. Critics of this trial suggest that as this is an invasive proce-dure with its own morbidity and mortality rate, the proposed programme may have a patient compliance problem.

It is hoped that the evidence from this research will attempt to answer the cost benefit analysis question, i.e. whether the yield of colonic cancers from a national screening programme would justify its cost.

At present, the agreed medical opinion is that surgical resection with possible radiotherapy and chemotherapy still offers the best hope of cure for the patient. As surgical procedures and treatments for bowel cancer are determined according to the position of the tumour, it is important to understand the different surgical opera-tions so that definitive advice and information can be given to the patient preoperatively.

Cancer of the right side of the colon

The majority of patients with a right-sided cancer of the colon will present with

- Anaemia
- Weight loss
- Abdominal mass
- Alteration in bowel function

These features could be suggestive of other gastrointestinal diseases such as cancer of the stomach or gastric ulcer. A palpable mass is sometimes evident but colonoscopy or barium enema should still be performed for a definitive diagnosis. More modern ultra-sound machines are able to identify typical appearances of colon cancer. Low obstruction of the bowel as the presenting symptom occurs only in 25% of right-sided colonic cancers. Abdominal X-rays would confirm this by showing loops of dilated small bowel.

Surgical intervention

This usually involves a performing a right hemicolectomy with a primary anastomosis (see Figure 5:2). This procedure is still under-taken even in the presence of hepatic metastases (Dukes D), as it is believed to give the best attempt at palliation (that is, the reduction of symptoms of the disease). It is not a curative procedure. Sometimes, the surgeon is unable to remove the tumour and therefore performs a bypass procedure by anatomizing the ileum to the transverse colon.

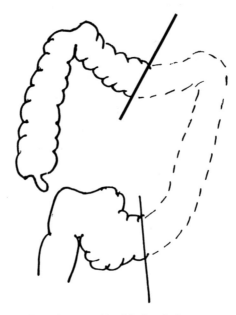

Figure 5.2 Section of bowel removed in right hemicolectomy.

The patient will be prepared for right hemicolectomy as per individual hospital consultant policies and guidelines. The nurse and patient, using the model of care that is used on the surgical ward, will plan preoperative and postoperative care.

It is important to allow time for questions as the age group will be predominantly elderly (over 65 years of age) and may have other disabilities. These can inhibit or distract from formulating necessary information and advice given by both the nursing and medical staff.

Postoperatively, the standard care of a major abdominal procedure will be undertaken. It is important to remember that one of the major functions of the large bowel is to reabsorb water, and this patient has had a significant part of his or her large bowel removed. Bowel motions after this procedure will usually be more fluid than before the operation. This should now be considered normal for this patient but may improve in time.

This change in bowel habit requires careful explanation so that the patient realizes it is to be expected. Otherwise, patients may believe that they have diarrhoea that is bacterial or viral induced or that the cancer may have returned.

Cancer of the left side of the colon

In patients who have not had previous surgery colon cancer is the most common cause of large bowel obstruction. In all, 30% of patients with bowel cancer of the left side will present with colonic obstruction and be admitted as a surgical emergency.

In order to obtain a definitive diagnosis and exclude other causes of colonic obstruction, the doctor will request either a water soluble or emergency flexible sigmoidoscopy. If the patient has perforated the bowel and has general peritonitis he or she will require urgent surgical intervention. Once a definitive diagnosis of a carcinoma in the region of the upper sigmoid to splenic flexture is made, the surgeon will usually proceed to a left hemicolectomy (see Figure 5.3). The nursing care will be the same as for a patient who has undergone a right hemicolectomy.

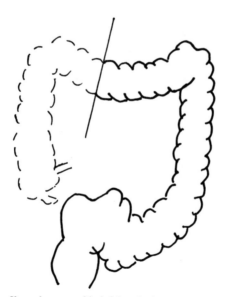

Figure 5.3 Section of bowel removed in left hemicolectomy.

Cancer of the sigmoid

In all, 21% of all colon cancers are found in the sigmoid; this is the second most common presenting form of colon cancer. The sigmoid colon is approximately 30 cm in length but can vary. As in the case of other left-sided colonic lesions, patients may present with alteration in bowel habit such as constipation, diarrhoea or blood with their stool. Weight loss can be a poor prognostic sign and sometimes an abdominal mass is palpable. If a lesion is found in the sigmoid then the surgeon will proceed to remove the sigmoid; in most cases a primary anastamosis is performed (see Figure 5.4).

In a small number of cases a primary anastomosis is still performed but the surgeon will form a loop ileostomy or loop colostomy. This is done to protect the patient against the effect of a leak by diverting the faeces away from the anastomosis. Assessment of the primary anastomosis is obtained by a radio opaque enema and once it has been determined that there is no anastomotic leak, then the second operation can proceed. This usually does not require another laparotomy but can be performed through the previous incision around the stoma. The patient's bowel function after reversal should return to semi-firm stool as before the operation.

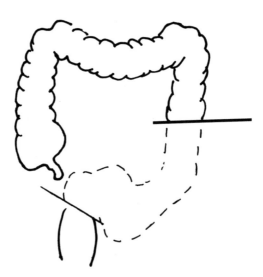

Figure 5.4 Section of bowel removed in sigmoid colectomy.

Cancer of the rectum

Cancer of the rectum is the most common form of colon cancer, accounting for 38% of all the colon cancers (CRC Factsheet, 18.1.93). The rectum has conventionally been divided into three sections. Position of the rectal tumour within the three sections is important when the surgeon is deciding upon the most appropriate type of surgical procedure.

The rectum can be divided into:

- Upper rectum   12–15 cm from the anal verge
- Middle rectum   8–11 cm from the anal verge
- Lower rectum   4–7 cm from the anal verge

Patients with rectal carcinoma will often present with symptoms of rectal bleeding, altered bowel habit and the distressing symptom of tenesmus. Tenesmus is described by patients as the feeling of never having completely emptied their bowel and of making repeated visits to the toilet to do so, often only passing slime and blood. Very few rectal cancers are admitted as emergencies. They are usually referred by their general practitioner to the hospital consultant in the outpatient department.

Confirmation of a rectal lesion can be obtained by a digital examination or, if the lesion is higher than 10 cm it can only be seen on sigmoidoscopy and a biopsy taken for histology. A small number of rectal carcinomas will extend out of the anus and are visible. A colonoscopy or a barium enema may also be required if no lesion is visible on sigmoidoscopy.

It is also important to recognize that normal anal function is required for continence. Any damage to the anal sphincter may result in the patient facing life with faecal incontinence, with both the physical and psychological distress of a permanent colostomy. Selection of the most effective surgical procedure will depend on the position of the lesion in relation to its position within the rectum.

Advances in sphincter-saving surgical procedures such as anterior resection have reduced the number of total excisions of the rectum now performed.

If a sphincter-saving procedure is not possible and the formation of a permanent stoma is suggested, the surgeon will refer the patient to the stoma care nurse. This nurse will provide support and advice on the possible lifestyle implications of a permanent colostomy. The discussion may involve the patient's partner if the patient so wishes. Concern about diagnosis and prognosis can add to anxiety about self concept with a stoma. Therefore, sensitive preoperative counselling and advice are necessary to enable the patient to progress to a positive alteration in self concept and self-esteem (Wade, 1989).

Research suggests that patients who are counselled before surgery have a more positive alteration in self concept and self-esteem (Wade, 1989). Simple clarification and discussion with the patient at this stage should lead to a reduction in the patient's anxiety and fear (Watson, 1989).

Cancer of the upper rectum

High anterior resection of the rectum is usually performed on patients who have a carcinoma in the upper half of the rectum (see Figure 5.5). In order for this procedure to be considered, the lesion must be suitable for adequate excision and anastomosis to remaining rectum.

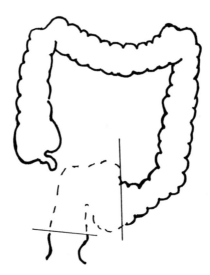

Figure 5.5 Section of bowel removed in anterior resection.

The surgeon will be aiming for 2–3 cm clearance below the tumour from the bowel margin for anastomosis to the remaining rectum (Pollett and Nicholls, 1983). On low rectal cancers, however, it is important to remove all of the mesorectum, or 5 cm distal to the tumour.

High anterior resection anastamoses are considered to be 10 cm or more above the anal verge whilst low anterior resections are anything below 6–7 cm from the anal verge.

The difference for the patient is that in low anterior resection, bowel function post-surgery may be poor; frequency, urgency and incontinence can be a problem for weeks or in some cases months (Bennett, 1976).

The surgeon establishes a loop ileostomy or loop colostomy to divert faeces away from the primary closure. This is considered necessary to reduce the systemic effect on the patient should the primary anastomosis develop a leak postoperatively.

The loop ileostomy or colostomy will remain until an X-ray has determined whether the primary anastomosis has healed or not. If there is evidence of anastomotic leak the ileostomy will not be closed and another X-ray will be taken in another six to eight weeks to determine then if it has then healed. If it is then still not resolved, further major surgery may be indicated at the primary anastomotic site.

Cancer of the lower rectum

In some cases the rectal lesion is so near the anal margin that removal of the tumour would damage the sphincter and therefore cause the patient to become incontinent. In these cases it is suggested to the patient that total excision of the rectum will be required in an attempt to cure them. This will necessitate the formation of a permanent colostomy (abdominal excision of rectum and formation of a permanent left iliac colostomy; see Figure 5.6). The patient should be offered an opportunity to discuss this with a stoma care nurse.

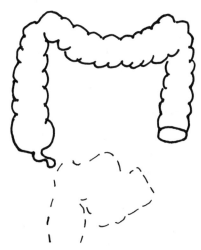

Figure 5.6 Abdominal perineal resection and formation of colostomy.

In males there is a possibility that due to proximity of the nerves that are involved with penile erection and ejaculation patients may subsequently experience impotency and retrograde ejaculation. It is reported that the risk of these complications may be as high as 43% (Joels, 1989). If the surgeon believes this may be the case then he or she will discuss these possible complications with the patient preoperatively.

Advances in colorectal surgery for patients with low rectal carcinoma

In London and Maastricht a pioneering surgical procedure has been created in which the neo-anal sphincter is electrically stimulated.

Anal cancer

Cancer of the anus accounts for about 4% of all colorectal malignancies. There is a higher incidence of anal carcinoma in women than in men, and the most common age for developing this form of cancer is 50 to 60. For many years these lesions were treated with radical surgery: an abdominal perineal excision of rectum and permanent colostomy. Recent evidence suggests that combination of radiotherapy and chemotherapy can achieve improved survival and prevent radical surgery.

Most patients are assessed by both a surgeon and a clinical oncologist and a course of radiotherapy is tried, with or without chemotherapy. Surgery will be considered if the above treatments do not achieve success (Jones and James, 1993).

Radiotherapy

Radiotherapy can be given either preoperatively or postoperatively in the treatment of colorectal cancer.

Preoperative radiotherapy

Patients who have rectal carcinoma are believed to benefit from a course of preoperative radiotherapy, which can achieve up to a 40% reduction in local recurrence at the rectal cancer sites. It is recommend in Cancer Guidance (1997) that patients with rectal carcinoma should be routinely offered preoperative radiotherapy, unless the surgeon can demonstrate a local recurrence rate of less than

10%. Local recurrence can be extremely painful and very difficult to manage. Surgeons who have a low recurrence rate of less than 10% may decide with the clinical oncologist to reserve the course of radiotherapy and use if further treatment is necessary.

The possibility of pre- or postoperative radiotherapy should be explained to the patient by a suitably experienced nurse, oncology/colorectal specialist nurse or stoma care nurse. This group of patients is likely to be elderly and may have previous personal knowledge or experience of patients and family who have undergone radiotherapy. They sometimes confuse comparable treatments such as chemotherapy with radiotherapy, which often leads to unrealistic fears and anxiety. The nurse and the doctors should be able to reduce these fears and give precise individual information about the effects of the radiotherapy in a manner the patient is able to understand and, based on that knowledge, make an informed decision whether to proceed with treatments offered.

Postoperative radiotherapy

Patients with recurrent metastatic tumours or patients who are judged to have a high risk of local recurrence may be offered a course of radiotherapy.

In cases of known advanced disease or bone metastases, a course of palliative radiotherapy is known to help reduce the local symptoms of the disease and may be offered. Radiotherapy can only be offered to patients who have not undergone radiotherapy in that area before.

Chemotherapy

Chemotherapy for colorectal patients can be divided in two groups: adjuvant chemotherapy and palliative chemotherapy (see Chapter 3).

Adjuvant chemotherapy (such as 5-fluorouracil and folinic acid – 5FU FA) is presently recommended for patients with a Dukes stage C colorectal cancer. Use of systematic adjuvant chemotherapy is believed to increase survival by about 6%, i.e. six deaths prevented per 100 patients treated (Cancer Guidance, 1997). The aim of adjuvant chemotherapy is to destroy any of the cancer cells that may have spread.

Palliative chemotherapy may be offered to patients with advanced disease. Its aim is to aid symptom control and improve the patient's overall quality of life. Palliative chemotherapy, if given at an early stage, has shown an increase in survival of about 3–6 months. Palliative chemotherapy is again based on a regime of 5-fluorouracil and folinic acid. The benefits and the possible side effects of the chemotherapy should be explained by the medical oncologist and the patient should be offered an opportunity to make an informed decision whether to proceed with the treatment

Elderly patients can often have very strong views on chemotherapy. They may be very much in favour of further treatment, or alternatively if unsymptomatic they may decline chemotherapy. It is important that the patient has an opportunity to discuss the proposed treatment with the oncologist and nurses to ensure that he or she can make the decision on the basis of up-to-date current practice and the effects of the specific drugs used in the treatment of colon cancer. In some cases, patients will have personal experience of relatives or friends who have had chemotherapy for other types of cancer and have suffered alopecia and or severe nausea/vomiting, and they may decline treatment based on this.

Research trials for colorectal cancer

At present various research trials are being undertaken in the UK.

The most significant and well known is the QUASAR study (Quick And Simple And Reliable). This trial is designed to compare no chemotherapy with high- and low-dose treatment. The decision-making process is by randomization, based on whether or not the doctor believes there to be a 'certain' or 'uncertain' indication for treatment with chemotherapy. So if the doctor is 'uncertain', the patient is randomized to treatment or not. If the doctor is 'certain' that he wants treatment, the randomization is between high-dose and low-dose treatment.

Case histories

Mrs Amos

Mrs Amos is a 78-year-old widow. She presented with acute intestinal obstruction and was in severe pain and vomiting faecal fluid. Her 50-year-old daughter accompanied her.

Mrs Amos was admitted to a general surgical ward as an acute surgical emergency. The house officer admitting her took a clinical history. She appeared to have no history of abdominal disease previous to the onset of her acute abdominal pain. An abdominal X-ray was performed and a diagnosis of left colonic obstruction made. The nurse admitting Mrs Amos was only able to take a short nursing history from her, due to her severe pain. Her daughter was, however, able to help provide general basic information. Once a definitive diagnosis had been made surgical intervention was discussed with Mrs Amos. As there was a possibility that a stoma might be necessary, the ward nurse contacted the stoma care nurse. The stoma care nurse visited Mrs Amos to offer preoperative information and advice and counselling on life with a stoma. In such cases, due to the amount of discomfort the patient is suffering, limited information and advice may be given and it will be determined by the patient herself.

It is necessary to mark the abdomen for the surgeon to indicate the most appropriate place for the stoma, so that the patient can manage the stoma postoperatively.

This decision can have a profound effect on the patient's postoperative rehabilitation, so it is of the utmost importance that a suitable site is chosen for the stoma (Elcoat, 1986; Bass et al., 1977).

Mrs Amos returned from theatre, where the tumour had been resected and a primary anastamosis achieved; stoma formation was not found to be necessary.

Mrs Amos was discharged from hospital after 12 days.

Mrs Amos attended an outpatient clinic with her daughter, where she asked the consultant whether she was cured of her cancer. The histology report indicated that her cancer had been classified as a Dukes C. The consultant asked Mrs Amos if she would prefer her daughter to be there whilst this was discussed, so her daughter was asked into the consultation room.

The consultant was able to tell Mrs Amos that they had been able to remove the entire tumour locally and that there had been no evidence of liver metastases at operation. Mrs Amos asked if any further treatment would be necessary. The consultant replied that she would be referred to the medical oncologist for consideration of chemotherapy.

The oncologist suggested that it was necessary to commence

chemotherapy. Mrs Amos discussed this with the oncologist and decided that she would agree.

Mrs Amos will be required to attend the hospital outpatient department for routine follow-up for up to five years. During one of these visits a full colonoscopy will be performed to ensure that there are no other lesions in her colon, as this procedure was not possible due to her presenting as a surgical emergency.

Mr Brown

Mr Brown is a 62-year-old married man who presented to his GP with rectal bleeding. He was referred to his local hospital and was seen by a colorectal surgeon who performed a sigmoidoscopy and was able to obtain a biopsy of a lesion that was found at approximately 15 cm from the anal margin. A barium enema was requested, and it confirmed a lesion in the descending colon. Mr Brown was admitted for anterior resection, as again there was a possibility of a stoma formation; the stoma care nurse was contacted for marking of his abdomen, preoperative counselling and advice to both the patient and his wife.

Mr Brown's tumour was completely removed and an anterior resection with primary anastamosis performed. The surgeon formed a loop ileostomy. Mr Brown remained in hospital for 12 days, during which time he was taught to manage his loop ileostomy. The stoma care nurse supported him and his wife in the community, by visiting him at his home and by outpatient appointment. His GP and district nurse also supported him.

The histology was found to be Dukes B classification. Therefore, no further treatment such as chemotherapy or radiotherapy was considered necessary. Mr Brown will be routinely seen at the hospital outpatient department for two to five years, where regular colonoscopy will be performed to examine the bowel for any evidence of recurrence of the cancer.

Mr Clark

Mr Clark is a 67-year-old married man. He presented to his GP with rectal bleeding and weight loss. In his district there is a rapid access clinic for rectal bleeding and he was referred there. At this clinic a flexible sigmoidoscopy was performed and a lesion was confirmed to be an adenocarcinoma on histology. Other investigations were requested and an ultrasound scan of his liver undertaken to check for any evidence of metastases.

He was referred to the colorectal team, where he was placed on the urgent waiting list to be admitted. The ultrasound showed no evidence of spread of the disease. Therefore Mr Clark was admitted for an abdominal excision of the rectum and formation of a permanent end colostomy. The stoma care nurse visited Mr Clark and his wife regularly both preoperatively and postoperatively to offer both education and support with management of the colostomy.

Mr Clark was discharged after 14 days and the histology and was found to be a Dukes C tumour. The consultant discussed the results with the patient, suggesting that Mr Clark consult the oncologist for an opinion on a course of radiotherapy or chemotherapy. After consultation Mr Clark decided to proceed with the oncologist's suggestion of a course of chemotherapy.

Mr Clark would be routinely followed up as an outpatient for up to five years by the surgeon and by the oncologists for any evidence of recurrence of the disease.

During a follow-up appointment with the surgeon at six months Mr Clark explained that he was now impotent and this was causing some problems for him and his wife. The surgeon was able to refer him to the urologist for review and treatment.

There are various options available, such as alprostadil, an intracavernous injection that will enable the patient to have an erection. There are also other treatments such as a penile implant or vacuum device. Recent developments in drug therapy may offer a benefit in the treatment of organic erectile dysfunction. After discussion with the urologist Mr Clark decided to carry out intracavernous injections and found them to be successful in enabling him to resume his previous sexual relationship with his wife.

Conclusions

Colorectal carcinoma is curable if diagnosed early, yet it is the second most common cause of cancer death in the UK. It remains one of the least talked about forms of cancer, and until that taboo is lifted patients will still literally be dying from embarrassment. The embarrassment associated with the discussion of the alteration of bowel habit or other symptoms such as noisy wind, which the patients also find socially inhibiting, often prevents them from going to their GP in time.

Development of an early detection process may prove successful in reducing mortality from this disease and it should reduce the number of stomas, thus limiting the effect this disease has on the patient's body image and sexuality (see Chapter 16).

The nurse involved with management of this group of patients can help reduce the patients' anxiety by being knowledgeable about the different types of surgical procedures, and the possible effects that the surgical procedure may have upon the patient's lifestyle. The nurse can offer psychological support by listening to patients' concerns and anxiety and assisting them through the different stages of their illness. Support from the patient's family and partner to adapt to a potentially devastating altered body image is very important. This can enable them to overcome their feelings of fear and isolation and return them to their preoperative perception of self worth and self-esteem.

Chapter 6
Lung cancer

CHRISTINE FEHRENBACH

Introduction

Lung cancer encompasses all phases of a chronic illness. Families and carers of lung cancer patients need particular support and attention. The majority of such patients are cared for at home with episodic hospitalizations for symptom management. The role of the nurse is crucial in conveying the diagnosis to sufferers honestly and sensitively. Realistic information should be given of the likely outcome and prognosis. Fears should be discussed and coping strategies should underpin good nursing practice. Public attitudes reflect that this is a disease of the poor and the old who have brought it upon themselves through their own smoking habits. Health professionals need to be instrumental in providing qualitative care to meet the complex needs of lung cancer patients and their carers.

There is no effective screening test and a limited range of treatment options, which means that lung cancer has a generally poor prognosis (Lowden, 1998). However poor the prognosis, patients benefit from accurate information regarding their disease process. Studies examined by Melville and Eastwood (1998) found that 90% of patients with lung cancer preferred to know the truth. As a cure is not an option, they will need to come to terms with the fact that their treatment may only be of a palliative nature. The Calman-Hine Report (1995) focused on evidence-based practice for the commissioning of cancer services.

Following on from this, the National Cancer Guidance Group (1998) looked at effective management of lung cancer. The recommendation deals with seven areas, with the obvious emphasis on prevention and palliative care. These areas include:

- Prevention
- Diagnosis and staging
- Multiprofessional teams
- Communication information and support
- Radical treatment for non-small cell lung cancer

Incidence and prognosis

Lung cancer is the most frequently occurring cancer in the UK, accounting for one in seven cancer cases (Cancer Research Campaign [CRC], 1994). It is estimated there are over 40,000 new lung cancer cases every year (CRC, 1996d). It is the commonest cancer in men, accounting for 22% of all new male cases, and in women the incidence is overtaking that of breast cancer (Murphy, 1997). The prognosis is generally poor; about 80% of patients die within one year of diagnosis (Northern and Yorkshire Cancer Registry, 1997) and 5.5% survive for five years (Berrino et al., 1995). Lung cancer is responsible for almost a quarter of all cancer mortality. It is the leading cause of cancer death in men and the second most common in women (CRC, 1996b). On average in the UK over 100 people die from lung cancer every day, or one person every 15 minutes (CRC, 1996d).

Predisposing factors

Smoking

Some 90% of lung cancer deaths are estimated to be caused by smoking. The risk of lung cancer in smokers is about 15 times that for those who have never smoked. It is highest for heavy smokers and increases with more years of smoking. The form in which tobacco is smoked and type of cigarette smoked also influences the risk. Non-smokers are at risk of developing lung cancer from passive smoking. A report from the Royal College of Physicians in 1992 indicated that about 300 people die of lung cancer in the UK each year as a result of passive smoking.

Occupational risk factors

Asbestosis is the most common occupation-related cause of lung cancer. The risk increases with cumulative exposure (Doll and Peto, 1981). Building workers, plumbers, gas fitters, carpenters, electricians, metal plate workers and fitters form the largest high-risk groups (Peto et al., 1995). Exposure to other substances known or believed to cause lung cancer include acetaldehyde, acrylonitrile, arsenic, beryllium bis(chloromethyl) ether, cadmium, chromium formaldehyde, nickel, polycyclic aromatic compounds (in diesel exhausts) silica, synthetic fibres, vinyl chloride and welding fumes (Coultas and Samet, 1992). Occupational groups who are at higher risk have been identified and guidelines have been developed to safeguard and protect their interests (Valanis, 1996).

Radon

Radon is a naturally occurring odourless radioactive gas which emanates from some types of rock. People who live in houses in which radon levels are high are more likely to develop lung cancer (Darby et al., 1998). Radon levels vary widely across Britain (NRPB, 1996), and information about all aspects of risk and prevention can be obtained from the National Radiological Protection Board.

Nutrition

Higher consumption of fruit and vegetables (in particular green vegetables and carrots) may halve the risk of lung cancer (World Cancer Research Fund, 1997). Genetic predisposition and alcohol consumption also are associated with increased risk (Valanis, 1996).

Types of lung cancer

Lung cancer can be divided into two categories. Small cell lung cancers (SCLC) and non-small cell lung cancers (NSCLC). The SCLC account for 25% of malignant tumours and are the most aggressive, growing rapidly and disseminating widely. They include oat cell tumours (20%). NSCLC account for the remaining 75% and are less aggressive. These are divided into squamous cell carcinoma (50%), adenocarcinoma 13% and large cell carcinoma 10%. Mesothelioma is a malignant tumour of the pleural mesothelium

sed by exposure to asbestos. At present it repre-
ratory cancers. Carcinoid tumours are usually
t like malignant tumours and when doing so are
ιt.

Presentation

A large percentage of patients with lung cancer present with symptoms directly related to the tumour but some put off coming to the
doctor despite their symptoms, thinking they may have flu (Krish-
nasmy and Wilkie, 1997). Table 6.1 lists the main signs and symptoms of lung cancer.

Table 6.1 The main signs and symptoms of lung cancer

Main signs and symptoms complained about	Percentage of complaints
Cough	80%
Haemoptysis	70%
Chest pain	70%
Dyspnoea	60%
Cyanosis wheeze	15%

The main presenting symptom is a cough due to the stimulation
of nerve endings by the tumour, especially if it is in the major
airways. The tumours are vascular and tend to bleed so haemoptysis
presents; this is often the most worrying symptom for the patient.
Prolonged haemoptysis can cause anaemia. Dyspnoea is caused by
occlusion and this can lead to atelectasis in the affected airway or
infection in the distal airways.

Central invasion of the tumour may affect the laryngeal nerve
and cause hoarseness from paralysis of the vocal cord. The phrenic
nerve may be involved, causing paralysis of the diaphragm resulting
in a decrease in ventilation. Enlarged lymph nodes in the mediastinum may compress the superior vena cava. This leads to enlargement of the face, neck and arms. Invasion of the chest wall and ribs

may involve the brachial plexus (Pancoast's tumour), presenting in shoulder pain. A third of patients present with symptoms due to metastatic spread. Bony metastases are common, presenting in pain and perhaps a fracture. Secondary deposits may present in the liver and brain. Headache and personality changes will be the presenting features. Secondary deposits may occur in the adrenal glands. Fatigue, anorexia and weight loss are common. Finger clubbing may also be present.

Investigation

Preliminary procedures include full physical examination, history, chest radiography and blood tests. The aim of diagnosis is both to identify the presence of lung cancer and to determine the tumour type. Histological confirmation is usually achieved using bronchoscopy, which involves introducing a flexible tube into the affected part of the lung and taking samples of the tumour by brushing, washing or biopsy. Bronchoscopy can have adverse effects (mortality rate 0.2%) and can be unpleasant for patients. Although tumour type can sometimes be identified from sputum cytology, this method cannot be used to exclude lung cancer because it has a high false-negative rate (Mehta et al., 1993).

Staging

Radical treatment, which may substantially increase life expectancy, is likely to be appropriate only for early-stage tumours. Staging assesses the pathological progress of the tumour. The international tumour, node and metastasis (TNM) classification is used. Apart from bronchoscopy, other means can be used to obtain specimens. They include fine-needle biopsy, often via CT scan. Chest aspiration and biopsy can be carried out if there is a pleural effusion. Mediastinoscopy allows direct visualization of the mediastinal nodes at the tracheo–bronchial junction. Mediastinotomy is a cut made over the second intercostal space on either side to gain access, usually to the left upper lobe, to take biopsies. Video assisted thoracoscopic (VAT) or open lung biopsy, and increasingly a thoracoscopy, enables biopsies to be taken to make a tissue diagnosis.

The staging process looks at the local intrathoracic extent, the extent of the disease ranging from tumour proven from presence of malignant cells to actual measurement and location of the tumour, whether it invades any local structure or whether atelectasis or malignant pleural effusions are present. The process also looks at nodal spread to local or regional nodes and whether there are distant metastases or metastases present, with the site specified. In NSCLC accurate staging is particularly important for decision-making about surgery.

Management

The management of patients with lung cancer should be the responsibility of specialist multiprofessional teams. A typical team in a cancer centre would consist of a chest physician, medical/clinical oncologist, pathologist, specialist nurse, thoracic surgeon and palliative care practitioners.

Non-small cell lung cancer

For those with early stage disease, first-line treatment is normally surgery or radiotherapy.

Surgery

Patients need to be carefully selected, as surgery is appropriate only for those who are relatively fit and who have adequate respiratory capacity. There is no evidence that selection should be based on the patient's age (Richelme et al., 1990). Lobectomy reduces FEV1/FVC by about 10–15% predicted and pneumonectomy by 20–30% predicted. Surgery carries an overall 5% mortality risk and causes significant morbidity. 10% of patients have major life-threatening complications and 50% have persistent incisional pain for 1– 4 years (Lederle, 1994).

Radiotherapy

Radiotherapy can be used if the tumour is localized and can be encompassed by a radiation field. Clinical oncologists treat the patient radically with the intention of cure. Medium-term survival appears to be improved by higher doses of radiotherapy, but the risk of serious adverse effects also increases.

Chemotherapy

Chemotherapy leads to a slight improvement in survival compared with no chemotherapy (NSCLC Collaborative Group, 1995).

Palliation

Many patients present with advanced/metastatic disease for which palliative interventions are likely to be appropriate. The main aim is to reduce the severity of symptoms. Chest symptoms such as breathlessness, cough and haemoptysis can be relieved by radiotherapy. Radiotherapy offers substantial relief in over 40% of patients with pain due to metastases.

Small cell lung cancer

The first-line treatment for SCLC is normally chemotherapy. Radiotherapy may be used in addition. Median survival without chemotherapy stands at 2–4 months, whereas reported survival with chemotherapy stands at around 12 months (Facchino and Spiro, 1998). Combination chemotherapy, usually cyclophosphamide, doxorubicin/vincristine (CAV), leads to better outcomes than single-agent treatment (Facchino and Spiro, 1998). Up to 10% of patients in some trials have died after chemotherapy, usually 1–2 weeks after treatment (Souhami et al., 1998). Nausea and vomiting peak at about three days with each cycle (of which there are usually six) and can cause marked impairment of quality of life. Patients who respond to chemotherapy may also benefit from radiotherapy to improve local tumour control and to the brain to reduce the risk of brain metastases.

Management of advanced disease

Patients with lung cancer experience more symptoms and often these are more severe and distressing in comparison to patients with other cancer sites (Ventafridda et al., 1990). The short prognosis of many patients means it is imperative that intervention is offered as soon as possible so that maximal quality of life can be maintained (Corner, 1997).

Symptom control

Lung cancer produces a wide range of symptoms which need to be managed to give the patient the best quality of life possible.

Respiratory symptoms will relate to the tumour and include dyspnoea, coughing, haemoptysis and increased sputum production. Pain will be related to chest wall involvement and bony metastases. Speech problems may be due to laryngeal nerve involvement. The oesophagus may be affected, leading to dysphagia. Fatigue and weight loss are also significant.

Dyspnoea

Breathlessness may be the symptom most feared by the patient. The cause is multifactorial. The care needs to concentrate on enabling the patient to express the emotions associated with breathlessness, to allow the physical and mental state to co-exist.

The breathlessness could be due to one or many of the following: airway calibre related to bronchial obstruction, and breathing pattern, which impairs gas exchanged. Panic attacks may occur as a consequence of hyperventilation and dyspnoeic fear. In a respiratory panic attack patients are very frightened, convinced they are suffocating to death. Coping strategies may involve breathing pattern training and relaxation techniques.

A study by Corner et al. (1996) demonstrated the usefulness of intervention strategies such as counselling and adaptation strategies in patients with lung cancer. Routine measures such as positioning the patient with arms resting on pillows and leaning forward can help chest expansion.

If the patient already has chronic obstructive pulmonary disease, high-dose bronchodilators may improve ventilation. Oxygen is only of benefit if the patient is hypoxic, otherwise cool air via a fan or open window may help.

Local anaesthetics may be inhaled or nebulized (Twycross and Lack, 1990). Eating and drinking must be avoided for several hours due to the local anaesthetic action.

Anxiolytic drugs such as diazepam are used for their sedative effects, and morphine leads to reduction in anxiety. Endobronchial therapies such as brachytherapy may be used to relieve airway obstruction (Grey, 1995). Tracheobronchial stents made of silicone are used for strictures due to external compression.

Anorexia, weight loss and fatigue are common in the advanced stages of lung cancer. Prednisolone may be useful in boosting appetite, and nutritional supplements may be helpful. Attention needs to be given to the patient's level of social support; help often needs to be given with the tasks of daily living.

Pain relief

When there is persistent pain, analgesics need to be given regularly and prophylactically in advance of the return of pain. Mild pain may be treated by non-opioid analgesics. More severe pain with a combination of a weak opioid (e.g. codeine) and a non-opioid should be used immediately for severe pain. Wherever opiates are used, it is essential to be aware of the side effect of constipation.

Smoking

Lung cancer patients experience immense fear, anxiety and distress, which is made worse by the knowledge that the causative factor of their disease has been self-induced. Some patients find the process to quit smoking at diagnosis very easy, others more difficult. Support should be given at this time by the nurse.

Health promotion

Screening

Screening using radiography and/or sputum cytology for asymptomatic men at high risk of cancer concluded that it was not effective (US Preventative Task Force, 1996).

Smoking

Clearly prevention is vastly better than cure for lung cancer, and much more cost effective. There would be a tremendous reduction in the number of patients requiring treatment for lung cancer if cigarette smoking were to be prevented. Smoking prevention is the only measure that can be expected to have a substantial impact on lung cancer incidence. The prevalence of cigarette smoking had been decreasing since about 1970 but has increased since 1994, particularly among young people and women under 35 (ONS, 1997). The powerful multinational tobacco industry has brought about a global smoking epidemic that will remain one of the greatest causes of disease, death and misery (Moxham, 1995). Effective interventions range from mass media campaigns to individual advice and support. Quit rates range from 2% from advice from a health professional to 12% from nicotine replacement plus advice, support and counselling. It appears that young people are not greatly influenced by fear of fatal or disabling disease caused by smoking. No-smoking policies on hospital premises and provision of smoking cessation counsellors may assist quit rates.

Case history

Sarah Smith

Sarah Smith, who was 72 and widowed, lived in a warden-controlled flat and was well supported by a very caring daughter. Although she used to be a smoker she had stopped around ten years previously.

Mrs Smith started to feel very tired, lost her appetite and developed a cough, even on occasion coughing up some blood. She attended her GP surgery and her doctor sent her for a chest X-ray (CXR), which showed a 'shadow' on her lung, leading to her being referred to the local chest physician. On attending the hospital she was advised to have a bronchoscopy and was admitted for the day; returning home following the procedure.

Mrs Smith returned to clinic the following week to have the bad news broken to her that she had lung cancer. The lung cancer specialist nurse was present at the consultation and supported Mrs Smith and her daughter afterwards. It was agreed between the doctor, patient and family that she should receive some palliative radiotherapy as this would suit the tumour type. She was also prescribed some oral steroids to help her appetite and weight loss, as Mrs Smith explained that these were her most worrying symptoms. In addition to suffering a great deal of anxiety, Mrs Smith felt extremely tired and therefore the consultation was based around determining which activities were most important to her so that she could concentrate her energy on them. During her radiotherapy, Mrs Smith felt tired and the chest pain she suffered was controlled with simple analgesia. Her daughter continued to be very supportive but found that her feelings about her mother's illness were difficult to come to terms with.

Mrs Smith was reviewed by the chest physician regularly but within six months had developed secondaries in her liver. She was referred by her GP to the palliative care team and later died peacefully in the local hospice.

Conclusions

Lung cancer is the most common form of cancer in the world, with patients over 65 accounting for more than half the new cases. Statistics show that the risk increases with age and this means that as life expectancy increases we can expect more cases of lung cancer.

The link between smoking and lung cancer means that there is a stigma attached to the disease and many people, including some health professionals, have negative views about it.

The management of lung cancer depends on histological cell type, performance status, patient choice, physician choice and treatment centre. Prognosis is usually poor because most patients have locally advanced or metastatic disease and 80% die in the first year.

Both the psychological and physical needs of a patient must be managed by a multidisciplinary team to promote supportive care for both patients and their carers.

Chapter 7
Gynaecological cancers

TRACEY WILSON

Introduction

This chapter will discuss the different types of gynaecological cancers. It will look at the more common types of malignancies such as ovarian, cervical and uterine, but it will also discuss the lesser known malignancies such as those of the endometrium, vagina, vulva and Fallopian tubes.

The chapter will also consider predisposing factors, detection, treatment and prevention of these cancers and support that is available to patients and their families, either within the NHS or from independent support groups and organizations.

Cancer of the cervix

This is the third most common malignancy in women. Although there is a decrease in incidence, there are about 4,500 cases in the UK each year (Hunter, 1994, Hancock, 1996a). the main predisposing factors are:

- Women in lower socioeconomic groups (groups 4–5)
- Commencing sexual intercourse at a young age
- Large number of sexual partners
- Viral infections such as human papilloma virus
- Smoking
- Multiparity ·
- Non-barrier methods of contraception
  (Barnes and Chamberlain, 1988)

At present the average age of women affected by carcinoma of the cervix is 50s to 60s, although the incidence of positive or abnormal smears through the 20s and 30s is increasing (McKie, 1993). In the 20–30 age group there is a higher proportion of adenocarcimona: 26% compared with an overall incidence of 10% (Slade et al., 1998).

Screening

The UK has a screening programme that helps detect changes on the cervix. The screening is in the form of a cervical smear, carried out routinely by GPs, practice nurses and the family planning service. All sexually active females should be offered a cervical smear every 3–5 years (Department of Public Health, 1993).

A cervical smear is not a test for cancer but a test to detect any changes that may have occurred to the cervix. Any such changes may be staged as cervical intra-epithelial neoplasia (CIN). CIN is then graded between I and III according to the degree of cytological abnormality. Women may also be recalled for a repeat cervical smear due to an inadequate sample, or if any bleeding occurred during the procedure, as this may contaminate the sample. Since the introduction of cervical screening there has been a great deal of debate over its accuracy and necessity. McPherson (1994) asks:

1. What number of positive smears progress to invasive carcinoma?
2. What numbers regress to normal?
3. How long do these changes take to occur?
4. What factors influence these changes?

Research by McIndoe et al. in 1984 and previously by Peterson in 1956 followed up a group of 131 women treated for CIN III who continued to have abnormal cytology for more than two years after initial treatment. After 20 years, 36% of these women had developed invasive disease (Soutter, 1993). Since the introduction of cervical screening in the developed world, mortality rates from cervical cancer have decreased by approximately 30% (between 1960 and 1980). This has been attributed directly to the screening programme and early treatment (Hunter, 1994).

Staging

Carcinoma in situ

Cervical intra-epithelial neoplasia (CIN) is graded from I to III, according to the degree of cytological abnormality.

CIN I: mild dysplasia/abnormality
CIN II: moderate dysplasia
CIN III: severe dysplasia

Cervical dysplasia is considered a premalignant condition that may require treatment or monitoring by annual cervical smears.

Treatment

The treatment for cervical dysplasia is by loop diathermy, cautery, laser vaporization, cone biopsy, cold coagulation, or laser loop excision.

Loop diathermy/cautery or cryocautery

A probe is inserted into the cervix which is then frozen at -56 °C for two minutes. This can be done as an outpatient, or, if deeper cautery is required, a general anaesthetic may be administered. After this treatment women should be warned that there may be some bleeding and discharge and also to avoid intercourse for at least 14 days (Barnes, 1988).

Laser vaporization

A laser is operated under colposcopy conditions, which allows for specific areas of the cervix to be treated. A carbon dioxide laser is commonly used in gynaecology – this works by the beam from the laser being absorbed by the tissue on the surface; the cells are disrupted and the tissue vaporized (Soutter, 1993).

Cone biopsy

This is not a substitute for colposcopy. A colposcopy should be performed prior to a biopsy to determine the margins for the biopsy. The biopsy itself involves the use of general or local anaesthetic, and a sample is taken from the cervix in the shape of a cone to be sent off for cytology (Soutter, 1993).

Cold coagulation

This treatment is not suitable for lesions that have extended to the vagina. For cold coagulation to work the whole lesion must be visible by colposcopy. It can take up to ten minutes, with specific sites having treatment of 20 seconds at a time (Soutter, 1993).

Laser loop excision

The transformation zone may be excised using a large cutting elec-trosurgical loop. The benefit of laser loop excision is that it combines diagnosis and treatment in one visit (McPherson, 1997).

A cervical smear should be taken six months after this treat-ment, and if necessary treatment should be repeated. Depending on the severity of the disease, a hysterectomy may be required. As with other diseases, an accurate diagnosis and appropriate staging of the carcinoma is imperative to give the woman the best treatment options and the best chance of survival.

Staging for carcinoma of the cervix follows the FIGO recommenda-tions (see Table 7.1)

The treatment for cancer of the cervix depends on the staging of the disease. Early diagnosis may require a hysterectomy but this carries a very high long-term survival rate. Stages II and III will require surgery, which may involve a hysterectomy and node sampling. The node sampling will aid with the staging of the disease, followed by radiotherapy and possibly chemotherapy.

Stage IV disease may require patients to undergo surgery, radio-therapy and chemotherapy. These treatments will probably only be able to offer palliation of symptoms at this stage.

Radiotherapy will be given either externally or internally. Exter-nal radiotherapy would require a number of visits to a radiotherapy department over a few weeks. Guidelines should be given on care of the skin around the radiotherapy site. Dietary advice should be given by the clinical oncologist, radiographers and nurses within the depart-ment. Internal or intracavity radiotherapy may be given as an outpa-tient using a machine known as a microselectron (see Chapter 2). This

Table 7.1 FIGO staging for cervical cancer

Stage	Description	5-year survival rate
Stage 0	Carcinoma in situ	79%
Stage I	Confined to cervix 1a microinvasive 1b others	
Stage II	Beyond cervix but not reaching pelvic side walls involves upper two-thirds of vagina	47%
Stage III	Cancer extends to pelvic side wall or to lower third of vagina There may be hydronephrosis or a non-functioning kidney	22%
Stage IV	Cancer extends beyond pelvis; involves the bladder or rectal mucosa Distant metastases	7%

type of treatment will require more than one visit to the radiotherapy department. If treatment is required over a few days, then a hospital admission will be necessary. The patient would have to be accommodated in a side room and limited visiting would be allowed due to the radiation. The applicators may be inserted in theatre under general anaesthetic and then the radioactive sources inserted later on in the ward, after the patient has been to the simulator to ensure the applicators are in the correct position (see Chapter 2).

Chemotherapy treatment can be given on an outpatient or inpatient basis, depending on which drugs are used.

There may not be any physical signs or symptoms when a woman presents with this disease. It may simply be found following a routine smear. The clinical features a patient may present with include:

- Postcoital bleeding
- Inter-menstrual bleeding
- Post-menopausal bleeding
- Vaginal discharge
- Pelvic pain or discomfort

If other organs are involved there may be tenesmus and diarrhoea, with the possibility of a fistula, haematuria and renal failure
(Sinclair and Webb, 1993).

Prevention

If we look at what are commonly perceived as the predisposing
factors of cancer of the cervix, perhaps information could be
included in school sex education lessons warning young girls that the
more sexual partners they have the more likely they are to develop
the disease (this is quite apart from the fact that they need to consider
the problem of unwanted pregnancies).

If teenagers could have access to appropriate information it may
lead to greater numbers attending for cervical screening. McKie
(1993) found that many women made negative links between cervical cancer and sexual promiscuity.

Cancer of the ovary

This is the fifth most common cancer in women; approximately 5,000
women are affected and there are 4,000 deaths from this disease annually in the UK. Ovarian cancer kills more women than endometrial
and uterine cervix cancers combined. Cancer of the ovary is more
common in women over the age of 40 (Hancock, 1996a).

Ovarian tumours can be benign, malignant, primary or
secondary, solid or cystic. This chapter will look at epithelial ovarian
cancer, the commonest form, which accounts for 90% of ovarian
cancers, as well as non-epithelial cancers such as germ cell tumours
and sex cord tumours.

Predisposing and protective factors

There is a strong indication that pregnancy and the oral contraceptive pill have protective features.

The risk factors for ovarian cancer are late menopause, nulliparity or infertility. Ovarian dysfunction may be responsible for the
infertility.

Screening

There are several tests available and in use, but if used in isolation they are not sensitive enough for a conclusive diagnosis. The tests that have been evaluated for ovarian cancer screening are bi-manual pelvic examinations, abdominal ultrasound and serum CA125 levels. A C125 test requires a sample of blood to be analysed in a laboratory. At present there is no simple, cost effective test that is accurate enough to be used in a screening programme for ovarian cancer. To date no single screening test for ovarian cancer has combined high enough levels of sensitivity and specificity to be considered suitable for use in population screening (David, 1995). A screening tool for the future may lie with chromosome 17, identified as one of the genes that predisposes to ovarian cancer (Hancock, 1996b).

Presentation

Late presentation is common as early symptoms tend to be non-specific, such as abdominal discomfort, indigestion, pelvic pain, urinary frequency or incontinence. Bowel actions may change and there may be some backache. Not all women will have these symptoms, if they have any at all. The vagueness of the symptoms may explain why 70% of cases have disseminated disease at the time of diagnosis (Hernandez and Rosenhein, 1989) (see Table 7.2).

Table 7. 2 FIGO staging for ovarian cancer

Stage	Description	5-year survival rate
Stage I	Confined to ovaries 1a one ovary – no ascites 1b two ovaries – no ascites 1c one or two ovaries with ascites or tumour on ovarian capsule	Between 60–77 %
Stage II	One or two ovaries with extensions to the pelvis	45%
Stage III	Widespread intraperitoneal metastases; omentum commonly involved or positive retroperitoneal nodes	17%
Stage IV	Distant metastases	5%

Treatment

Some women will be referred for treatment via general surgery or medicine, having presented with non-gynaecological symptoms. In the case of any women over the age of 40 with gastrointestinal symptoms or bowel problems, ovarian cancer should be ruled out (Sinclair and Webb, 1993).

The primary treatment for ovarian cancer is surgery. The extent of the surgery will depend on the stage of the disease. For advanced stage disease, debaulking surgery is routine, and should ideally be carried out by an oncological gynaecologist. The surgery will involve total abdominal hysterectomy, bilateral salpingo–oöphorectomy and removal of the omentum. The smaller the amount of residual disease remaining at the end of surgery, the better the prognosis (Hancock, 1996b).

Chemotherapy may follow surgery. Blood tests will be carried out before each course of chemotherapy to ensure that haemoglobin, white blood cells and neutrophils are within 'safe' limits to continue with treatment. A serum CA125 may also be taken. Although a CA125 is not adequate as a screening tool for ovarian cancer, it can be used as a tumour marker in some patients, i.e. in those where it is elevated preoperatively. Serum CA125 tumour marker is elevated in 80% of patients with advanced epithelial ovarian cancer. The rapidity of the CA125 drop under chemotherapy is an independent prognostic variable, and the marker rises in the event of a relapse (Piccart, 1993). Following relapse second-line chemotherapy may be required.

A patient with terminal ovarian cancer may present at any time with abdominal ascites. This may require drainage on more than one occasion, and a shunt may be used to improve the quality of life for those women who require frequent drainage. There is also the possibility of bowel obstruction, which will initially require admission to hospital. The patient may also have vomiting associated with the obstruction. Surgery is not an option for women with end-stage disease. Many women with advanced disease may well be cachexic. This can be a very distressing time for their families. The patient may have an extended abdomen due to her ascites, but otherwise be wasting away before their eyes.

Prevention

As the risk factors for ovarian cancer are late menopause, no pregnancies and possible infertility, there appears to be little an individual can do to prevent this type of cancer. Not all women want children and the timing of the menopause is out of our control.

Germ cell tumours of the ovaries

Germ cell tumours are uncommon tumours of the ovary. They include endodermal sinus tumours (yolk sac), embryomal carcinomas, malignant teratomas, mixed germ cell tumours, choriocarcinomas and gonadoblastomas.

These tumours respond extremely well to chemotherapy. Germ cell tumours are more common in younger women, and chemotherapy rather than surgery or radiotherapy offers greater potential for continued fertility (Early, 1995). Sex cord stromal tumours or granulosa cell tumours are very rare, and the cell of origin is uncertain. These tumours often secrete hormones, most commonly oestrogens, with oestrogen-related symptoms such as post-menopausal bleeding, menorrhagia and breast tenderness.

Endometrial cancer

There are approximately 3,000 new cases of endometrial cancer in the UK each year. About 3% of women over the age of 30 will develop this disease, and it is becoming more common (Slade et al., 1998). In the United States, 34,0000 new cases were diagnosed in 1989 (Hernandez and Rosenhein, 1989).

Endometrial cancer generally affects post-menopausal women, with the average age ranging from 60 to 70 years.

Aetiological factors

The aetiological factors associated with endometrial carcinoma are nulliparity or low parity, obesity, diabetes, hypertension and prolonged use of oestrogen therapy. There is concern over the use of tamoxifen for breast cancer, as there has been a slight increase in the incidence of women taking tamoxifen and being diagnosed with endometrial cancer (Hancock, 1996a). Slade et al. (1998) also mentions a positive family history in about 15% of endometrial carcinoma cases.

Screening

At present there is no screening programme, but this disease has a good prognosis, with 85% survival rate at five years for stage I (Hancock, 1996b).

Signs and symptoms

Endometrial cancer usually presents with the clinical features of post-menopausal bleeding, which may be heavy and include clots. In pre-menopausal women there may be irregular bleeding, as well as a vaginal discharge, but this is less common. Table 7.3 illustrates the FIGO stages of endometrial cancer.

Table 7.3 FIGO staging for endometrial cancer

Stage	Description	5-year survival rate
Stage I	Confined to endometrium	76%
Stage II	Cancer spread to cervix	51%
Stage III	Cancer spread to surrounding pelvic tissue	26%
Stage IV	Cancer spread to bladder or rectum and possibly distant metastases	9%

Treatment

Endometrial carcinoma is generally treated by surgery and a total abdominal hysterectomy, and bilateral salpingo–oöphorectomy is recommended if the disease is at stage I. For stage II a Wertheim's hysterectomy is recommended. A Wertheim's hysterectomy involves the removal of a 2–3 cm cuff of vagina and supporting tissues along with a total hysterectomy.

If a patient is considered unfit for surgery, external beam radiotherapy and intracavity radiation (brachytherapy) are options that can be effective (see Chapter 2). Following surgery, radiotherapy is recommended for patients with significant invasion of the myometrium or lymph node involvement. External beam radiotherapy may be given over a few weeks, and requires daily attendance. Intracavity treatments require an admission to hospital. The patient may be treated in a single room and have limited visitors (see Chapter 2).

The patient will have a urinary catheter and be on bed rest for the duration of the treatment. The intracavity device may require an anaesthetic in theatre or, if a 'dobbie' tube is used, this can be inserted on the ward.

If a patient has a relapse with endometrial carcinoma the most common systemic treatments are progestational agents, which give remission rates in 29% of patients. The women who respond to progestogens have a survival period of 23–29 months compared with six months for the women who do not respond (Earl, 1995).

Prevention

The factors associated with endometrial carcinoma are obesity and hypertension. Obesity is something that with hard work and determination can be overcome in the majority of us, although it may require the help of a dietitian or leisure club to help change the way a person cooks, shops or perceives food.

Levi et al. (1993) concluded from research into endometrial carcinoma that 'some qualitative aspects of the habitual diet may also be associated with the risk of endometrial cancer, chiefly the intake of animal proteins and fat (directly) and of fresh fruit, vegetables and fibres (inversely)'. A reduction in weight may help to reduce blood pressure, which again is a predisposing factor to endometrial cancer.

Follow-up

A patient who has had either surgery or radiotherapy would ideally be followed up in a joint gynaecology/oncology clinic. Initially the appointments would be about 4–6 weeks after treatment, at 3-monthly intervals for 2 years, then 6-monthly until the fifth year then annually (Hernandez and Rosenhein, 1989).

Cancer of the vagina

Carcinoma of the vagina is very uncommon, accounting for approximately 1–2% of female genital cancers (Sinclair and Webb, 1993). It is usually associated with elderly women but there have been reports of this disease in young women and children. It accounts for 150 deaths in the UK per year.

Predisposing factors

Squamous carcinomas account for the majority of vaginal carcinomas, at over 90%. The predisposing factors of this disease include a previous CIN, irritation due either to a prolapse of the uterus – which may mean that the cervix protrudes through the vagina – or a ring pessary. There may also be a relationship between this disease and chronic infection or previous radiotherapy (Slade et al., 1998). Squamous carcinoma of the vagina presents as a lump or an ulcerative mass. There may be some vaginal bleeding and occasionally a vaginal discharge. There are rarely any reports of pain, and any spread of this disease is usually via the lymphatics or localized. If the disease has spread via the lymphatics then this may involve pelvic and para-aortic lymph nodes and nodes in the groin.

Treatment

The treatment of choice for vaginal carcinoma is radical radiotherapy. Care has to be taken with radiotherapy, as the rectum and bladder are in close proximity to the area being treated (Sinclair and Webb, 1993). Although radiotherapy is the treatment most units choose, surgery may be required in some cases. Surgery may also be required for recurrent or resistant disease (Slade et al., 1998).

Chamberlain (1995) indicates that surgery gives a better prognosis, although the treatment is radical and involves the removal of the vagina, uterus and pelvic lymph nodes.

Radiotherapy does not provide such a good prognosis and should be used for recurrent and local spread. It is difficult to predict survival rates as the number of women suffering from this disease is so small and figures vary, although Slade et al. (1998) suggest a 75% survival rate at stage I at five years, and 0–20% survival rate at stage IV at five years.

Rare vaginal carcinomas

Clear cell adenocarcinomas

Rare tumours of the vagina include clear cell adenocarcinoma, which is more common in the USA than the UK. It is associated with young women whose mothers were treated with stilboestrol during pregnancy. If a woman has been treated with stilboestrol during pregnancy and delivers a girl, the child should be tested for clear cell carcinoma during her teenage years with vaginal smears and colposcopic examination. Radical surgery is the main course of treatment (Chamberlain, 1995).

Sarcoma botryoids

This type of tumour presents with bleeding or haematoma at the entrance to the vagina, affecting very young girls at about the age of two. The treatment of choice is chemotherapy, with long-term survival increasing (Slade et al., 1998).

Malignant melanomas

This type of tumour is extremely rare and accounts for about 1% of vaginal tumours; treatment is the same as for malignant melanomas elsewhere on the body with a similar prognosis (see Chapter 8).

Carcinoma of the vulva

Carcinoma of the vulva accounts for approximately 5% of female genital cancers and there are around 800 new cases each year in England and Wales. This disease affects mainly elderly women although there have been cases of women being affected in their 20s and 30s (Slade, 1998). Squamous carcinoma accounts for approximately 85%, melanoma 10% and other more rare conditions account for the remaining 5% of reported cases.

The presenting features for carcinoma of the vulva are similar to carcinoma of the vagina. Women may present with a lump or an ulcer which may be bleeding or infected. Some women may have a history of vulval intra-epithelial neoplasia (VIN) and lichen sclerosus. VIN is associated with strains of the human papilloma virus, and lichen sclerosus is a term used to describe an inflammatory process of unknown aetiology. Lichen sclerosus is also associated with VIN, although it is not proven to be a premalignant condition. Pruritus is also a common feature of this disease, with the intense irritation causing some women to scratch the area and cause some local trauma. Diagnosis of carcinoma of the vulva is made by biopsy.

Treatment for carcinoma of the vulva depends on the extent of the disease at diagnosis; the tumour may spread to the inguinal or lymph nodes in the groin. Surgery involves triple incision vulvectomy and bilateral node dissection, while large tumours may require more extensive surgery. This type of treatment may also be offered as a palliative measure. Radiotherapy may be offered to patients who are unfit for surgery, but the area of skin involving the vulva tends to be intolerant to radiotherapy (Hancock, 1996a). One of the possible side effects of node dissection is lymphoedema. This can lead to swelling of the lower limbs, but early mobilization and physiotherapy post-surgery may help.

The prognosis for carcinoma of the vulva depends on the stage that the diagnosis was made, with lesions of less than 2 cm having a better prognosis than larger tumours. For tumours that are small and with no evidence of spread to the inguinal nodes, a prognosis of about 90% of women surviving five years is not uncommon (Chamberlain, 1995).

Rare carcinomas of the vulva

Rare carcinomas of the vulva include malignant melanomas and basal cell carcinomas, with malignant melanomas of the vulva having a very poor prognosis as spread via the lymphatic system can lead to distant metastases in the lungs or brain. Treatment of this disease is by radical surgery which involves radical vulvectomy with dissection of lymph nodes. Basal cell carcinoma is a very rare, slow-growing tumour that does not metastasize. Treatment is by surgery, which involves a localized excision of the affected area (Chamberlain, 1995).

Carcinoma of the fallopian tubes

Carcinoma of the fallopian tubes is extremely rare, accounting for fewer than 1% of genital malignancies in women. There are approximately 40 new cases per year in England and Wales. The type of cancer is usually an adenocarcinoma and one or both tubes can be affected. The women affected are mostly between 40 and 60 years of age (Chamberlain, 1995).

This type of cancer usually presents late because there are no symptoms at the early stage. During the later stages there may be abnormal vaginal bleeding/discharge which may be watery, usually in post-menopausal women (Slade et al., 1998). If there has been any metastatic spread to the surrounding organs, there may be an abdominal or pelvic mass which can be felt on examination. There may also be some ascites and pain.

The treatment for carcinoma of the fallopian tubes is similar to ovarian cancer, with surgery being required and the ovaries, the uterus and both fallopian tubes being removed. The prognosis is poor because a diagnosis may not previously have been made and only confirmed at surgery (laparotomy).

Chemotherapy may be given following surgery; again the treatment would be similar to ovarian cancer.

Staging of this disease is usually carried out at laparotomy, although FIGO does not have a classification for carcinoma of the fallopian tubes (Hernandez and Rosenhein, 1989), so the TNM classification would be used.

Cancer during pregnancy

Cancer during pregnancy is extremely rare, accounting for approximately 0.8% of all cancer cases in women. In the USA about one in 1,000 cases of cancer occur in pregnancies annually (Bonner, 1995). In the UK hydatidiform moles occur in about one in 700 pregnancies, with choriocarcinoma occurring in 1 in 30,000. The incidence of choriocarcinoma is higher in Asia (Hancock, 1996a). Gestational trophoblastic disease in the UK is managed by regional centres. Any patients with a hydatidiform mole should be referred to one of these units for specialist care/management.

Hydatidiform moles

Hydatidiform moles usually occur during the first 18 weeks of pregnancy and the cause is unknown. Patients may present with excessive nausea and vomiting, absent foetal heart beat and a 'snowstorm' appearance on ultrasound scan. Approximately 20% of hydatidiform moles will become malignant, that is choriocarcinoma (Sinclair and Webb, 1993). Choriocarcinoma is diagnosed by histology. This disease is curable if detected early, and the treatment is by chemotherapy.

Staging of this disease depends on the level of β-HCG in both the urine and the blood serum levels. The patient will also have a pelvic examination and a chest X-ray. Chemotherapy offers a good prognosis, and will cure about 85% of patients. Following successful treatment many women will have pregnancies, but there is an increased risk of molar pregnancy in women who have previously suffered trophoblastic disease (Hancock, 1996 a).

Cervical cancer and pregnancy

Women who are diagnosed as having cervical carcinoma during pregnancy usually present at stage 1.

Treatment of cervical cancer during pregnancy presents a dilemma. The mother may wish to delay any treatment until after the birth of her baby. Each case needs to be assessed individually and take into account the site, the stage of the disease and the health of both mother and foetus.

Early treatment with radiotherapy may result in spontaneous abortion of the foetus, which can then be followed by internal radiotherapy (Chamberlain, 1995). If the pregnancy is in the later stages, a short delay may be considered if a viable birth is feasible. A vaginal delivery is contradindicated due to the possibility of dissemination of malignant cells via the lymphatic system, therefore a caesarean and Wertheim's hysterectomy may be performed, followed by radiotherapy if indicated. Slade (1998) mentions a report that describes the use of chemotherapy at 22, 25 and 28 weeks gestation with no adverse effects on the foetus. The prognosis for women with cervical cancer during pregnancy remains the same as for women who are not pregnant when the diagnosis is made.

Case histories

Sarah

Sarah is a 28-year-old who, although unmarried, has been in a relationship for nine years. She and her partner have no children but plan to have a family in the future. Sarah is a teacher and was called by her GP to make an appointment following her cervical smear. Sarah was referred to the local hospital for colposcopy, the results of which indicated that a cone biopsy was required. This involves the excision, under anesthetic, of the transformation zone. This biopsy subsequently showed carcinoma of the cervix stage II and a hysterectomy was advised. Sarah was devastated by this news. She had shown no symptoms, had been with her present partner for many years, did not smoke and did not consider herself promiscuous. She discussed her fears and anger with the gynaecology/oncology nurse specialist and contacted BACUP for more information.

Sarah and her partner also had to accept that they were now unable to have children of their own.

Sarah had her surgery and spent a few days in hospital. On discharge she had a follow-up appointment in a joint oncology/gynaecology clinic, and in future will be reviewed regularly in this clinic.

Sue

Sue was a 48-year-old part-time shop assistant. She was married to Dave and they had three children, two of whom had left home. The youngest was in her final year at school taking her GCSEs.

Sue presented at her GP with what she thought was probably irritable bowel syndrome. She had been having altering bowel actions with some discomfort for a few months. She was referred to a gynaecologist, who at the initial consultation decided to send her for further investigations which included serum CA125 and an abdominal ultrasound. Sue's CA125 was raised and the ultrasound showed a large mass. A date was arranged for surgery.

Sue had a laparotomy which proceeded on to a total abdominal hysterectomy, bilateral salpingo-oöphorectomy and debaulking. Biopsy and an abdominal lavage were performed and samples sent to the laboratory for histology. The histology indicated that Sue had stage III ovarian cancer.

Her treatment was chemotherapy once a month for six months. Between each course she would have a full blood count (FBC), and regular CA125 measurements were also undertaken.

Five months after completing her chemotherapy Sue unfortunately had a relapse. Her CA125 was once again rising and she had abdominal ascites, which required her admission to hospital so that the ascites could be drained. Sue was to receive second-line chemotherapy, which was given every two weeks. This was undertaken as an outpatient.

Sue's condition continued to decline, but although she knew that the only treatment available was to control her symptoms she was still very much in control of her own life. During this time Sue had the support of her Macmillan nurse and refused admission to a hospice, choosing to spend her remaining time at home but keeping open the option of respite care at the hospice. With the support of her family Sue was able to arrange her own funeral. She had time to say goodbye to her family and remained positive to the end. For her last few days a syringe driver was commenced to help with the pain and nausea, which enabled Sue to die peacefully at home with her family around her.

Doris

Doris is a 68-year-old housewife, married with two children and three grandchildren. Doris is overweight by about four stone, hypertensive and recently diagnosed with diabetes.

She has had some vaginal bleeding and, as she went through the menopause approximately 13 years ago, she made an appointment at her GP. Her GP referred her to the local hospital, where an appointment was made for an overnight stay for an examination under anaesthetic (EUA) and dilation of the cervix with uterine curettage (D&C). Prior to the EUA and D&C Doris also had a chest X-ray, which was clear, and a full blood count to check her haemoglobin. Following the EUA and D&C Doris had a follow-up appointment with the gynaecologist to discuss the results and possible treatment. She was advised that a total abdominal hysterectomy was required, followed by radiotherapy. Due to her other medical conditions, i.e. her diabetes, obesity and hypertension, the doctors were reluctant to consider a long anaesthetic and therefore offered the alternative treatment of radiotherapy. Doris was admitted to a single room and went to theatre the following morning for insertion of intracavity devices, i.e. uterine tubes and ovoids. The caesium was inserted later on the ward. Doris also had an indwelling urinary catheter. The caesium was left in situ and Doris was to remain on her bed. Visitors were restricted to a few minutes per day and her grandchildren were not allowed to visit. On removal of the caesium and catheter, Doris's urine output was monitored, together with her vaginal loss for a few hours. She was then allowed home. Doris was followed up in the joint oncology/gynaecology clinic six weeks later, and continued to be followed up in this clinic at regular intervals.

Conclusions

Gynaecological cancers can bring additional specific concerns, including the effects of surgery and treatment that may affect fertility, sexual functioning and self image. For cervical cancer there is a national screening programme that can detect any changes to the cervix and is available to all women within the UK, but it is up to the individual woman to attend for her cervical smear. Many women associate cervical cancer with being promiscuous, but a recent study looked at a number of women who had only had one sexual partner, and it was found that the more sexual partners these men had in the past, the more likely their present partners were to develop cervical cancer.

For younger women, a diagnosis of a gynaecological cancer may bring the possibility of loss of fertility following hysterectomy. This may exacerbate feelings of losing control of oneself and one's bodily functions, and may magnify any body image problems. Any woman who has an early menopause due either to surgery or radiotherapy will then have to consider what treatment, if any, she will accept. Generally some form of hormone replacement therapy is recommended: by patches, implants or oral medication.

All women need to be aware of their natural body functions, and any abnormal bleeding or pelvic discomfort needs to be investigated. Any gynaecological condition can involve embarrassment and women's perceptions of any disease need to be treated with empathy. Women must be encouraged to attend their GP surgeries for cervical screening and where possible attend well women clinics. Education needs to start early and should include such subjects as predisposing factors associated with different types of cancer. Prevention is better than cure and early diagnosis gives a better prognosis. Once a gynaecological cancer has been diagnosed women require respect for their own feelings. The distress engendered arises from many sources, whether a fear of dying, pain, mutilation or simply fear of the unknown, resulting in a feeling of utter helplessness.

Medical and nursing staff have a duty to treat the whole patient – to give holistic care. The medical profession may have a tendency to focus selectively on the life-threatening aspects of the disease at the expense of other factors. Many health workers find it embarrassing to use sexual vocabulary but it is necessary and will be required from the initial stage of identification onwards.

Chapter 8
Skin cancers

JANICE GABRIEL

Introduction

Skin cancers are a group of malignant conditions which include basal cell carcinoma (BCC), squamous cell carcinoma (SCC) and malignant melanoma (MM). BCC is the most common type of skin cancer, accounting for approximately 75% of skin cancers in the UK. It is followed by SCC, accounting for approximately 20% of skin malignancies, followed by malignant melanomas, which account for the remaining 5% (Ketcham and Loescher, 1993).

This chapter will look at the different types of skin cancers, predisposing factors for developing these malignancies and how they can present. The prevention, detection and management of these cancers will also be discussed, together with the support available to patients.

The skin

The skin comprises two layers, the epidermis and the dermis (Figure 8.1). Squamous cells are found below the keratin layer of the epidermis and basal cells are situated beneath the squamous cells (Gibson, 1975).

The skin has multiple functions. Not only does it protect an individual from injury and infection, but it also regulates body temperature and stores water, fat and vitamin D.

There are six different skin types, depending upon how much melanin is contained within the layers of an individual's epidermis. The more melanin someone's skin contains, the less likely they are to burn when they are exposed to the sun (Gibson, 1975; Morton, 1993). Morton (1993) has highlighted the six different types of skin; these are summarized in Table 8.1.

Table 8.1 Skin types

Celtic ancestry	{ Skin type 1: hardly ever tans, and always burns Skin type 2: tans with difficulty and burns easily
Mediterranean ancestry	{ Skin type 3 : tans and does not burn easily Skin type 4 : tans easily and does not burn
Asian or African ancestry	{ Skin type 5 : darkens easily and does not burn Skin type 6 : resists burning. Naturally very darkly pigmented skin

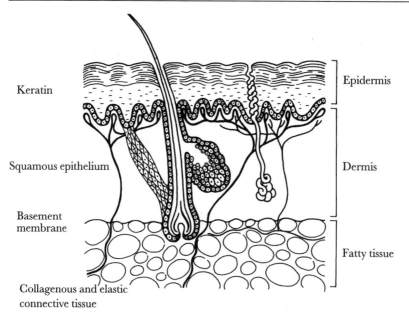

Figure 8.1 The skin.

Aetiology

Ultraviolet radiation (UVR) is believed to be the most common cause of skin cancers. Because of this, most skin cancers are found on sun-exposed areas of an individual's skin. Common sites include the face, ears, neck, upper back, arms and legs (Ketcham and Loescher,

1993). UVR is produced by the sun and contains two types of rays which are harmful to our skins, i.e. UVA and UVB (Ketcham and Loescher, 1993; Morton, 1993). UVA rays penetrate deeply into the skin, while UVB rays are shorter and cause superficial damage, i.e. burning.

It is believed that the UVR leads to damage of the skin cells' DNA, which can result in malignant changes occurring at a later date (Ketcham and Loescher, 1993; Morton, 1993). There has been much debate regarding the depletion of the earth's ozone layer and the possible effects that this will have on the incidence of skin cancers (Mason, 1992; Ketcham and Loescher, 1993). In the USA, the Environmental Protection Agency estimated that a 1% decrease in the ozone layer would correlate to a 1–3% increase in skin cancers per annum (Ketcham and Loescher, 1993). In the UK various organizations have campaigned for the public to be made aware of the potential risk of burning from UVR on a regular basis, and this is now a regular feature of summer weather forecasts (Mason, 1992).

The majority of us, regardless of our skin type, have some pigmented lesions on our bodies. We may have been born with a mole or birthmark, but as we get older these benign lesions increase in number. If we are familiar with our 'normal' moles, freckles and birthmarks, any additional lesions or changes in existing marks can be investigated sooner rather than later.

The more melanin an individual's skin contains, the lower their incidence of skin cancer is likely to be. However, that is not to say that people with naturally dark skins, e.g. people of Asian and African descent, are immune to skin cancer. They can develop skin cancers on the less densely pigmented areas of their body, such as the soles of their feet.

Apart from an individual's skin type and exposure to UVR, other risk factors contributing to developing skin cancer can include past exposure to ionizing radiation, past exposure to chemicals, previous trauma to the skin and long-term use of immunosuppressive agents. Previous damage to the skin can also cause DNA changes to take place. This can give rise to malignant changes in the area of previously damaged skin (Ketcham and Loescher, 1993).

Types of skin cancers

Basal cell carcinomas

Basal cell carcinomas (BCC) or 'rodent ulcers' are the commonest form of skin cancer in the UK, accounting for 75% of all skin cancers registered each year.

A BCC arises from the basal cell layer of the epidermis and is commonly found on sun-exposed areas of an individual's body. Common sites include the face, ears, neck, upper back, legs and arms (Ketcham and Loescher, 1993). These lesions usually enlarge locally, destroying tissue as they increase in size, which is why they are commonly referred to as 'rodent ulcers'. As the lesion enlarges it usually ulcerates. The ulcers are commonly characterized by their smooth, well defined borders (Figure 8.2).

BCCs generally do not metastasize, due to their superficial nature, but if left untreated, or inadequately treated, they can go on to cause widespread local damage (Figure 8.3). There is, however, an aggressive sub type of a BCC known as a 'basosquamous cell carcinoma'. This tumour contains basal cells and squamoid-like cells which can go on to metastasize if left untreated or inadequately treated.

Treatment

Treatment can consist of:

Surgery

Surgical excision of the BCC needs to be complete to ensure that the patient does not experience a recurrence of the cancer at a later date. The actual extent of the surgery will depend upon how large the lesion is and where it is situated (Ketcham and Loescher, 1993). A small lesion on the back or the face may well be removed under local anaesthetic, and the incision closed with sutures. A small lesion on the inner canthus may involve a more complicated procedure requiring reconstruction by a skin graft.

Radiotherapy

Radiotherapy can be used successfully for the treatment of some BCCs, depending upon where they are situated. It is not a treatment

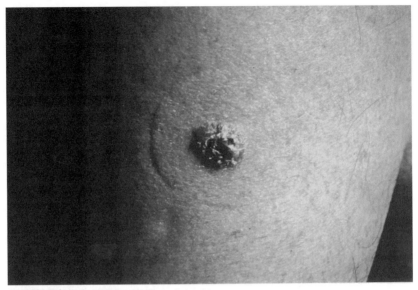

Figure 8.2 A typical basal cell carcinoma.

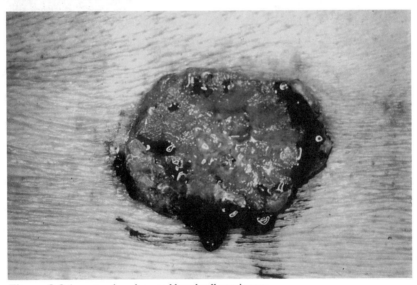

Figure 8.3 An extensive ulcerated basal cell carcinoma.

to be considered when the BCC is situated close to underlying bone or cartilage, e.g. the outer ear, as a late side effect of the radiotherapy could be necrosis of the bone or cartilage. In order to exert its maximum effect on the malignant cells, the radiotherapy is usually administered in several fractions. The radiotherapy can be administered by conventional superficial radiotherapy or by use of 'high dose rate microselectron moulds' at specialist oncology centres (see Chapter 2) (Svoboda et al., 1995).

Some specialist centres treat lesions on the hands and lower legs by the use of a silicone rubber or perspex mould. The mould is attached to a radiotherapy afterloading machine. This machine delivers a radioactive source into the mould, which is fixed to the patient's skin overlying the lesion to be treated (Figure 8.4). The exposure time for each fraction is very short and well tolerated by the patient. It also achieves a good cosmetic result (Svoboda et al., 1995).

A moist reaction (moist desquamation) commonly occurs in the treated area. It usually peaks about ten days after the commencement of the radiotherapy, and can take up to six weeks to settle, with the area becoming dry and sloughy (Svoboda et al., 1995).

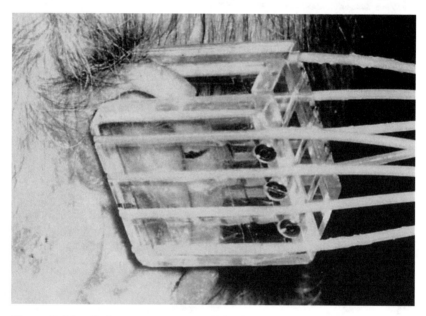

Figure 8.4 A radiotherapy treatment mould for skin cancer.

Cryotherapy

Cryotherapy is a treatment using liquid nitrogen that is normally used for superficial lesions. The liquid nitrogen, usually sprayed or 'dabbed' on to the lesion, causes freezing of the tissues. The tissue then thaws and the process is immediately repeated. The rapid freezing and then thawing of the cells results in their destruction (Ketcham and Loescher, 1993). The cryotherapy causes necrosis of the tumour, which will leave the patient with a 'scab' over the treated area. As the 'scab' dries, healing occurs. This treatment is initially uncomfortable. Indeed, some patients have likened it to a burning sensation, but the discomfort soon passes.

This treatment can easily and quickly be undertaken in the outpatient setting for superficial lesions. It is, however, unsuitable for BCCs situated close to underlying cartilage. This is because the cryotherapy damages the cells of the cartilage and during the healing process, which can take up to six weeks, the cartilage can become buckled. This will not only achieve a poor cosmetic result for the patient, but can also lead to a higher recurrence rate (Ketcham and Loescher, 1993).

Chemotherapy

Topical cytotoxic chemotherapy agents can be used for the treatment of BCCs. As these treatments are applied locally they do not have a systematic effect on the patient.

Currettage

Curretting can be used for the treatment of small superficial BCCs, usually those with an overall diameter not exceeding 2 cm (Ketcham and Loescher, 1993). The procedure, which is commonly undertaken in the outpatient setting, involves 'scraping out' the cells in the BCC. The advantages and disadvantages of the main treatments for BCCs are summarized in Table 8.2.

Due to the range of treatments available for the management of BCCs, it is helpful if the patient is seen in a 'combined skin cancer clinic', where discussions concerning treatment options can include the clinical oncologist, dermatologist and surgeon.

Follow-up

It is generally accepted that the total follow-up period for patients with BCC should not extend beyond two years. This is because any local recurrence is likely to occur within 18 months of treatment (Holt, 1988).

Table 8.2 Advantages and disadvantages of various treatments for BCCs

	Quick	Discomfort	Likely recurrence	Cosmetic result
Surgery	✓	++	very minimal	depends upon area being treated
Radiotherapy	Can involve several visits	+	very minimal	depends upon area being treated
Cryotherapy	✓	++	possible	good
Curettage	✓	+	possible to moderate	good to reasonable

Squamous cell carcinomas

Squamous cell carcinomas (SCC) account for approximately 20% of all skin cancers in the UK. They arise from the epithelium, are more aggressive and grow rapidly compared to BCCs. They can metastasize, depending on how deep the lesion is. A superficial SCC is less likely to metastasize than a deeper lesion. Metastatic spread is usually first identified in the regional lymph glands (Ketcham and Loescher, 1993).

SCCs located on areas of skin exposed to UVR, e.g. nose, lip, ears, etc., are less likely to give rise to metastatic spread than lesions located on other parts of the body. Despite this, exposure to UVR is by far the commonest cause of SCCs (Edwards and Levine, 1986; Stegman, 1986).

In contrast with BCCs, there are several other predisposing factors to developing SCCs. These can include:

- past exposure of the skin to ionizing radiation
- long-term use of immunosuppressive agent
- previously burned skin (either as a result of heat or chemicals)

SCCs resulting from any of these causes tend to have a higher incidence of metastatic spread (Ketcham and Loescher, 1993). These lesions are commonly characterized by elevated, firm papulae in their early stages. They may then ulcerate and become haemorrhagic (Figure 8.5). Due to the risk of metastatic spread, treatment should be adequate, so as to minimize the likelihood of recurrence. Therefore surgery or radiotherapy tend to be the treatments of

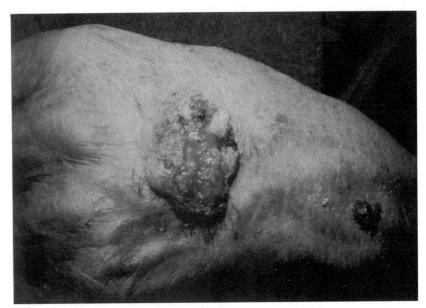

Figure 8.5 A squamous cell carcinoma.

choice, depending upon where the lesion is situated. In order to offer the individual patient the most appropriate treatment, on both curative and cosmetic grounds, it is helpful if they can attend a combined skin cancer clinic.

Melanomas

Melanomas arise from the pigment-producing cells of the skin, i.e. melanocytes. Melanocytes are found not only in the skin but also in the eye, gastrointestinal tract, respiratory tract, meninges and lymph nodes (Balch et al., 1989). They account for approximately 5% of skin cancers in the UK. There are more than 2,000 million melanocytes in the skin of an average individual (Weaver, 1976). Malignant changes can occur in an existing mole (naevus) or any melanocyte. The main factor that differentiates malignant melanomas from BCCs and SCCs is their ability to metastasize rapidly via the blood and lymphatic system (Dryden and Whyte, 1997).

In 1967 an American clinician by the name of Clark identified three types of malignant melanoma (Dryden and Whyte, 1997). A fourth type has subsequently been added.

These four types are:

Superficial spreading melanoma

This accounts for 70% of all cases of melanoma. It spreads outwardly, occasionally leaving an area of white skin as it increases in size (Figure 8.6).

Nodular melanoma

This carries the worst prognosis of all melanomas, with an average five-year survival rate of only 30% (Figure 8.7). It accounts for between 15% and 30% of all melanomas.

Lentigo melanoma (Hutchinson's freckle)

This commonly occurs on sun-exposed areas, e.g. the face, in older people. It is slow-growing with a favourable prognosis (Figure 8.8).

Acral lentiginous melanoma

This is rare in fair-skinned individuals. It accounts for between 4% and 10% of all melanomas.

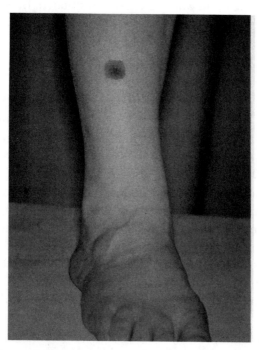

Figure 8.6 A superficial spreading malignant melanoma.

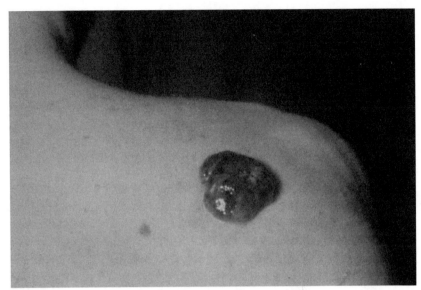

Figure 8.7 A nodular malignant melanoma.

Uveal melanoma

This is also a rare type of melanoma affecting the eye. It is more common in later life and thought to be linked to exposure to UVR. Treatment of choice tends to be enucleation. Prognosis is influenced by how advanced the lesion is when the patient presents.

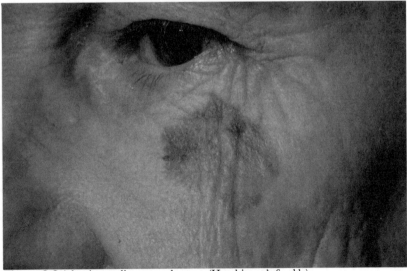

Figure 8.8 A lentigo malignant melanoma (Hutchinson's freckle).

Survival rate is influenced by the type of malignant melanoma, the degree of spread (stage) and sex of the individual (Weaver, 1976; Dryden and Whyte, 1997). Males have a worse prognosis for two main reasons. Firstly, males tend to present with their melanomas on less obvious anatomical sites than females, e.g. the trunk and back. Secondly, men commonly present with more advanced lesions than females (Dryden and Whyte, 1997). Melanomas are staged according to the level (depth) of invasion (Table 8.3). This is known as the 'Clark level' (Ketcham and Loescher, 1993).

Table 8.3 Clark level staging of melanomas

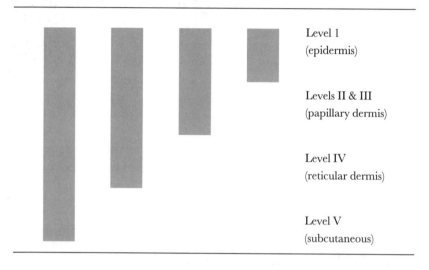

Level 1
(epidermis)

Levels II & III
(papillary dermis)

Level IV
(reticular dermis)

Level V
(subcutaneous)

Predisposing factors to developing malignant melanoma are undoubtedly linked to an individual's skin type and exposure to the sun. It has been known for some time that fair-skinned emigrants, from northern Europe to Australia have a high incidence of melanoma (Shukla and Hughes, 1990). We have also seen that more recreational time, and changes in social habits, can also increase an individual's risk of developing skin cancers, including melanomas. Boyle et al. (1995) have highlighted an increased incidence of melanomas in northern Europe compared with southern Europe. It is believed that the lighter skin types of the native populations of northern Europe provide very little protection for modern, outdoor recreational activities and annual holidays to hotter climates.

Treatment

If a patient is thought to have a malignant melanoma, referral to a specialist combined skin cancer clinic can be helpful in confirming the diagnosis and advising the individual on the treatment available. As already discussed, malignant melanoma can readily metastasize via the blood and lymphatic system (Dryden and Whyte, 1997). To minimize the risk of metastatic spread, a wide surgical excision of the lesion should be undertaken if the surgeon is suspicious of malignant melanoma (Weaver, 1976).

Surgery is unquestionably the most appropriate first-line treatment for malignant melanoma. Its success will depend upon the type of melanoma, how deep it is and if there is any metastatic spread present at the time of initial surgery. Metastatic melanoma is not very sensitive to the current range of cytotoxic drugs available (Ketcham and Loescher, 1993). If the patient's melanoma is confined to a limb, isolated limb perfusion can be used with a limited degree of success (see Chapter 3) (Weaver, 1976).

Radiotherapy has a positive role to play in the management of locally advanced disease, but has no place as a first-line treatment. Palliation of brain metastases with radiotherapy can bring considerable short-term relief for many patients, as can the use of radiotherapy for the palliation of subcutaneous and nodal metastases (Overgaard, 1986).

Prevention of skin cancer

Prevention is obviously better than cure and there are a number of steps that can be taken to minimize an individual's risk of developing skin cancer.

Firstly, we must be aware of our individual skin type (see Table 8.1) and take appropriate preventative measures to protect it from UVR damage (Ketcham and Loescher, 1993; Morton, 1993). These preventative measures must start in childhood, as our ability to withstand the harmful effects of UVR are not fully developed until we reach our teens. Young babies should be fully protected from UVR. Older children should wear protective clothing, such as a wide-brimmed hat, T-shirt and high factor sunscreen (Ketcham and Loescher, 1993; Morton, 1993).

Many individuals do not appreciate the need for sunscreen, or understand how the sun protection factor (SPF) of a sunscreen actually works. Morton (1993) describes how sunscreens have been developed specifically for an individual's skin type. He developed a test whereby an individual's skin was exposed to a sunlamp to ascertain how long it would take to redden. If it took five minutes, the test was repeated, but this time a specified amount of sunscreen was applied. If it now took 50 minutes for the skin to redden, Morton (1993) stated that the Sun Protection Factor (SPF) was 50. This was then divided by the original 'reddening' time of five minutes, i.e. $50 \div 5 = 10$. This means a sunscreen with a factor of 10 would provide an individual with 10 times more protection for their skin than if they did not use a sunscreen. This does not mean that once a sunscreen is applied for the day no further precautions need to he taken. The UVR is strongest between 10 am and 2 pm, and surfaces such as snow, water and sand reflect UVR on to the skin. Therefore, care should be taken to minimize activities during the hottest part of the day, and/or involving surfaces that reflect UVR (Ketcham and Loescher, 1993).

By using a sunscreen, as opposed to a sunblock (which provides maximum protection for the skin against burning), it is possible to develop a tan, if so desired. This will, however, depend upon the individual's skin type. People with skin type 1 burn very easily, so will have to use a high factor sunscreen to minimize the risk of damage to their skins. Individuals with skin types 2 and 3 can develop a tan by starting off with a high factor sunscreen. After a few days a lower factor sunscreen can then be substituted for the higher one. As the skin naturally darkens (tans) to provide some of its own protection against the sun, an even lower factor can be substituted, but this process should not be rushed. Even individuals with naturally dark skins can burn, especially if they live in cool climates and visit hot, sunny countries for their holidays. So individuals should be advised not only to use sunscreens, but how to use them. People with darker skin types only need to use a low factor sunscreen for the first few days of their holiday, i.e. until their skin starts to darken naturally.

Case histories

Sam

Sam, a 50-year-old local solicitor who enjoys sailing at the weekends, has presented at his local hospital with a small lesion above his upper lip. He has had it for a number of weeks and noticed that it has been slowly increasing in size. His hospital doctor has advised him that, in view of his history and lifestyle, the lesion is likely to be an easily treatable form of skin cancer known as basal cell carcinoma (BCC). The doctor has suggested two forms of treatment to Sam: either surgery, or radiotherapy daily for ten days, following an initial diagnostic biopsy of the lesion. In view of his busy professional lifestyle, Sam has decided to opt for surgical removal of the entire lesion under local anaesthetic.

Apart from wearing a hat when sailing, Sam has not been using any other forms of sun protection. He has been advised to continue to wear wide-brimmed hats and to use sunscreens. He has also been advised of the dangers of exposure to the sun during the hottest part of the day, i.e. between 10 am and 2 pm, and the reflection on to the skin of UVR from the water.

After removal of the lesion Sam will be required to see his hospital doctor at specified time intervals for up to two years following his initial treatment.

Mike

Mike, a 66-year-old retired council gardener, has presented at his local hospital with a large, ulcerated lesion on the upper part of his ear. It has been present for only a few weeks and is rapidly increasing in size. His hospital doctor has advised him that, in view of his history and previous occupation, he suspects the lesion is a squamous cell carcinoma (SCC). As the lesion is situated very closely to underlying cartilage, Mike is advised that the treatment of choice should be wide surgical excision under a general anaesthetic.

As there is a likelihood that this lesion could metastasize, Mike will be followed up regularly by his hospital doctor for between two and five years.

Jane

Jane, a 20-year-old student teacher, presents to her GP complaining that a mole she has had on her leg for many years has started to increase in size. She has also noticed that it has become quite lumpy. As Jane's GP is suspicious that this could be a malignant melanoma he decides to refer her to the local hospital. When Jane sees the hospital consultant he is highly suspicious that Jane's mole could be a nodular malignant melanoma. He takes a personal and family history, together with a general physical examination, documenting Jane's other moles. Jane does not have any enlarged inguinal lymph glands, which could be evidence of metastatic disease. She also has a chest X-ray performed, which is reported as 'normal'. Jane is informed of the hospital doctor's suspicions and advised to undergo wide, deep surgical excision of the mole under a general anaesthetic.

The histology from the excised mole does confirm a diagnosis of nodular malignant melanoma. In view of this Jane is informed that she will require long-term follow-up at the hospital for up to ten years. She is also advised if she notices any changes in existing moles to seek an earlier appointment, and not to wait for her pre-arranged follow-up visit. Although Jane stated that she was aware of the precautions required to minimize her risks of developing skin cancers in the future, she was given some general literature and an initial appointment was made for her to see the hospital Macmillan nurse regarding general psychological support.

Conclusions

Sunshine undoubtedly gives us all a sense of wellbeing. However, we must be aware of its potential invisible dangers as one of the commonest causes of skin cancer. If prevention fails to stop an individual developing a skin cancer, then early detection can play an important role in influencing their prognosis. Education of healthcare professionals and the general population has to be of paramount importance in preventing and reducing the incidence of skin cancers.

Although many skin cancers have a good prognosis, their effect on the patient can be devastating. The patient has, after all, been diagnosed with a 'cancer'. Nurses can play a vital role in supporting patients and helping them to minimize their risks of developing future skin cancers.

Chapter 9
Haematological malignancies

JOANNE TODD

Introduction

This chapter will examine the most common haematological malignancies. However, it is not possible to discuss malignant haemato-oncology without first considering blood cell maturation (haemopoiesis).

The bone marrow is the most important site of haemopoiesis from around six to seven months of foetal life through childhood and into adult life. In early infancy the bone marrow is entirely haemopoietic but during childhood fat replaces much of the marrow in the long bones. In adulthood, haemopoietic marrow is confined to the central skeleton and the proximal ends of the femurs and humeri (Hoffbrand and Pettit, 1993).

Figure 9.1 represents the cell divisions that occur from the pluripotent stem cell in the bone marrow through the cell lines that give rise to the circulating blood cells. The diagrammatic representation of haemopoiesis can be referred to throughout this chapter to enable the reader to visualize where in the cell line the disease process begins.

Acute and chronic leukaemia

Leukaemia can be defined as a group of disorders characterized by an accumulation of abnormal white cells in the bone marrow (Hoffbrand and Pettit, 1993). As a result of overcrowding in the bone marrow of abnormal cells, bone marrow failure occurs. Patients present with features of marrow failure such as neutropenia

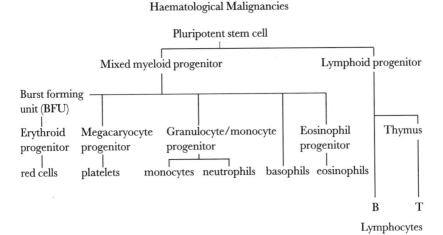

Figure 9.1 Haemopoiesis.

(neutrophil count of <2.0 x 10^9/l), anaemia (haemoglobin <10g/l) and thrombocytopenia (platelet count of <50 x 10^9/l). Refer to Table 9.1 for normal haematological blood values.

Aetiology

Although the aetiology of leukaemia is unknown there are a number of predisposing factors, for example, exposure to benzene and ionizing radiation. There is also a genetic predisposition, with a twenty-fold increase in the rate of leukaemia in children with Down's syndrome (Hoffbrand and Pettit, 1994).

Classification

The leukaemias are classified into acute and chronic forms of the disease. Classification is based upon morphology, cell maturity and speed of onset. Acute leukaemia is subdivided into acute myeloid leukaemia (AML) and acute lymphoblastic leukaemia (ALL). Acute lymphoblastic leukemia is sub-divided according to immunological markers into L_1, L_2 and L_3 types. Acute myeloid leukaemia is subdivided into eight types based upon where in the cell line the abnormal cells proliferate (M0–M7).

    The chronic leukaemias form two main groups: chronic myeloid leukaemia and chronic lymphoblastic leukaemia.

Table 9.1 Normal haematological values

	SI unit
Haemoglobin	13.0–18.0 g/dl (M) 11.5–15.5 g/dl (F)
Mean corpuscular haemoglobin (MCH)	27–34 pg
MCH concentration	30–35 g/dl
Mean corpuscular volume (MCV)	78–98 fl
Packed cell volume (PCV) or haematocrit	0.40–0.54 (M) 0.35–0.47 (F)
Red cell count	$4.5–6.5 \times 10^{12}/l$ (M) $3.8–5.8 \times 10^{12}/l$ (F)
Reticulocyte count	$10–100 \times 10^{9}/l$
Leucocytes (adult)	$4.0–11.0 \times 10^{9}/l$
Differential white count: neutrophils lymphocytes monocytes eosinophils basophils	$2.5–7.5 \times 10^{9}/l$ $1.0–3.5 \times 10^{9}/l$ $0.2–0.8 \times 10^{9}/l$ $0.04–0.4 \times 10^{9}/l$ $0.01–0.1 \times 10^{9}/l$
Platelets	$150–400 \times 10$
Erythrocyte sedimentation rate (ESR)	0–6 mm/hr = normal 7–20 mm/hr = doubtful >20 mm/hr = abnormal

Incidence

Of the leukaemias diagnosed, over half fall into the acute classification. ALL is most common in children, with a higher incidence at four years of age. AML occurs in all age groups and is the most common form of leukaemia in adults. AML forms only 15% of leukaemia found in children (Williams, 1996).

Presenting symptoms

Patients present with symptoms resulting from bone marrow failure and/or organ infiltration. The signs of anaemia include pallor, lethargy and dyspnoea. Persistent fevers, infections and malaise are features of neutropenia. Thrombocytopenia gives rise to spontaneous bruising, purpura, bleeding gums and menorrhagia. Children often present with aching and tender bones due to overproductive

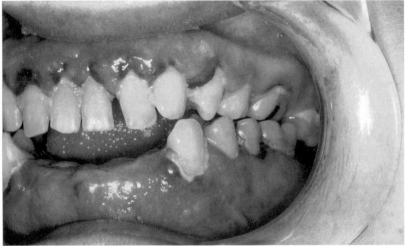

Figure 9.2 Gum hypertrophy.

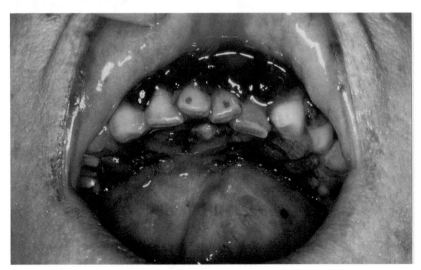

Figure 9.3 Gum hypertrophy and bleeding.

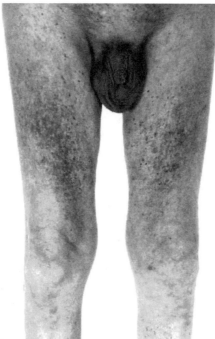

Figure 9.4 Thrombocytopenic purpura.

bone marrow. Enlarged lymph nodes, spleen and liver can be features of ALL. Gum hypertrophy, skin infiltration, central nervous system involvement and testicular infiltration can also be features of the disease (Figures 9.2, 9.3 and 9.4).

Diagnosis

A diagnosis of leukaemia is made by the examination of bone marrow under the microscope. This involves the removal of bone marrow and other tissue from the iliac crest, sternum or tibia.

Fluid bone marrow is removed by *aspiration*, and the examination of such bone marrow gives information about the development of cells. A *trephine biopsy* involves the removal of a core of bone including marrow, which provides details of the marrow structure.

Management

Once the diagnosis of leukaemia has been made, supportive treatment for bone marrow failure is commenced. In most situations it is necessary to insert a central venous catheter, for example a skin-tunnelled catheter or peripherally inserted central venous catheter (PICC) for the delivery of blood products, intravenous fluids, antibiotics and chemotherapy. It is important that the catheter is placed with its tip terminating in the superior vena cava, i.e. central circulation, as many of the drugs used to treat patients with hematological malignancies are vesicant and irritant and thus can cause damage to peripheral veins and tissues (see Figure 9.5) (Todd, 1998).

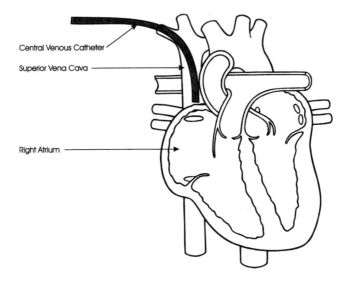

Central Venous Catheter

Superior Vena Cava

Right Atrium

Figure 9.5 Central venous catheter tip position.

Patients also require frequent blood sampling, and therefore an access device that permits easy entry for blood samples minimizes the distress and discomfort associated with venepuncture. Treatment for bone marrow failure often involves blood and platelet transfusions to lessen the symptoms associated with anaemia and thrombocytopenia. The use of intravenous antibiotics is required where persistent, unresolved infection exists. In most situations patients will require intravenous fluids to prepare the kidneys for the onslaught of nephrotoxic chemotherapy.

As a result of neutropenia, patients are severely at risk of infection and this risk is increased once treatment with chemotherapy has begun (Wilson, 1995). Patients are most at risk from their own commensal bacterial flora, for example Gram-positive skin organisms such as Staphylococcus and Streptococcus (Wade et al., 1982). There is also risk of infection from Gram-negative bacteria that exist within the patients own gastrointestinal system, for example Pseudomonas aeruginosa and Escherichia coli. Such organisms, which are not normally pathogenic, can cause life-threatening septicaemia in the absence of neutrophils. Viral, fungal and protozoal infections can also occur, particularly when neutropenia is prolonged or when patients have been subjected to long courses of antibiotics.

In order to minimize the risks from such infections, it is advisable that patients are nursed in single rooms with reverse barrier nursing techniques such as aprons, stringent handwashing and the use of alcohol hand rub (Brandt, 1994; Carter, 1994; Fenlon, 1995; Nauseef et al., 1981; Wilson, 1995). Due to the risk of ingesting bacteria from certain foods, most hospitals advocate the use of a 'clean diet' (Wilson, 1995).

Patients are educated regarding effective general hygiene measures (Wade et al., 1982), such as daily showering and a strict oral hygiene programme to decrease the risk of oral infection. The risk of infection via the mucous membranes is increased due to breeches in the body's defence mechanisms due to mucositis. Good oral hygiene significantly decreases the risks of oral infection (Richardson, 1987). Patients are monitored regularly and routinely by nursing staff for signs of infection such as pyrexia and areas of inflammation. A thorough continuing assessment of the patient is essential in order to recognise the first signs of infection (Reheis, 1985) (see Figure 9.6). Intravenous catheter sites, the mouth, throat, perianal and perineal areas are particularly likely areas for a focus of infection. It is important to remember that due to a lack of neutrophils patients do not form pus at the site of infection.

Patients are treated prophylactically with antibacterial and anti-fungal agents in an attempt to prevent the occurrence of infection. Possible infection is treated promptly and blindly with broad-spectrum intravenous antibiotics after blood cultures, urine samples and swabs from potential sites of infection have been obtained in an attempt to isolate the organisms involved. Diligent attention to detail by nurses caring for neutropenic patients is essential to reduce the risk of death from septicemia.

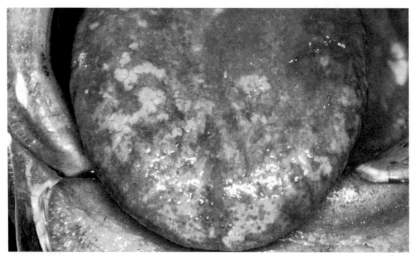

Figure 9.6 Oral candida infection.

Chemotherapy

Chemotherapy is administered with the aim of destroying the capacity for leukaemic cell reproduction. Drugs are given in combination to increase the cytotoxic effect and reduce drug resistance. Years of clinical trials involving different combinations of drugs at varying doses have produced today's regimens, with improved remission and long-term survival rates. Most centres continue to treat patients within clinical trials in an attempt to make further advances in the management of leukaemia.

The first course of chemotherapy can often initiate hyperkalaemia (high serum potassium levels) and hyperuricaemia (high serum uric acid levels) due to tumour lysis syndrome. Tumour lysis is the result of tumour breakdown following chemotherapy, and uric acid is the byproduct of this process in patients with a high tumour burden. The rise in serum uric acid levels can cause renal failure due to precipitation in the distal tubule and collecting ducts of the nephron. For this reason patients are prescribed allopurinol prior to starting chemotherapy. Intravenous fluids and alkalization of the urine is often recommended with the addition of sodium bicarbonate to the infusion.

Chemotherapy for leukaemia is given in cycles. The first cycle aims to induce a remission (absence of any clinical or conventional evidence of the disease) (Hoffbrand and Pettitt, 1993). Subsequent cycles are then given to destroy any hidden leukaemic cells, with the aim of preventing the disease from relapsing. The drugs are given in intervals to reduce toxicity and allow normal bone marrow cells to recover.

In acute lymphoblastic leukaemia it is known that a long duration of treatment reduces the risk of relapse (Hoffbrand and Pettit, 1994). Therefore, patients undergo up to two years of maintenance therapy. It is also well established that in ALL there is a significant risk of disease relapse in the central nervous system and testicles (Williams, 1996). For this reason, patients are subjected to prophylactic cranial irradiation and intrathecal (via lumbar puncture) chemotherapy. As yet prophylactic testicular radiotherapy is not routinely administered, and patients are only treated when testicular relapse occurs.

Patients with AML usually undergo a remission–induction course of therapy followed by two or three consolidation courses if remission is obtained. Maintenance treatment is not given, but in some circumstances patients go on to receive a bone marrow transplant to achieve the best chance of disease-free survival. This is discussed in more detail later in this chapter.

Prognosis

The prognosis of children with good-prognosis ALL following chemotherapy alone can be as high as 60–80% long-term disease-free survival. However in adults, who frequently have poor prognosis disease, the long-term disease-free survival can be as low as 20–30%.

In AML in the under 60 age group, the long-term disease-free survival with chemotherapy alone is approximately 30%. This figure rises to 50–60% in specifically selected cases that undergo bone marrow transplantation (Hoffbrand and Pettit, 1994).

Support

To be faced suddenly with a life-threatening illness is a source of severe mental anguish. The diagnosis of leukaemia is often totally unexpected and comes from 'out of the blue' (Bertero and Ek, 1993). This obviously affects not only the patient but his or her family and network of friends. Leukaemia is a complex disease to understand and the treatment is equally foreboding in its possible effects, duration and intricacy. It is the role of the nurse caring for such patients to provide information at a pace that can be coped with and in a format that aids understanding (Calman and Hine, 1995). Caring for the patient with leukaemia is truly a collaborative, multidisciplinary effort and it is the nurse's role to coordinate care, ensuring a seamless treatment trajectory.

Not only does the patient face a multitude of physical problems; he or she also has to learn to cope with an altered body image, loss of role within the family, stress and boredom. This is complicated by the realization that there is a high chance of facing mortality (Bertero and Ek, 1993).

Chronic myeloid leukaemia

Chronic myeloid leukaemia (CML) comprises fewer than 20% of all leukaemias, and is most common in middle age. Patients often present with vague symptoms of weight loss, malaise, anorexia and night sweats. The spleen is frequently enlarged and this causes pain and indigestion. Patients may show signs of anaemia (pallor, dyspnoea and tachycardia) and thrombocytopenia (bruising, petechial rash, epistaxis or haemorrhage). Blood tests identify leucocytosis (high white count), often greater than $50 \times 10^9/l$, and frequently the presence of an abnormal chromosome, 'Philadelphia', on cytogenetic analysis.

Treatment

CML often remains in its chronic phase for up to ten years and during this stage can be treated with oral chemotherapy and/or alpha interferon. These strategies help to control the white count and curtail the disease. In younger patients following stabilization, intensive chemotherapy is often utilized with bone marrow transplantation in the hope of achieving long-term disease-free survival and a possible cure.

In 70% of patients the disease transforms into an acute leukaemia (often referred to as blast crisis) that results in a swift deterioration of the patient, with worsening bone marrow failure. Survival following transformation of CML is often brief, rarely exceeding one year.

Chronic lymphocytic leukaemia

Chronic lymphocytic leukaemia (CLL) accounts for approximately

2% of leukaemias. The disease occurs in the older age group and is more common in males. Patients often present incidentally with a raised lymphocyte count. There is often enlargement of the cervical, axillary and inguinal lymph nodes and in the later stages it is accompanied by an enlarged spleen and liver. Patients frequently experience bacterial and fungal infections due to immunosuppression.

Many patients with slowly progressing disease survive for more than ten years and frequently succumb to ailments other than CLL. Most patients survive in excess of 3–5 years. Death occurs due to progressive bone marrow failure and immunosuppression, usually through overwhelming infection.

Treatment

Patients with low-grade disease often require no treatment. However, patients with bone marrow failure, symptoms of lymphadenopathy and/or enlarged spleen are treated with corticosteroids and oral chemotherapy. There are newer cytotoxic drugs available for patients who do not respond initially to such therapy, and some undergo radiotherapy to enlarged lymph nodes and spleens. Such treatments are accompanied by active treatment of infection with antibiotics and antifungal agents. In the end stages of the disease patients are supported with transfusions of blood and platelets as required.

Multiple myeloma

Multiple myeloma is a malignancy associated with a proliferation of plasma cells in the bone marrow. It is characterized by lytic lesions in the bone, abnormal accumulation of plasma cells in the bone marrow and the presence of a paraprotein in the blood and urine. Most cases of myeloma occur in patients over the age of 40.

Presenting symptoms

Bone pain and pathological fractures due to the presence of lytic lesions are the most common features at diagnosis. Some patients present with some degree of marrow failure, for example lethargy and weakness associated with anaemia. Patients often experience repeated infections as a result of depleted antibody production and/or neutropenia in advanced disease. Renal impairment is not uncommon due to the presence of heavy protein molecules in the blood causing damage to the renal tubules. Symptoms of hypercalcaemia may also be present with thirst, polyuria, nausea, constipation and confusion. This occurs due to the destruction of bone by lytic lesions. In rare situations patients present with a hyperviscosity syndrome (raised plasma volume), causing bruising, haemorrhage, visual disturbances and heart failure.

Diagnosis of myeloma is dependent on the presence of three abnormalities:

- Presence of paraprotein in the urine and/or blood
- Increased plasma cells in the bone marrow (>15% in the marrow aspirate sample)
- Osteolytic lesions on skeletal survey (see Figures 9.7 and 9.8)

Treatment

On diagnosis emergency treatment is often indicated for the following situations:

Uraemia

Patients may be hyperuricaemic and therefore require rehydration and in some situations haemodialysis. In the presence of a high serum calcium (hypercalcaemia), rehydration is performed with

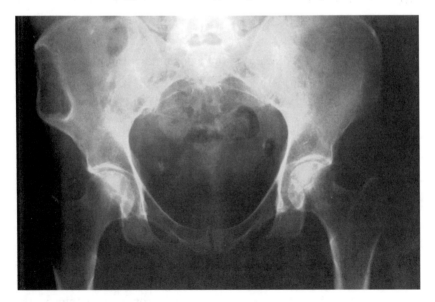

Figure 9.7 Osteolytic lesions: pelvis.

isotonic saline and drugs such as pamidronate are given to reduce the blood calcium levels and prevent further bone absorption.

Osteolytic lesions

In the presence of lytic lesions in the vertebral column there may be evidence of spinal cord compression and this is treated with radiotherapy or surgery to the affected area. Lytic lesions are frequently responsible for severe pain and this is addressed with potent analgesia and radiotherapy to the affected area when appropriate.

Anaemia

Patients with severe anaemia are transfused with packed red cells.

Hyperviscosity (high plasma viscosity levels)

Those patients who present with hyperviscosity syndrome and are experiencing haemorrhage may be treated with plasmapheresis (the removal of excess circulating plasma).

Once the patient's general condition has been stabilized, treatment is instigated to destroy the excess plasma cells and hence reduce the production of paraprotein. In the elderly patient oral

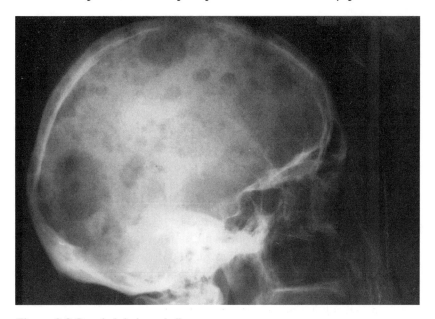

Figure 9.8 Osteolytic lesions: skull.

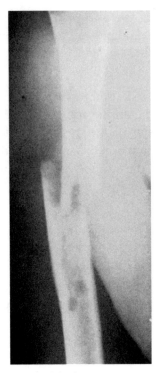

Figure 9.9 Pathological fracture of the femur.

Photographs in Figures 9.2 to 9.9 reproduced by kind permisswion of Dr C N Simpson, Consultant Haematologist, Ipswich Hospital NHS Trust.

chemotherapy agents such as melphalan and cyclophosphamide are given, often alongside a steroid such as prednisolone. This is usually given for four to seven days in cycles of varying time spans, for example monthly. Such treatment is often given as an outpatient with little upset to the patient. Due to the myelosuppressive nature of the drugs and the disease patients are advised of, and observed for, the risk of acquiring infections, which need to be treated without delay.

In the younger patient chemotherapy treatment is more intensive, with the use of cycles of a combination of drugs; for example, vincristine and adriamycin by slow continuous infusion for four days on a monthly basis. Up to six courses are often given to reduce the disease to a minimum and then in some situations autologous bone marrow transplantation following high-dose chemotherapy is performed. This can sometimes result in disease remission for several years.

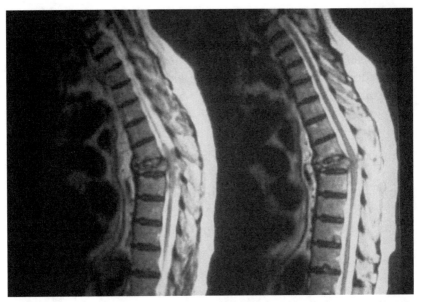

Figure 9.10 Magnetic resonance image illustrating spinal cord compression due to tumour invading vertebral column (coronal view).

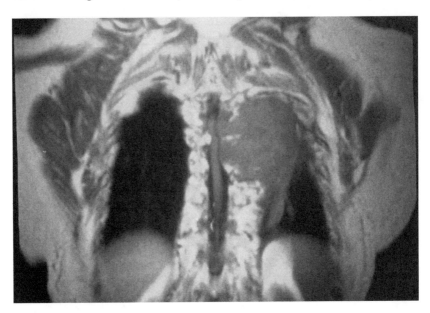

Figure 9.11 Magnetic resonance image as above illustrating tumour compressing spinal cord (sagittal view).

© Medical Illustration, Ipswich Hospital NHS Trust (both pictures).

Prognosis

Multiple myeloma is generally considered to be incurable. The median survival is two years with only about 20% of patients surviving for four years. Patients who present with renal failure have a particularly poor prognosis of only a few months (Williams, 1996).

Malignant lymphomas

Lymphomas are divided into Hodgkin's and non-Hodgkin's disease. They result from the replacement of normal lymph tissue with abnormal cells. Microscopically in Hodgkin's disease there is a presence of Reed-Sternberg cells (RS) and in non-Hodgkin's disease, diffuse or nodular abnormal lymphocytes (Williams, 1996).

Hodgkin's disease

This disease can present in any age group but peaks in young adults (20–30 years) and again in middle to old age (over 50 years). There is a 2:1 male predominance ratio (Williams, 1996).

Clinical features

- Painless, non-tender, asymmetrical, rubbery enlarged lymph nodes in the neck, axilla or groin
- Enlarged spleen
- Enlarged liver
- Mediastinal lymph node involvement with associated pleural effusions and/or superior vena cava obstruction
- Swinging fever
- Pruritus
- Alcohol-induced pain in the affected area
- Weight loss
- Profuse, drenching night sweats
- Fatigue

Haematological findings

- Anaemia
- Raised white cell count
- Raised eosinophil count
- Reduced lymphocyte count in advanced disease

- Raised erythrocyte sedimentation rate (ESR is used to monitor progress)
- Bone marrow involvement in advanced disease
- Raised lactate dehydrogenase (LDH) in 40% of cases; indicates a poor prognosis

Diagnosis

Diagnosis is made by removal of an affected lymph node and histological examination. There are four main histological classifications of Hodgkin's disease: lymphocyte predominant, nodular sclerosing, mixed cellularity and lymphocyte depleted. The disease is then staged by thorough examination including chest X-ray, bone marrow trephine and CT scan.

There are four stages:

Stage I indicates lymph node involvement in one area only.

Stage II indicates lymph node involvement in two or more lymph nodes confined to one side of the diaphragm.

Stage III indicates lymph node involvement both sides of the diaphragm.

Stage IV indicates diffuse involvement outside the lymph nodes such as the bone marrow and liver.

The disease is then further classified according to the presence of symptoms such as fever, night sweats or weight loss; 'A' being absence and 'B' presence.

Treatment

Patients with early stage I or II disease can be treated with *radiotherapy* only to the affected lymph nodes. This treatment can cure Hodgkin's disease in a large number of patients. Radiotherapy is also used in combination with chemotherapy for patients with stage III or IV disease. It is often the treatment recommended for bulky tumour masses of the mediastinum or skin lesions.

Patients with stage III or IV disease and those with stage I and II with B symptoms receive cyclical *chemotherapy*. This often involves a combination of three or four drugs such as vincristine, adriamycin, bleomycin and prednisolone. This treatment is normally given as an outpatient and it is usual to give up to six cycles.

Treatment with such drugs will cause alopecia, nausea and

vomiting, bone marrow suppression and possible long-term sterility. For this reason, young men are offered the opportunity of sperm storage prior to commencing treatment. Unfortunately in young women there is little to offer, as oocyte cryopreservation is unsuccessful. However research is underway examining the benefit of cryopreservation of ovarian tissue for later re-implantation. In some centres this is offered but with informed consent regarding the limited research in this area. To date there have been no live births from this method of fertility preservation.

Relapsed disease

In this situation the patient is often treated with an alternative combination chemotherapy regimen and often in combination with radiotherapy. Once remission has been achieved these patients frequently go on to receive autologous bone marrow transplant (where appropriate) as a technique to deliver high doses of chemotherapy in an attempt to achieve cure.

Prognosis

Approximate 5-year survival rates are:

- Stage I 85%
- Stage II 85%
- Stage IIIA 70%
- Stage IIIB 50%
- Stage IV 50%

Non-Hodgkin's lymphoma

The non-Hodgkin's lymphomas are a disparate group of diseases that range from high-grade and rapidly fatal to the low-grade and indolent forms of the disease. Figure 9.12 helps to describe the developments of lymphocytes and thus explain the classification system.

The Kiel classification system is most commonly followed; this is shown in Table 9.2 (Hoffbrand and Pettit, 1993).

There are some diseases that can predispose to the development of NHL, for example AIDS. In some situations patients who have undergone previous chemotherapy or radiotherapy and those who have received immunosuppressive treatment following organ transplantation have an increased risk of developing the disease.

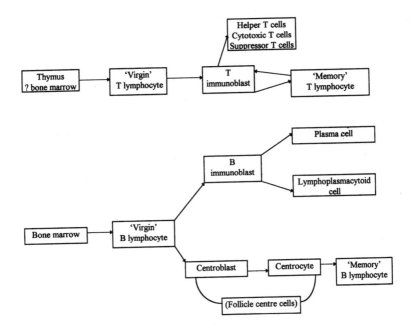

Figure 9.12 Lymphocyte maturation.

Clinical features

- Enlarged lymph nodes – asymmetric and painless
- Fever
- Night sweats
- Weight loss
- Anaemia, neutropenia with recurrent infections and thrombocytopenia in patients with bone marrow disease
- Splenomegaly
- Hepatomegaly
- Enlarged retroperitoneal or mesenteric nodes
- Other organs: Skin, brain, testis, gastrointestinal tract
- Abnormal blood chemistry: raised uric acid and abnormal liver function tests
- Raised serum LDH in extensive disease; this can be used as a prognostic marker

Table 9.2 Kiel classification of non-Hodgkin's lymphoma

B cell	T cell
Low-grade malignancy	**Low-grade malignancy**
Lymphocyte	Lymphocyte
Lymphoplasmacytic	Small cerebriform cell mycosis fungoides Sezary's syndrome
Plasmacytic	Lymphoepitheloid
Centroblastic/centrocytic follicular diffuse	Angioimmunoblastic
Centrocytic	T zone
	Plemorphic medium and large cell
High-grade malignancy	**High-grade malignancy**
Centroblastic	Pleomorphic medium and large cell
Immunoblastic	Immunoblastic
Large cell anaplastic	Large cell anaplastic
Burkitt's	Lymphoblastic
Lymphoblastic	

Diagnosis

Diagnosis is made through histological examination of lymph nodes. Staging procedures include chest X-ray, CT scan, bone marrow aspirate and trephine.

Treatment

In some situations patients with *low-grade and indolent disease* require no therapy if they are experiencing no effects from the disease. Local radiotherapy to enlarged lymph nodes can be used for early stage disease.

Those who require treatment often receive oral chemotherapy in the form of chlorambucil or cyclophosphamide. Patients with advancing disease and systemic symptoms can be treated with intravenous combinations of cytotoxic chemotherapy or a relatively new drug called Fludarabine. Trials are underway in some centres examining the benefit of antibody therapy and high-dose chemotherapy with bone marrow transplantation.

In the case of *intermediate grade disease*, patients with localized disease can be treated with combination chemotherapy, for example a regime known as CHOP that consists of cyclophosphamide, hydroxydaunorubacin, vincristine (oncovin) and prednisolone. radiotherapy is also given to localized areas of tumour bulk. Patients with advanced disease are often treated with high-dose combination chemotherapy to achieve remission.

Patients with large cell lymphomas that are localized can be cured with radiotherapy. In most situations the disease is widespread and systemic chemotherapy is required. Chemotherapy is usually intensive with high early remission rates; however, early relapse is common. As central nervous system relapse is common, most patients are treated prophylactically with intrathecal chemotherapy and high-dose methotrexate. Methotrexate is a chemotherapeutic agent that is known to cross the blood–brain barrier and is therefore of use in this situation. In young patients, prophylactic cranial radiation is often used. Bone marrow transplantation in first remission is often considered in patients with poor prognostic disease.

Relapsed disease

As with Hodgkin's disease, reinduction chemotherapy is used to achieve a second remission followed by intensive, high-dose chemotherapy and subsequent bone marrow or peripheral blood stem cell rescue in order to attempt to achieve a cure.

Prognosis

In the case of low-grade disease, most patients survive for more than five years and many are alive ten years after diagnosis. Patients with localized high-grade disease are cured with radiotherapy. Patients with widespread disease treated with intensive chemotherapy have a 40–50% disease-free survival at two years (Hoffbrand and Pettit, 1994).

Bone marrow transplantation

Bone marrow transplantation (BMT) is a therapy in which ablative doses of chemotherapy and/or radiotherapy are given to patients with diseases involving the bone marrow to eradicate their existing marrow and disease (Tiffany, 1988). BMT was first shown to be possible in humans in 1959 (Mathe et al., 1959), when donor marrow was given to four victims of radiation exposure. Over the years it became evident that patients who received marrow from twin siblings did well and it was from here that the histocompatible locus antigens (HLA) were identified. The HLA system is situated on chromosome six and is now widely used as a means of tissue typing for BMT.

There are four main types of BMT:

- Syngeneic: where the donor and recipient are identical twins
- Allogeneic: where the donor and recipient are of the same species and HLA matched
- Autologous: where the patient's own bone marrow is used following cytotoxic therapy
- Peripheral blood stem cell: where progenitor stem cells are purged from the marrow of the patient or a donor into the peripheral blood and collected

Diseases treated by BMT

- Acute leukaemia
- Chronic myeloid leukaemia
- Myelodysplastic syndromes
- Lymphoma and Hodgkin's disease
- Neuroblastoma
- Multiple myeloma
- Breast cancer
- Testicular teratoma
- Genetic diseases of the bone marrow
- Aplastic anaemia

Patients with haematological malignancies are treated with BMT to eradicate diseased bone marrow. Patients with solid tumours are treated with BMT as a means of rescue following high doses of toxic, myeloablative treatment. Due to the intensive nature of this form of treatment it is rarely carried out on patients over the age of 55 years. BMT is usually embarked upon when the patient is in full remission from the disease and following rigorous examination for underlying organ damage. It is important to ascertain that the patient has satisfactory cardiac, respiratory, renal and liver function as the high-dose therapy given during BMT may damage such organs.

Management

Due to the profoundly myelosuppresive nature of bone marrow transplantation, the patient is nursed in protective isolation. The degree of isolation varies from centre to centre and is dependent upon the disease being treated and the type of transplant undertaken. This means that some patients may simply be nursed in single rooms with staff and visitors donning plastic aprons and adopting a rigorous handwashing policy, while others will be nursed in laminar flow cubicles with staff wearing theatre clothing, hats and masks (Brandt, 1994; Carter, 1994; Fenlon, 1995; Nauseef et al., 1981, Wilson, 1995).

Patients undergo conditioning myeloablative treatment with chemotherapy, and possibly total body irradiation, with the aim of totally destroying their bone marrow and any residual disease. In allogeneic transplant the destruction of the patient's immune system through myeloablative treatment reduces the risks of engraftment failure due to rejection of the donor marrow cells.

Approximately one to two days following chemotherapy the marrow cells are infused intravenously via an indwelling central venous catheter.

Post-transplant management

Following a period of two to three weeks of severe pancytopenia the first signs of engraftment may occur. This is usually indicated by a slow and gradual rise in the blood count.

Prior to engraftment the patient is at severe risk of infection due to pancytopenia. The risk of infection is significantly reduced by protective isolation techniques but the patients remain at risk from bacterial, viral and fungal *infection*. For this reason they receive numerous prophylactic oral antiseptics, antibiotics, antifungal and antiviral agents. When fever occurs the patient is treated immediately with broad-spectrum antibiotics, after blood cultures and other microbiological specimens have been obtained in an attempt to isolate the causative organisms. Untreated infection in the BMT patient can be rapidly fatal and therefore rigorous observation on the part of the nurse caring for the patient is vital.

Platelet counts frequently drop to below $10 \times 10^9/l$ during the pancytopenic phase of BMT. Platelet concentrates are given to prevent *haemorrhage* until the patient's platelet production maintains a count of above $20 \times 10^9/l$.

In most situations patients become severely *anaemic* during the pancytopenic phase. Blood transfusion is required to maintain a haemoglobin of 10g/dl or above to minimize the symptoms of anaemia.

In allogeneic BMT *graft versus host disease* (GVHD) is caused by the donor-derived immune cells, particularly the T lymphocytes, reacting against the recipient tissues (Hoffbrand and Pettit, 1993). Acute GVHD occurs within 100 days of transplant and is characterized by skin rashes, gastrointestinal tract disturbances and deteriorating liver function. The skin rash often affects the palms of the hands, soles of the feet, ears and face. Chronic GVHD occurs after 100 days and usually evolves from acute GVHD. Joints and the lacrimal glands can also be involved.

GVHD can be treated and/or prevented by the use of immunosuppressive drugs such as cyclosporin, methotrexate and steroids. Severe acute GVHD can be fatal.

Interstitial pneumonitis is one of the most frequent causes of death post-BMT. In some situations the cause is identified as infection but sometimes the only factor thought to be indicated is the conditioning radiotherapy and chemotherapy.

Failure to engraft is a rare but nonetheless devastating risk associated with BMT. In allogeneic BMT patients, previously stored bone marrow, where available, is infused to rescue the patient from the risks of pancytopenia.

Veno-occlusive disease of the liver is an acute complication that arises as a result of the chemotherapy and/or radiotherapy. It is characterized by rapidly deteriorating liver function and can often be a fatal complication.

Aplastic anaemia

Definition

- Pancytopenia with a hypocellular bone marrow (Williams, 1996)
- Neutrophil count of <0.5 x 10^9/l
- Platelet count of <20 x 10^9/l
- Corrected reticulocyte index of <1

Aetiology

- Acquired by exposure to chemicals, for example benzene, drugs, radiation and viruses
- Hereditary conditions known to be associated with aplastic anaemia are: Fanconi anaemia, dyskeratosis congenita and Schwachman diamond syndrome
- Aplastic anaemia can also be idiopathic, i.e. no known cause, in about 65% of cases

Features

- Fatigue
- Bleeding
- Infections

  all as a result of bone marrow failure.

Diagnosis

The diagnosis of aplastic anaemia is made through bone marrow aspirate and cytogenetic tests.

Treatment

Bone marrow transplant is the only curative form of treatment for patients with aplastic anaemia. This is only possible in younger patients who have a matched sibling or volunteer unrelated donor. Only one-third of patients have a suitable donor (Williams, 1996).

Immunosuppressive treatment is an option but not a curative form of management for this condition. This can involve the use of drugs such as cyclosporin. The use of cyclosporin carries risks for the

Table 9.3 Late complications of bone marrow transplants

Relapse of original disease

Chronic GVHD

Infection: bacterial, fungal and viral. Prophylactic antibiotics and antiviral agents are used for several months post-BMT as the immune system often takes this time to recover.

Delayed pulmonary complications due to total body irradiation or infection

Endocrine disorders, e.g. hypothyroidism, growth failure in children and impaired sexual development, particularly related to the use of total body irradiation (TBI).

Cataracts due to TBI

Central nervous system disturbances due to TBI

Sterility

Impotence

---

patient, particularly in relation to renal impairment. About 25% of patients treated with cyclosporin will respond.

Antithymocyte globulin, derived from rabbits or horses, is often used as a means of treating aplastic anaemia. The use of such agents can lead to quite substantial reactions such as fever, chills and a rash, known as serum sickness.

Supportive care

On diagnosis, younger patients should immediately undergo HLA tissue typing along with any siblings.

Patients should receive only minimal transfusions if they are to undergo bone marrow transplant. Any blood products given should be leucocyte-depleted to prevent sensitization and refractoriness during the subsequent transplant phase of treatment.

Patients are cared for with respect to their degree of neutropenia and risk of infection.

Case histories

William (acute leukaemia)

William was a 51-year-old married man with two grown up children. William had worked all his life and for the past 15 years had been employed as a factory foreman. His wife worked part-time as an office cleaner and William was therefore the main wage earner.

William was admitted to hospital under the care of the haematology team with severe pancytopenia (below normal white cell, red cell and platelet count). This was identified on a full blood count sample taken by his GP to investigate persistent lethargy, weakness and depression. William had been to his GP four times prior to this episode with these vague but consistent complaints, but his symptoms had been put down to depression.

On presentation William was pale, lethargic and dyspnoeic. He had persistent oral mucosal ulceration and was covered in diffuse thrombocytopenic purpura. Haematological investigations identified a normochromic, normocytic anaemia with a white cell count of $45 \times 10^9/l$, haemoglobin 6.2 g/dl and platelet count of $7 \times 10^9/l$. His blood film, when examined microscopically, showed 89% leukaemic blasts and a confirmed diagnosis of acute myelomonocytic leukaemia was made. This was classed as type M4 according to the French–American–British Group Classification (FAB). Chromosomal analysis identified a translocation between chromosomes six and nine. The features of William's disease indicated that he was classified within the poor prognosis group.

Following his hospital admission the team spent a lot of time with William and his family explaining his presumed diagnosis of acute leukaemia and supporting him through a variety of investigations, for example, bone marrow aspirate and trephine, lumbar puncture and a wide range of blood tests. This was naturally a time of intense anxiety and the provision of up-to-date and accurate information was of prime importance to enable William and his family to gain some sense of control over the situation that was rapidly running away from them. Calman and Hine (1995) recommended that: 'Patients, families and carers should be given clear information and assistance in a form that they can understand about treatment options and outcomes available to them at all stages of treatment from diagnosis onwards.' The most immediate problems identified were his lethargy and dyspnoea associated with a haemoglobin of 6.2 g/dl, thrombocytopenia, a need for information and his fear associated with his sudden life-threatening diagnosis. Following the investigations and within 24 hours of admission a diagnosis of acute myeloid leukaemia, type M4 was made. The speed of diagnosis is of extreme importance in the haematology patient to facilitate speedy initiation of treatment in a disease that can become uncontrollable within days. In such a case it is ideal to treat within a Medical Research Council trial if the patient meets all the inclusion criteria. The medical management of acute leukaemia is complex and it is only through MRC clinical trials that treatment has advanced. William's treatment within the AML 12 trial was composed of four courses of chemotherapy. These four courses of treatment combined took eight months to complete, with only short breaks of a week at home between each course. The main side effects of this combination of drugs were:

- severe myelosuppression (neutropenia, anaemia and thrombocytopenia)
- alopecia
- nausea and vomiting
- cardiotoxicity
- mucositis
- thrombophlebitis

Due to the degree of irritation produced by these drugs and the level of intravenous support required through such treatment, patients such as William require long-term tunnelled central venous access.

William went on to receive a fourth course of chemotherapy followed by autologous bone marrow transplantation at the nearest cancer centre 60 miles from his home. He required a great deal of ongoing support through this period and in fact was returned to the district general hospital early due to his emotional fragility whilst in the bone marrow transplant unit. He remained pancytopenic four months from BMT, and found it very difficult to distance himself from the hospital team.

Matthew (lymphoma)

Matthew, a 19-year-old delivery person, was admitted via his GP to the medical admissions unit with a diagnosis of pneumonia. He was treated with intravenous antibiotics for several days with no response. The persistence of his symptoms and worsening features on his chest X-ray worried his doctors and a CT scan of his chest was performed. This showed that Matthew had massively enlarged mediastinal lymph nodes and a pleural effusion. Pleural aspiration was performed and after two weeks in hospital the pleural fluid was found to contain lymphoblasts. Bone marrow aspirate and trephine confirmed a diagnosis of T cell lymphoblastic lymphoma.

Once the diagnosis had been explained to Matthew and his parents he was transferred to the oncology ward and treatment for his high-grade lymphoma commenced. Prior to starting treatment Matthew was offered the opportunity to store sperm, as long-term sterility can follow treatment with chemotherapy. Matthew's treatment consisted of two cycles of combination chemotherapy and prednisolone, each lasting 28 days. The first course of therapy was given as an inpatient in order to stabilize Matthew's condition. It was also important that Matthew was protected against tumour lysis. Hyperuricaemia (excessively high serum uric acid levels) can occur as an end result of purine catabolism due to tumour breakdown. As uric acid is excreted through the kidneys, excess can accumulate in the distal tubules and collecting ducts of the nephron and this can lead to irreversible renal failure. In order to prevent this, patients are given allopurinol orally during the first course of treatment. It is also possible to alkalinize the urine with sodium bicarbonate added to intravenous fluids maintaining a urine output of at least two litres per 24 hours. During this phase of therapy it is important to monitor patients' fluid balance, blood pressure and weight, observing for fluid overload. Within these treatment cycles Matthew was also subjected to lumbar punctures with intrathecal methotrexate as prophylaxis (prevention) against central nervous system disease spread. Matthew's third chemotherapy cycle consisted of three courses of high-dose methotrexate over a period of one month. Again, this was not only to treat the disease but also to protect against central nervous system spread. This is possible with high-dose methotrexate as it is one of the few drugs that is able to cross the blood/brain barrier.

Although the first course of treatment was given as an inpatient the majority of the second course could be given as an outpatient. With effective anti-emetics against nausea, Matthew experienced few side effects to his treatment. The main problem he faced during his treatment was emotional distress due to the nature of his diagnosis and the frustration at not being able to lead the normal life of a young adult. Matthew felt very repressed and consequently frequently attempted to rebel against parental concern and protection.

Matthew responded well to his treatment and achieved a full remission; however, due to the nature of his presenting features of the lymphoma (i.e. bone marrow involvement) he had to undergo a sibling allogeneic stem cell transplant in order to improve his long-term survival chances. In all his treatment programme lasted longer than six months and it was more than a year from diagnosis before he was able to truly lead a normal life.

John (myeloma)

John, a 51-year-old builder, had been attending his GP's surgery on numerous occasions with back pain. As his pain persisted despite treatment, his doctor sent him to hospital for an X-ray that revealed crushed vertebrae at L2 and L3. A full blood count later showed a haemoglobin of 10g/dl with normal white count and platelets. Biochemistry investigations revealed a raised creatinine and urea, indicating renal impairment. John was also found to be producing a serum paraprotein, and bone marrow aspirate showed that his bone marrow contained 60% plasma cells. These features combined indicated that John had multiple myeloma.

John commenced his first course of combination chemotherapy by continuous infusion for four days, with a course of high-dose dexamethasone. The drugs included in this regimen were adriamycin and vincristine, which are highly vesicant (cause tissue necrosis), and therefore a long-term tunnelled central venous catheter was inserted to facilitate the safe delivery of John's treatment. The first course of chemotherapy was given with intravenous fluids and allopurinol in order to reverse his renal impairment and prevent tumour lysis. A single fraction of radiotherapy was given to L2 and L3 to relieve pain and stabilize the vertebral column.

John was given six courses of treatment in monthly cycles and over this period his paraprotein levels were monitored to observe his progress. At the end of his final course of therapy his paraprotein level had plateaued to 4 g/dl. This was considered to be a good response to treatment. Once John had achieved a remission it was necessary to attempt to delay disease relapse and progression, and this was done using subcutaneous interferon injections. Interferon is a protein that the human body produces in response to viral infections. It has a variety of effects on the immune system, enhancing natural killer cell and other cytotoxic properties thus inhibiting some tumour cell multiplication (Hoffbrand and Pettit, 1994). John was taught how to self administer his interferon and this enabled him to lead a life independent of the hospital. He was unable to work due to his persistent weakness in his back but enjoyed his painting and family life until he died from progressive disease five years from diagnosis.

Conclusions

The diagnosis of cancer is devastating for any patient and their family. However, haematological malignancies also create an extra burden due to the acute nature of the illnesses and the extreme youth of many of the patients affected. Treatment is frequently long term, if cure is the aim, and sometimes the fight is futile when patients succumb to the disease or treatment itself.

Caring for such patients is therefore challenging for the nurse. A multiprofessional and truly holistic approach to patient care is paramount to meet such complex needs. It is because of this approach to patient management that haematology nursing is so rewarding.

Chapter 10
Urological cancers

AUDREY HAYWARD

Introduction

This chapter will look at the more common genito-urinary cancers which are found in the kidney, ureters, prostate, testicle and penis. The bladder and the prostate have a significantly higher incident rate than other urinary tract cancers, and according to statistics are about the fifth and sixth most prevalent tumours amongst male cancers. The aetiology can vary and may often be unknown. Many aspects of management are different, and so each type of urological cancer will be discussed individually in terms of aetiology, predisposing factors, diagnosis and relevant investigations, along with appropriate management of the disease.

Prostate cancer

Incidence

This is the second most common cancer in men, with about 10,000 new cases a year in the UK. Although this malignancy may present at an earlier age, it is most prevalent in men between the ages of 65 and 85. Research has found that small foci can be detected in 37% of men 50–60 years old, and in 77% of men over 80 years old who appeared to be asymptomatic, on post mortem (Bullock et al., 1995). Despite improvements in early detection and efforts to find cures, the death rate has not changed significantly.

Predisposing factors

Many aspects are being investigated to identify causes of the disease, and at present family links demonstrate that there is a 2:1 increase in incidence amongst immediate relatives. Racial and geographical influences are being compared, as well as cultural issues such as traditional types of food consumed and high fat diets, such as those eaten in the Western developed countries (Ekman et al., 1997).

A racial association has been identified in African Americans, who develop much higher levels of prostatic cancer than Asian men, for example. There is evidence to show that they have poorer survival rates than white men. This is believed to be as a result of not seeking treatment until the disease has progressed (Ben-Joseph et al., 1998).

Presentation

The symptoms are similar to those for benign prostatic enlargement, such as frequency, poor stream, urge incontinence, nocturia, and retention of urine (Rous, 1996).

In up to 25% of men, advanced disease symptoms may be found on presentation, including bone pain, weight loss, anaemia, shortness of breath, lymphoedema, lymphadenopathy and neurological problems (MacFarlane, 1988).

Prostatic cancer is thought to be caused by 'a disturbance of the androgen–oestrogen balance which, with age, leads to over growth of prostatic epithelium' (Bullock et al., 1995). The cancer arises in the periphery of the posterior aspect of the gland, which has a different embryonical origin from the central tissue where benign enlargement occurs, where isolated or multiple nodules in the tissue may be found on examination. There may be direct local spread through the capsule to the seminal vesicles and the base of the bladder as well as to distant organs and tissue by the lymphatics and the vascular channels (MacFarlane, 1988).

Many centres have developed prostatic assessment clinics, often run by urology nurse practitioners/nurse specialists, where the patient is assessed and essential investigations carried out. This makes it easier for the surgeon and the GP to offer appropriate treatment.

The nurse practitioner/specialist initiates the investigations.

Investigations

An International Prostate Symptom Score (IPSS) questionnaire is frequently used. It can be completed by patients while they wait for the investigations.

Digital rectal examination may demonstrate a small, hard irregular palpable nodule, which is indicative of a cancerous lesion. At a more advanced stage the whole gland may obliterate the median sulcus and be felt outside in the seminal vesicles or encircling the rectum.

Serum prostatic specific antigen (PSA) is commonly raised, especially if metastatic lesions have occurred, although a normal level (4 ug/ml) cannot exclude the possibility of cancer. The antigen is a serine protease made by the epithelial cells of the prostate and is secreted into the prostatic ducts. Infections, infarctions and carcinoma may cause the PSA to diffuse from the acini and the ducts into the stroma which pass into the general circulation, hence the serum levels are raised. This increase can be as much as ten times per gram of the usual amount of PSA produced in the benign gland (Rous, 1996).

Transrectal ultrasound is able to identify tumours and aid in the assessment of extra-capsular metastases by emitting inaudible soundwaves through the prostate tissue; these then bounce back to produce an image of the prostate gland visually on the screen. This can facilitate access to the tumour when taking a transrectal or transperineal biopsy of the prostate by passing a biopsy needle directly through the rectal wall or the perineal tissue. Although the procedure is momentarily uncomfortable, analgesia is rarely used. Preceding the biopsy a prophylactic antibiotic injection of gentamicin 80 mg to 120 mg is given to reduce the incidence of infection, and observation is carried out to ensure that there is no post-biopsy bleeding. The patient is advised to check and report any blood found in the urine or semen, or with bowel actions.

Prostatic chips are sent for histology at the time of a transurethral resection of prostate (TURP). A TURP will relieve obstructive symptoms, of which approximately 15–25% are diagnosed as cancerous. When a positive diagnosis is made the patient needs to have staging established so that appropriate treatment can commence or continued checks kept to monitor any progression of the cancer (see Chapter 1).

Staging

An ultrasound of the prostate is required, or if more detail is required then a CT scan or MRI scan should be taken. Several pictures can be obtained at different sections through the body, to identify or exclude distant metastases.

Pelvic lymphadectomy may be necessary to provide an accurate nodal staging, if the MRI scan is omitted or if the urologist is considering a radical prostatectomy operation as the most suitable treatment.

A bone scan will help to identify lesions by highlighting areas of increased uptake of isotope in the bones, usually showing an increased distribution of blood vessels, and a chest X-ray to identify or exclude metastatic lung involvement (Rous, 1996). Abnormal liver function tests are also indicative of further metastases.

Transurethral resection of the prostate would be indicated if there were obstructive symptoms or retention of urine; however, if this was not a problem then the grade, stage and clinical condition of the patient would be evaluated.

International staging for prostatic cancer is done by evaluating tumour, nodes, metastases and histology (T, N, M&H). The Gleason score quantifies the tumour aggressiveness. This score is obtained by estimating the degree of glandular differentiation under magnification of the areas of the tumour most represented in biopsy; each of these is then graded 1–4 and the totals are added together (MacFarlane, 1988). The Mostofi staging system is also used (see Table 10.1).

Treatment

Bilateral orchidectomy, total or subtotal (subcapsular): approximately 70%–80% of cases respond to this treatment and symptoms such as bone pain are eliminated or greatly reduced almost immediately.

There are differing views on treatment for metastatic cancer. *Hormone manipulation* poses the problem of which drugs to use and when to start the treatment. Generally hormone manipulation is commenced when symptoms develop. Some urologists favour observation if the patient is asymptomatic; however the evaluation of hormone manipulation efficacy to delay onset of symptoms has not been completed and is ongoing.

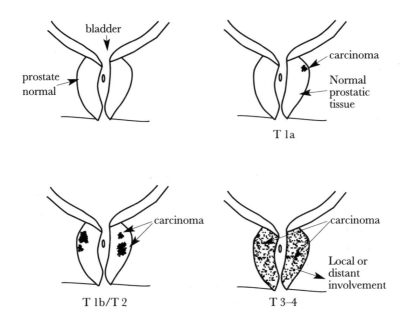

Figure 10.1 Prostatic staging.

Table 10.1 Gleason score and Mostofi staging for prostate tumours

Gleason score		Mostofi staging	
2–4	15% risk nodal metastases	Well differentiated	Grade I
6	30% risk nodal metastases	Moderately differentiated	Grade II
7	50% risk nodal metastases	Moderately differentiated	Grade II
8	75% risk nodal metastases	Poorly differentiated	Grade III
9–10	90–100% risk nodal metastases	Poorly differentiated	Grade III

T1a Well differentiated; less than 5% of the gland. Good prognosis without treatment. Follow-up and treat as symptoms occur.

T1b Diffuse/multifocal disease, a risk of metastatic development especially if less well differentiated. Radiotherapy may be considered: laser or radioactive seeds. Brachytherapy being trialled in some hospitals but not widely available at present.

T2 (NxM0) Well differentiated; in the case of a good prognosis may observe or give radical treatment. If poorly differentiated with local invasion or other metastases, radiotherapy is the most effective treatment.

T3/T4 (NxM0) Locally advanced, and involvement of the pelvic node may be present in up to 50% of the patients. Radiotherapy is effective with local advancement, or hormonal manipulation may be considered.

Anti-androgens such as cyproterone acetate and flutamide can be taken orally, and gonadotrophin-releasing hormone analogues such as goserelin (Zoladex) inhibit the release of pituitary hormones, which stimulate the production of testosterone in the testicle. Zoladex is given in the form of one or three monthly injections and appears to be effective for at least 18 months or longer.

In some instances the patient may not respond or may even relapse when hormone manipulation therapy is being administered. This can indicate that the prognosis is very poor.

The tumour can spread by direct local extension and into the prostatic capsule, although the fascia denonvillier acts as a barrier to the rectum. If the lymph nodes are involved then the condition is advanced and further haematogenous spread to the lumbar spine, pelvis, liver and lungs can occur.

Radical prostatectomy may be considered in the patient under 70 years of age if the investigations indicate that the cancer is confined to the prostatic gland. This procedure can offer a cure but there are possible side effects to consider; impotence and incontinence may be difficult to cope with in some instances. Nerve-sparing surgical techniques are usually attempted but are not always successful in preventing impotence or incontinence.

Prostatic screening for cancer

This is a contentious subject in that there are differing views as to the benefits. Many urologists think that this does not influence the treatment offered or the prognosis of the disease stage, except in younger males without metastatic lesions who choose radical surgery. Chamberlain (1998) says there is little evidence that early detection of malignancy improves or extends overall survival.

Advantages of screening

- Screening may detect abnormalities, and this may be beneficial to the patient if these are caught at an early stage
- Negative test result can reduce anxiety
- Prostatic specific antigen (blood test) screening is an acceptable investigation
- Screening of some other types of cancer has demonstrated benefits; therefore this could lead to similar developments in the field of prostate cancer

Disadvantages of screening

- A raised prostatic specific antigen result may not be caused by prostatic cancer; its discovery may therefore cause unnecessary anxiety and the need for further investigations
- A false negative result can give a false sense of reassurance
- Not all tests are hazard-free, and experienced operators are required for taking biopsies
- Financial resource implications

Bladder cancer

Incidence

Cancer of the bladder is one of the most common urological malignancies, with 20 people in every 100,000 developing the disease. About 8,000 new cases are diagnosed each year in the UK (Bullock et al., 1995). Bladder cancers are more common in developed industrial countries than the underdeveloped areas, except in Egypt where schistosomiasis is prevalent and predisposes to bladder cancer (Laker, 1994).

The peak incidence of this type of urological cancer occurs around the age of 65 years. It appears to have links with occupational exposures to certain chemicals, aromatic amines, dyes, and smoking. Chronic cystitis, bladder stones and schistosomiasis causing inflammatory tissue may increase the risk of malignant cell changes.

Table 10.2 Bladder cancer: types of tumour

Urothelial tumours	Benign papilloma – fibro-epithelial polyp Malignant transitional cell carcinoma 90%
Squamous cell carcinoma	5%–8%
Adenocarcinoma	1%–2%
Sarcoma	<1% an undifferentiated, highly anaplastic cancer

Presentation

This is often delayed and the disease may be at an advanced stage at the time of diagnosis, which will increase the risk of a poorer prognosis. Clinical features can include painless haematuria. The tumour can affect the whole of the collecting system since the transitional cell epithelium, a specialized waterproof tissue, extends from the renal papillae of the kidney along the ureter. This includes the lining of the bladder and approximately two-thirds of the urethra in the male and only halfway along the female urethra. A malignant growth can arise at any point in the collecting system and also be multifocal.

Investigations

Clinical history of episodes of haematuria, including the frequency and estimated amount of blood loss, is essential. Some 10% of patients over 45 years experiencing haematuria will have a bladder tumour causing this symptom.

Urine tests by a 'dipstick' to check for the presence of blood and infection are necessary. A midstream specimen of urine can be sent for culture if nitrates and red blood cells are present.

Ultrasound of the bladder will help to identify a tumour.

Flexible cystoscopy will allow visual examination of the bladder and access for taking a biopsy for histological examination. These investigations are now available at one-stop clinics in some hospitals. These clinics are managed by nurse practitioners working with senior medical staff. Patients can attend within the week of reporting their symptoms to the GP. It is possible to give a diagnosis on completion of these investigations before the patient goes home. It is therefore important to give the patient time to ask questions and provide appropriate information and ongoing support.

Differentiation of diagnosis needs to be made at this time, since a bladder tumour is not the only cause of haematuria and other investigations of the upper tract may be necessary if the bladder is excluded. On some occasions this may be idiopathic, as seen in the 'march' haematuria experienced by young soldiers in training.

Staging

International staging of bladder cancers is done by assessment of tumour, node and metastases (TNM) (see Table 10.3; Figure 10.2). The tissue type, depth, number of tumours, amount of nodal involvement and metastases are assessed, along with the degree of differentiation of tumour tissue on histological examination. Accurate staging of metastatic disease can be difficult since this cannot be assessed microscopically and is confirmed by the absence of symptoms within five years (see Chapter 1).

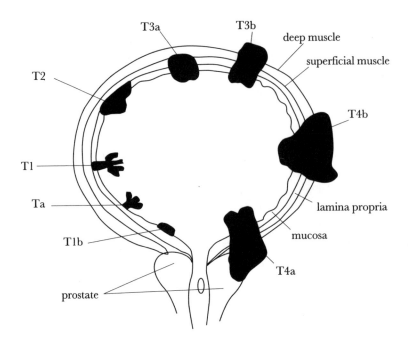

Figure 10.2 Bladder cancer staging.

Table 10.3 Staging of bladder tumours

Tis	Carcinoma in situ usually flat in appearance
Ta	Confined to the mucosa papillary
T1	Invasion of the lamina propria
T2	Invasion of the superficial muscle
T3a	Invasion of the deep muscle
T3b	Invasion of the perivesical tissue
T4 a	Tumour fixed to the prostate
T4b	Tumour fixed to other pelvic structures
M0	No evidence of metastases
M1	Metastasis present
MX	Metastasis
N0	No nodal involvement
N1	Single node involved (ipsilateral)
N2	Bilateral nodal, contralateral or multiple regional involvement
N3	Regional nodes involved, fixed and spreading to adjacent structures
N4	Regional nodes involved, wider metastatic disease
NX	Nodal status unknown

Management

A patient who has a diagnosed bladder tumour requires constant surveillance to monitor potential recurrences. Flexible cystoscopy is necessary at 3-, 6- or 12-monthly intervals depending on the previous findings and the time span between recurrent growths. Approximately 80% of bladder tumours are superficial, and no further treatment is required in up to 30% of these patients (Bullock et al., 1995). The remaining group would require treatment at a later stage, and of these patients 70% with invasive bladder tumour would have a prognosis of less than five years.

Recurrent growths may need more aggressive treatment, of cysto-diathermy, laser coagulation, transurethral resection of the tumour and further biopsies. If multiple superficial tumours have developed then intravesical chemotherapy can be effective in delaying the need for more radical treatments: mitomycin C and BCG (Bacillus Calmette-Guerin) are two of the drugs commonly used to treat this stage of the disease. Bladder instillations of the drugs are given weekly for several sessions and followed up by cystoscopy assessment.

Tumours that have deeply invaded the muscle are preferably treated by primary cystectomy, but a course of radiotherapy may be offered as an alternative treatment, which is usually given daily for up to six weeks. External beam radiotherapy treatment will need to be followed up by cystoscopy to reassess the bladder. In some cases side effects may develop, such as bleeding, incontinence and a contractile bladder. Salvage cystectomy may be necessary for some patients who develop recurrences. Major surgical techniques are used either to provide a diversion, as in a cystectomy and formation of ileal conduit, or in reconstruction to substitute a bladder. A length of the intestine is anastomosed directly on to the membranous urethra, and there is a need for straining or self-catheterization to empty the new bladder. Developments in the surgical techniques have helped to reduce the psychological effects on the patient of altered body image and lowered self-esteem.

Systemic chemotherapy may be used for metastatic disease in conjunction with other radical treatments. Palliative radiotherapy may relieve symptoms such as haematuria when the prognosis is poor due to metastatic disease.

Renal cancer

Incidence

Annual deaths from urological malignancies around the world are estimated to be 100,000. Tumours arising from the kidney, renal
parenchyma and urothelial lining of the collecting system account for
approximately 3% of all cancers (Bullock et al., 1995). 80% of renal
tumours are parenchymal (adenocarcinoma) and the incidence
appears to be slowly increasing. The Wilm's tumour (a nephroblastoma) occurs in children and accounts for 10% of childhood malignancies; of these 80% are detected under the age of five years. Renal cell
carcinoma (RCC), also known as hypernephroma or Grawitz tumour,
arises from the tubular epithelial cells and may present in various ways,
often whilst the patient is being screened for other conditions.

The incidence increases with age and reaches the peak at about
65 to 75 years at a rate of two men to every woman; 3% can have
bilateral involvement.

Predisposing factors

There are some implications from previous exposure to viruses and
certain carcinogens such as cadmium, and it is thought that
hormones and diet may also influence the onset (Dreicer and
Williams, 1992). Certain rare familial diseases such as Von Hippel-
Lindau disease and tuberous sclerosis predispose to renal cell carcinoma, of which 30% of patients present with metastatic disease. The
prognosis for this disease is poor, with less than a two-year survival
rate. Transitional cell carcinoma of the renal collecting system
accounts for 5–10% of renal cancers. Smoking is thought to be the
most likely carcinogen for this particular malignancy.

Presenting features

Many patients present with haematuria, although a mass may be
found in the loin, along with signs of anaemia, fatigue, anorexia, and
weight loss, probably caused by toxic substances called toxohormones produced by the tumour. Approximately 20% of renal
tumours present incidentally. Occasionally enlarged nodes in the left
supraclavicular fossa or a left varicocele may also be present in 1–2%

as a result of renal vein invasion. Other metastatic presentations may be with pathological fractures, pulmonary deposits and neurological symptoms due to brain metastasis or bilateral oedema and collateral venous circulation due to obstruction by vena caval involvement.

Investigations

A detailed history and physical examination will give some indication of the diagnosis, but this will need to be confirmed by specific tests.

Observation of the urine for obvious or microscopic presence of blood is essential.

Ultrasound of the kidney can also be done to highlight the tumour and help to distinguish between a cyst and a solid mass.

A CT scan helps in the staging by showing the degree of spread, including distant metastases such as the lungs and mediastinum, as well as an intact unaffected other kidney.

Bone scan will help confirm or eliminate infiltration into the bone.

All of these investigations assist in an accurate diagnosis and contribute to the staging process which will then help to determine the most effective treatments to be considered.

Staging

The tumour, node and metastases (TNM) method is usually used (see Table 10.4; Figure 10.3).

Table 10.4 Staging of renal cancer

Tumour	
T1	Kidney structure not distorted, small tumour identified
T2	Kidney structure distorted, larger tumour identified within the renal capsule
T3	Renal capsule and perinephric tissue involved
T4	Tumour spread to the adjacent organs and abdominal wall
Nodal status	
N0	Regional nodes not involved
N1	Single regional node involved
N2	Multiple regional nodes involved
N3	Nodes fixed, caused by tumour invasion to adjacent organs
N4	Lymphatic involvement beyond regional nodes
Metastases	
M0	Distant metastatic disease not present
M1	Distant metastatic disease present

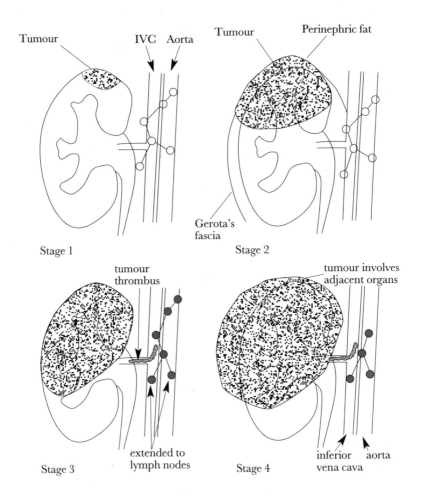

Figure 10.3 Renal cell carcinoma stages.

Management

Radical nephrectomy is advised for renal cell cancers if there is no evidence of metastases. This involves ligation of the pedicle and removal of the kidney, adjacent adrenal gland, and perinephric fat inside the intact Gerota's fascia. The upper ureter and enlarged para-aortic nodes may also be removed if there is further spread of the cancer. However if the patient has only one kidney functioning then a partial nephrectomy may be considered. This type of tumour tends to be resistant to radiotherapy, but may benefit the patient following surgery if the nodes are involved.

Transitional cell carcinoma

Investigations

Positive microscopy is required as well as an intravenous urogram which will confirm a filling defect or negative shadow, but this needs to differentiate from a blood clot or non-radiopaque stone. In order to diagnose carcinoma, a cystoscopy and retrograde pyelogram should be undertaken, or a ureteroscopy which will allow direct vision of the lesion.

Treatment

A radical nephrectomy, ureterectomy along with a cuff of bladder at the ureteric insertion would be advised since the tumour could easily spread along the transitional cell lining that extends from the pelvis of the kidney to the urethra including the bladder. In certain circumstances, such as a single kidney, a local excision may be made. These patients would need to have long-term follow-up.

Testicular cancer

Incidence

This occurs most frequently in young men ranging from 15 to 35 years of age, the peak time being in the 20s. It accounts for 19% of all male deaths caused by carcinoma in this age group (Stanford, 1988). Testicular cancer represents 1% of all male cancers and 14% of urological cancers (Stadva et al., 1983).

Predisposing factors

The cause is not known but there are factors of significance related to this condition. Males who have had late descent, undescended testicles or infertility are 11% to 15% more likely to develop testicular cancer. Testicular trauma and infection of the testicles, especially viral, and testicular atrophy following mumps may also be contributory factors.

Types of testicular cancer

The tumours may be described as seminomas or non-seminomatous germ cell tumours. Further classifications commonly used are:

- Seminoma – the most common testicular tumour which has the best prognosis
- Differentiated teratoma (DT)
- Malignant teratoma intermediate (MTI)
- Malignant teratoma undifferentiated (MTU) – rapid growth
- Sub-variant: malignant trophoblastic teratoma (MTT) – has a poor prognosis
- Teratoma with seminoma (MTU+ S)

It is possible to have mixed histological tumours with mixed characteristics. Patients are up to 700 times more likely to develop a second tumour in the other testicle if testicular cancer has been diagnosed (Laker, 1994).

Symptoms

A painless lump is the most common clinical feature, but 10% of patients experience discomfort and other problems such as redness, pain, inflammation, scrotal ache, heaviness and swelling which may have developed slowly. There is evidence to suggest that 10% of cases develop after injury and 30% have metastases on presentation or sudden pain, which occurs due to bleeding into the tumour (Dawson, 1996).

Diagnosis and investigations

A history of the onset of symptoms is essential, along with a clinical examination of the patient's testicle. A tumour will have a hard induration or firmer tissue in the centre than the surrounding tissue or collateral testicle, but differential diagnosis of other testicular conditions is important. Epididymitis, orchitis, hydrocele, spermatocele, torsion, and inguinal hernia – all of which should be separate from the actual testicle – have to be excluded or may be considered to be co-existent and require further investigations. Sometimes these conditions can contribute to a delay in diagnosis; hydroceles may specifically be associated with a testicular tumour.

Examination of the patient is best in the dorsal recumbent position. The epididymis needs to be identified before confirming the lump in the testicle and the abdomen and neck must be checked for lymph node metastases. If a lump is established then a series of investigations are required. The tumours can produce specific markers. These are substances found only in negligible amounts or undetectable in the absence of tumours. Blood samples are assayed for levels of alpha fetoprotein (AFP), human chorionic gonadotrophin (HCG) and placental alkaline phosphatase (PLAP). This helps in staging the tumour and monitoring treatment response, or recurrence of cancer cells (Dawson and Whitfield, 1996).

Ultrasonography can assist in distinguishing lesions of the testicle and epididymis, demonstrating a normal testicle with a high level of accuracy. Once the tumour is suspected the patient will need support and information, an understanding of the processes of investigations to confirm the diagnosis and discussion of the options for treatment. If surgery is to be considered then aspects such as body image, losing a testicle, concern for masculinity as well as sexual activity, potency, and capability have to be addressed. Since many patients will be young they face a difficult time adjusting to partners and family response as well as their own concerns, including the possibility of fatherhood and side effects. 'Education, psychological support and encouragement to work through the sense of loss and to look to the future' are essential aspects of care required (Bullock et al., 1995). It is extremely important to promote early detection by self-examination so that the treatment is commenced immediately to ensure best prognosis (see Table 10.5).

Staging

See Table 10.6.

Treatment

Orchidectomy is the most effective treatment, and can be performed as a day case. Counselling must be given so that the patient considers he has sufficient information to make the decision.

Table 10.5 Testicular self-examination

Frequency	Once a month
Check	Scrotal skin when relaxed; ideally after a bath or shower.
Technique	Hold testicles in the palm of the hand, look at the size and weight. If one is larger or heavier they need to be checked by your doctor. Looking at both testicles and using both hands, roll the testicle between the thumb and fingers. Identify the epididymus at the back of the testicle. It should be soft, spongy and tender to touch. Look for lumps, irregularities, enlargement, change in firmness or swelling. If any abnormality is found a medical check is essential.

Table 10.6 Staging of testicular cancer

STAGE 1	No evidence of spread outside the testis
STAGE 2	Spread of tumour to glands and the back of the abdomen A – <2 cm, B >2 cm, C >7 cm
STAGE 3	Spread to glands in the chest and neck. Supra-diaphragmatic
STAGE 4	Spread outside glands – commonly wings L1 Lung metastases <3 in number L2 Lung metastases >3 in number <2 cm L3 Lung metastases >3 in number >2 cm

When the histology is confirmed, further treatment may be indicated, such as chemotherapy or radiotherapy. The follow-up of the patient will be the responsibility of the oncologist. However, occasionally the urologist may need to operate to excise a mass or nodes in the abdomen following a course of chemotherapy or radiotherapy.

Cancer of the penis

Incidence

This type of cancer constitutes 2% of all male cancers, and is more common after the age of 45 years. The incidence increases with age but is most prevalent in the 60–70 age group. It is less likely to occur in circumcised males, as smegma may be carcinogenic (Bullock et al., 1995). This malignancy is commonly found in Africa, where it is often associated with erythroplasia of queyrat, a precancerous condition forming red plaques on the penile shaft that may be invasive.

Predisposing factors

Skin diseases or penile irritation, such as balanitis, will increase the risk of cancer developing if chronic inflammation persists of which may be related to poor hygiene and phimosis occurring. Patients with diabetes are more vulnerable.

Presentation

A warty growth, ulceration or fungating lesion develops on the glans penis or coronal sulcus which can be covered by foreskin, delaying discovery until there is pain, bleeding or even a discharge if at a later stage. There appears to be a lack of awareness, or embarrassment, which may cause delays in seeking help, and it is thought that up to 50% of cases delay for a year.

Squamous cell carcinoma is found in 97% of penile cancers and approximately 90% are found on the glans or prepuce. It is almost nonexistent in men circumcised as children (Corriere, 1986). The lesion needs to be differentiated from verrucous carcinoma.

Investigations

Lymphatic inguinal nodes need to be checked as infection and inflammation can cause enlarged nodes. About 80% of patients have lymphadenopathy at the time of diagnosis and half of them will have metastases. A course of antibiotics and reassessment before a biopsy will be necessary. Further investigations such as chest X-rays, urogram and CT scan will be required to assess the stage of the cancer.

Staging

- Stage 1   Confined to the foreskin or glans penis
- Stage 2   Invading the shaft of penis
- Stage 3   Invading as far as the scrotum
- Stage 4   Inguinal nodes involved

The tumour, node and metastases (TNM) method may also be used to stage the tumour.

Management

Radiotherapy is best if the lesion is a localized lesion to the penile shaft.

Partial amputation may be considered for recurrence, but it will shorten the penis considerably since a 2 cm proximal clearance of the tumour is essential.

Advanced carcinoma involving the shaft and scrotal skin is treated with a radical amputation involving removal of the penis and scrotal contents and the reconstruction of the urethra to form a perineal urethrostomy.

Palliative radiotherapy may be an alternative.

Counselling for body image changes and psychosexual problems may be required, and follow-up of all aspects will be necessary at intervals.

Support for the patient, family and close friends

Genito-urinary malignancies frequently cause distress, since giving detailed history of symptoms, intimate physical examinations and invasive tests are embarrassing for many patients. The fear of confirmation of a cancerous disease and prognosis all contribute to the delay in seeking treatment, and many patients already have metastases when initially diagnosed. The clinical features, such as haematuria, incontinence, retention and pain, disrupt the normal urinary elimination function and may cause sexual dysfunction. This can contribute to a lowered self-esteem and change of body image. The patient may be affected both physically and psychologically and will need help to adjust to the changes. More support has become available recently from specialist trained urological nursing staff, nurse practitioners, stoma therapists, psychosexual counsellors, urological cancer counsellors and continence nurse advisors. All of these nurses are able to give knowledgeable information and education to the patient and carers, to help them to develop a coping mechanism during treatment and recovery time or when receiving palliative care. The role of urological cancer nurse counsellors has been identified as essential in meeting the standards expected of specialist centres in supporting the patient. Support groups are another source of help for patients, relatives and friends.

Occupational acquired disease

Although there are some indications that occupational carcinogens may cause certain malignancies, conclusive evidence is generally not available. It is therefore difficult to obtain sufficient information to support such claims in urological malignancies to obtain compensation for occupational acquired disease. Generally it is advisable to take a detailed history of work and contact with such carcinogens, even though working practices have improved to reduce or eliminate suspected causes. It is more likely to be suspected in the older age group who may not be able to recall or obtain sufficient information to substantiate a claim.

The introduction of the Health and Safety at Work Act in 1974 made the employer responsible for ensuring that employees were not exposed to hazardous substances in the workplace. This act also introduced the concept of health and medical surveillance for employees and the maintenance of records. The Control of Substances Hazardous to Health regulations (COSHH, 1988, updated 1994) have been in force and are regularly monitored. The risks in the workplace must be assessed and adequate precautions must be taken.

Case histories

Mr Smith

Fifty-seven-year-old Mr Smith was admitted for further investigations, having experienced an episode of frank haematuria several weeks earlier and noticing some blood in his urine following this occurrence. Mr Smith gave a history of having lost a few pounds in weight and had reduced his cigarette smoking to only ten a day. An intravenous urogram had already been done and the results showed that both kidneys were excreting promptly, and nothing abnormal was found in the pelvicalyceals system or the ureters, but it confirmed that the bladder had an irregularity of the left side in keeping with the suspected tumour.

A full depth resection of the bladder tumour was performed at this time. Two months later a cystoscopy was repeated and further biopsies were taken of the bladder and prostate. This demonstrated an aggressive, invasive semi-solid tumour. Once the nature of the tumour had been established, a CT scan was arranged to check the chest and abdomen in advance of major surgery. Mr Smith had been given the opportunity to discuss his diagnosis and the possible treatments on each admission and decided to reject reconstructive surgery. Instead, he agreed to be prepared for a cystoprotatectomy. The CT scan showed that there was no metastasis or lymphoedema in the pelvis or para-aortic region. The stoma care nurse specialist counselled Mr Smith about the surgery and the aftercare of the stoma, and worked out the most suitable position for this to be placed considering the patient's lifestyle and dexterity. The surgery was carried out uneventfully.

After the operation Mr Smith was taught how to care for his stoma and change the stoma bag so that he was able to cope by himself in preparation for discharge home. Mr Smith would return to the outpatient clinic for the first of his follow-up appointments in a few weeks time. The stoma therapist would support and offer psychosexual counselling if the patient so wished. Mr Smith will need to be reviewed regularly and if no metastatic disease develops then only an annual follow-up is required. However, a joint follow-up with both the urologist and the oncologist may be necessary if metastatic disease is identified.

Mr Street

Mr Street (58) was seen by his doctor after suffering two episodes of haematuria, each lasting a few days, with bleeding at the beginning of the urine stream and low back pain. Mr Street was sent to the haematuria clinic a few days later. All the diagnostic tests were done during that visit and the results were available before he left the clinic. Mr Street's urine was dark red and he gave a history of urgency and nocturia. Blood samples were therefore taken for urea and electrolytes and haemoglobin estimation, and an abdominal ultrasound and flexible cystoscopy were arranged for that morning. The ultrasound demonstrated a possible mass on the right side of the bladder but the KUB (kidney, ureter and bladder) X-ray appeared normal. However the flexible cystoscopy confirmed the mass, and a resection would be necessary under a general anaesthetic. Mr Street was given the results of the investigations and the possible treatments were discussed. Mr Street went home that day and an urgent admission date for a bladder tumour resection was arranged, since he was in agreement with the proposed treatment. A cystoscopy to examine the bladder revealed a large tumour and on bimanual examination a thickened bladder wall could be felt. Tumours observed were resected from all over the wall and biopsies were obtained for histological examination.

The biopsy results showed that the tumour was predominantly well differentiated with variable grades, although focally moderately differentiated grade papillary transitional cell carcinoma with superficial stromal invasion was present. Treatments were discussed and intravesical chemotherapy was accepted as the best option at this stage. Mitomycin C was given at weekly intervals for six weeks, and then another cystoscopy was done to evaluate the effect of the instillations. The treatment appeared to be successful and Mr Street would continue to have check cystoscopies. Three- or six-monthly cystoscopies would need to be carried out as a follow-up. If there were recurrences, more radical treatment might be required. A 12-monthly 'check cystoscopy' may be the only follow-up required if the bladder is clear of tumour and the patient has no other symptoms associated with the malignancy.

Mr White

Mr White, aged 65, was seen by his doctor complaining of a poor stream with some urgency and having to get up at least five times every night to urinate. On examination a small smooth prostate was felt, but his prostatic specific antigen (PSA) was slightly raised and he was referred to the urologist to have further investigations. The investigations confirmed that the prostate was small and flat and the flow rate was reduced, but the prostatic biopsy showed a moderately differentiated adenocarcinoma, probably early stage and confined to the prostate.

The biopsy result and possible treatment options were discussed with the patient, the choices being offered were either radical radiotherapy or a radical prostatectomy. The treatments both have potential side effects including impotence and continence problems. Leaflets were given to support the information given by the consultant and Mr White was asked to try to decide over the next two weeks what treatment he wished to receive.

Mr White decided to have a radical prostatectomy since he was advised that this could offer him a 70% chance of a cure. Surgery was arranged urgently for two weeks ahead. Mr White was seen at a pre-clerking clinic where all the necessary preparations were made, and further discussion took place about what the operation involved and aftercare. The surgery was uneventful and recovery progressed satisfactorily so that by the twelfth day Mr White was ready for discharge home. It was necessary to leave a catheter in his bladder to allow the anastomosis of the urethra and bladder neck to heal. Three weeks later the catheter was removed and maintenance of continence was assessed. Although Mr White was able to pass urine, he experienced frequent leakage. A urinary sheath and drainage bag were worn to contain the leakage and pelvic floor exercises were taught at this time.

The histology results confirmed the tumour and clear excision margins, so Mr White was seen by the urologist four months later. The PSA levels were 0.5 ng/l and the incontinence problems were almost resolved, so that only one small disposable pouch was worn daily as a precaution. Several months later Mr White was continuing to make a good recovery. After requesting help with impotence problems he was referred to a sexual dysfunction clinic. Six-monthly checks of the PSA and potential symptoms would continue.

Mr Brown

Mr Brown (55) was seen by his doctor complaining of haematuria and passing blood clots on two occasions in the previous few weeks. He had severe pain for several hours which was not relieved with analgesia. The pain was intermittent, sometimes sharp and other times an ache. When he was examined a large tender mass was felt in the hyperchondrium, and obvious haematuria was noted.

Mr Brown was seen urgently by the urologist and a flexible cystoscopy, an abdominal/renal ultrasound and KUB (kidney, ureter and bladder X-ray) were arranged. The X-ray showed a mass on the left side. The ultrasound scan demonstrated a mass arising from the kidney which had the appearance of a hypernephroma. The right kidney and adjacent organs appeared to be normal, except the bladder which contained echogenic material assumed to be blood. A CT scan was ordered for the next week and this confirmed a large tumour in the upper pole of the kidney with some streaks of density of soft tissue extending into the perinephric fat, although other organs and nodes did not appear to be involved.

The results of the investigations were discussed with Mr Brown, who was offered a radical nephrectomy as the best option for treatment, and he agreed to undergo the surgery. Routine preoperative preparations were made and informed consent was obtained. The removal of the kidney and perinephric fat was difficult since the tumour was large, fixed and involved the renal vein. Postoperatively Mr Brown progressed without further complications although the histological findings demonstrated that there had been some infiltration beyond the renal capsule, and he was discharged the following week. Some six months later Mr Brown appeared to be making a good recovery and there were no obvious signs of disease progression. Long-term follow-up will be necessary to ensure that any recurrence will be treated at the earliest opportunity at the combined oncology and urology clinic.

Conclusions

Urological malignancies encompass a range of cancers, each necessitating different treatment. Health promotion and education can help to ensure that early detection is made where possible, as with testicular cancers. Screening for early detection is currently controversial, particularly in the case of prostatic cancer, because early diagnosis may not always affect the prognosis. Auditing outcomes and continued research is essential to achieve best standards of care and clinical effectiveness. The specialist nurse practitioner is recognised as making a significant contribution to best care practices, leading clinics for patients with haematuria, prostatic assessment and pre-clerking the patient. The length of time that patients stay in hospital is greatly reduced nowadays, so it is essential to have a knowledgeable nursing team with good communication skills. Nurses play a key role in ensuring that their patients receive the optimum level of care and support from the time of referral throughout treatment and during the follow-up period.

Chapter 11
Head and neck malignancies

KAY HOWARD

Introduction

Approximately 3,000 cases of head and neck cancer are reported in the UK each year, with an associated death rate of 25–30% (OPCS, 1994). The term 'head and neck cancer' can encompass many different structures including larynx, upper oesophagus, lip, tongue, floor of mouth, jaw, oral mucosa, palate, oropharynx, postnasal space, nasal cavity, paranasal sinuses, ear and salivary glands. Tumours of the skin and thyroid may also come under the definition of head and neck cancer but will not be discussed in this chapter. Anatomy of the head and neck will not be covered here but knowledge of this is necessary to enable us to understand the morbidity of this disease and its treatment, and the possible detrimental effects on an individual's quality of life.

This chapter will commence with a description of the most common tumour types and sites within the head and neck, together with their associated aetiology, epidemiology and signs and symptoms. It will also describe investigations carried out following presentation, the staging of disease and subsequent treatment options. Surgery and radiotherapy are the main options for curative treatment, but the role of chemotherapy will also be considered. Thereafter the chapter will focus on patient and family support and on the importance of a multidisciplinary team approach in the care of individuals with head and neck cancer. In conclusion, three brief case histories will be presented in order to clarify the text.

Types of head and neck malignancies

Head and neck cancer is most commonly taken to mean squamous carcinoma arising from the mucosa of the upper aerodigestive tract, which accounts for 95% of head and neck malignancies (Muir and Weiland, 1995), although a variety of tumour types can arise. Tumours of the larynx are the commonest, with the highest incidence occurring in males in a ratio of 10 men to one woman, although an abnormally high incidence has been reported in Scottish women (Maran et al., 1993).

Adenocarcinomas of the head and neck are uncommon but may arise from the surface epithelium or from salivary tissue (Wax et al., 1995). Primary malignant melanoma may affect the upper aerodigestive tract, in particular the oral and nasal cavities. Other rare tumours of the head and neck include the group of neuroendocrine neoplasms, which includes carcinoid tumours and small cell carcinomas. Histologically salivary gland malignancies include adenocarcinoma, acinic cell, mucoepidermoid and adenoid cystic carcinomas (Maran, 1988).

Head and neck malignancies are typically characterized by extensive local tissue destruction, involvement of regional lymph nodes and a low incidence of distant metastases. Prognosis is dependent on tumour type and stage, the number of pathologically positive nodes, surgical excision margins, and treatment options (Maran et al., 1993).

Aetiology/predisposing factors

Tobacco and alcohol consumption

The aetiology of head and neck cancers is clearly related to cigarette smoking and to a lesser extent alcohol consumption (Maran et al., 1993). Cancer of the larynx has been directly related to the number of cigarettes smoked, with an incidence risk of 2.4 for seven cigarettes a day, increasing to a risk factor of 16.4 for 25+ cigarettes a day (Maran et al., 1993).

Alcohol appears to have a synergistic role with tobacco in the incidence of cancers of the oral cavity, oesophagus, hypopharynx and larynx. Oral cancer is the eighth most common cancer in developed countries, has a ratio of five males to one female and is more common in the lower social classes (Boyle et al., 1998). The risk of oral cancer has been shown to rise with increased cigarette consumption and independently with increased alcohol consumption (Blot et al., 1988), but the effects of alcohol are multiplicative rather than additive (Boyle et al., 1998). The risk is increased 35 times with consumption of >40 cigarettes and >4 units of alcohol daily (Blot et al., 1988). There is also an association between the use of oral tobacco and oral cancer (Boyle et al., 1998).

Industry and occupation

Cancer of the larynx is twice as common in industrialized areas and exposure to asbestos, coal dust, mustard gas and sulphuric acid have all been implicated as risk factors. Nickel and chromate dust can cause lesions in the nose, larynx and paranasal sinuses (Maran et al., 1993). The development of carcinomas of the nose, nasal cavity and nasal sinuses has been linked to exposure to wood dust – particularly hard wood dust to adenocarcinomas and soft wood dust to squamous cell carcinomas (Maran et al., 1993). Links have also been made between head and neck cancers and exposure to formaldehyde and nickel compounds (Boyle et al., 1998).

Past medical history

There have been conflicting reports of the association of human papilloma virus with head and neck cancers, but this virus and the herpes simplex virus have been found in raised levels in oral cancer tissue (Tanaka, 1995). Paterson-Brown Kelly syndrome, characterized by iron deficiency, glossitis, kolonychia and upper oesophageal web, has been linked with the development of post-cricoid carcinomas (Maran et al., 1993).

Betel

Chewing betel (leaves from the betel vine and nuts from the betel palm) is widespread in South East Asia and is linked to the development of oral cancer, especially when combined with tobacco (Boyle et al., 1998).

Diet

High levels of nasopharyngeal cancers are found in South East Asia and South East China, and although this is a rare disease in

Caucasians, high rates are also found in Chinese migrants to Western countries. It has been suggested that early exposure to Epstein-Barr virus and childhood consumption of salted fish, particularly during weaning, may be aetiological factors (Boyle et al., 1998).

Presentation/symptoms

Due to the wide variety of tumour sites, symptoms of head and neck cancer obviously vary, but many early signs are similar to symptoms of benign illnesses, e.g. hoarse voice, mouth ulcer and sore throat, which may be a factor in the late presentation or referral of some individuals. Symptoms and signs are described by tumour location.

Larynx and hypopharynx

Symptoms reflect localization, size and degree of invasion. Early glottic (vocal cord) lesions present with painless hoarse voice, whilst larger tumours may present with severe hoarseness, odynophagia (painful swallow), dysphagia (difficulty swallowing), dyspnoea (breathlessness) and stridor (wheeze and noisy breathing on inspiration), referred otalgia (ear pain in the absence of ear disease) and neck masses. Otalgia is a common symptom of piriform fossa tumours. On direct/indirect laryngoscopy ulcerative lesions may be seen, together with reduced vocal cord mobility or fixation and pooling of saliva in the hypopharynx or piriform sinus.

Oral cavity and oropharynx

(Includes tonsils, soft palate, lateral posterior pharyngeal wall and base of tongue.)

Early lesions are often asymptomatic. May present as leukoplakia or unilateral localized pain, often secondary to infection, or as a painless neck lump. Larger lesions may be characterized by referred otalgia, bloodstained saliva, voice disorders, odynophagia, dysphagia, trismus (impaired jaw opening), reduced tongue movements, or ulceration.

Nose and paranasal sinuses

These often present as unilateral nasal obstruction, watery/purulent discharge, epistaxis, poor dental occlusion, trismus, antral fistula, ulceration, visual disturbances (diplopia/impairment), cheek swelling, numbness and paraesthesia. Neurologic symptoms are indicative of advanced disease.

Nasopharynx

These are often 'silent' tumours; patients may present with unilateral hearing loss and middle ear effusion due to occlusion of the Eustachian tube, or with a painless neck lump. Nasal obstruction is uncommon until the tumour involves the nasal cavity. Neurologic signs can occur due to compromised cranial nerves.

Ear

Malignancies of the ear may present with discharge, pain, hearing loss, or impaired facial nerve function.

Neck

Some patients with head and neck malignancies present with neck node metastases. There is a close relationship between the site of the primary tumour and the level/site of lymph node metastases.

Investigations

Ideally, diagnosis should be made in a multidisciplinary head and neck cancer clinic where a team approach is likely to promote high standards of physical and psychosocial care; this is highlighted as a recommendation by recent reports (Calman-Hine, 1995; Edwards, 1997). Investigation begins with a history and a full ear, nose and throat (ENT) examination including indirect laryngoscopy/flexible nasoendoscopy and palpation of neck. Examination, panendoscopy and biopsy under general anaesthetic is usually undertaken. CT and MRI scans can be valuable in assessing tumour volume and operability. Chest X-ray is performed as 10–15% of patients present with synchronous tumours in the head and neck region, lung and oesophagus (Manni, 1998).

Staging

Head and neck malignancies are staged using the TNM classification developed by the International Union Against Cancer and the

American Joint Committee on Cancer (see Chapter 1).

    T = Extent of primary tumour
    N = Regional lymph nodes
    M = Presence/absence of distant metastases

The T categories are specific to each tumour site within the head and neck region and examples are given of the classification for oropharynx and larynx tumours in Table 11.1.

Table 11.1 TNM classification for oropharynx and larynx tumours

Oropharynx	T1	Tumour 2 cm or less
	T2	Tumour more than 2 cm but not more than 4 cm
	T3	Tumour more than 4 cm
	T4	Tumour invades adjacent structures
Larynx	T1	Tumour limited to vocal cord(s) with normal mobility
(glottis)	T2	Tumour extends to supraglottis and/or subglottis, and/or impaired cord mobility
	T3	Tumour limited to larynx with vocal cord fixation
	T4	Tumour invades through thyroid cartilage and/or extends to other tissues beyond the larynx

(UICC, 1997)

T1 cancers of the head and neck can be cured in a high proportion of patients, whilst T4 tumours have a rather poor prognosis (Maier, 1998). The main determinant of prognosis in the TNM system is the presence of cervical lymph node metastases and distant metastases. For instance, a single positive lymph node in oral cancer reduces five-year survival by 45% (Ditroia, 1972). When three or more nodes are found in oral cancers the five-year survival rate is decreased from 49% (rate for single node) to 13% (Kalnins et al., 1977). The classification of metastases is depicted in Table 11.2.

The lung is the most common distant site of metastatic head and neck cancer, with liver and bone metastases being less common (Maier, 1998). Less well differentiated tumours are associated with a poorer prognosis (Henson, 1988), but even amongst tumours of the same histological type and site there are variations in prognosis that are dependent on the stage of disease. The current stage grouping for head and neck cancers is detailed in Table 11.3.

Table 11.2 Classification for the incidence of metastases in head and neck malignancies

Lymph node metastases

Nx	Regional lymph nodes cannot be assessed
N0	No regional lymph nodes
N1	Metastasis in single ipsilateral node, 3 cm or less
N2a	Metastasis in a single ipsilateral node more than 3 cm but less than 6 cm
N2b	Metastasis in multiple ipsilateral nodes, none more than 6 cm
N2c	Metastasis in bilateral or contralateral nodes, none more than 6 cm
N3	Metastasis in lymph node more than 6 cm

Distant metastases

Mx	Presence of distant metastases cannot be assessed
M0	No distant metastases
M1	Distant metastases

(UICC, 1997)

Table 11.3 Stage grouping for head and neck cancers

Stage 0	Tis	N0	M0
Stage I	T1	N0	M0
Stage II	T2	N0	M0
Stage III	T3	N0	M0
	T1	N1	M0
	T2	N1	M0
	T3	N1	M0
Stage IVa	T4	N0	M0
	T4	N1	M0
	Any T	N2	M0
Stage IVb	Any T	N3	M0
Stage IVc	Any T	Any N	M1

Management

Early stage oral cavity, oropharynx and larynx cancers are usually curable by surgery or radiotherapy. These are the main curative options for head and neck cancer, although chemotherapy does have a role in the management of some tumours. Tumour size is the main factor in deciding treatment options. Jones (1998) suggests the following as management guidelines:

- Early oral cavity: surgery
- Oropharyngeal up to and including T2: radiotherapy
- Larynx up to T3: radiotherapy with surgical salvage if necessary

- Piriform fossa up to and including T2: radiotherapy
- Small post-cricoid: radiotherapy or surgery
- Sinonasal tumours (often present late): surgery

Neck node metastases are usually treated by neck dissection at the appropriate levels. If extracapsular spread or multiple neck nodes are present then postoperative radiotherapy is usually indicated. Tumours with positive neck nodes carry a more than 20% chance of recurrence (Jones, 1998).

Surgery

As the term 'head and neck cancer' incorporates so many possible tumour sites, it is very difficult to describe surgical procedures within the confines of this chapter; therefore general principles will be outlined, and reference made to the most common tumour sites, i.e. the larynx and the oral cavity.

Surgery for head and neck cancer can result in severe dysfunction and disfigurement and multidisciplinary involvement in treatment planning is essential to maximize quality of life and achieve best possible rehabilitation. It is essential to understand the anatomy of the head and neck in order to be able to predict subsequent deficits and plan rehabilitation. Ideally, the multidisciplinary team should consist of surgeons (ENT, maxillofacial and plastic/reconstructive), oncologist, speech and swallowing therapist, dietitian, and nurses specializing in the care of head and neck cancer patients, with access to an extended team of palliative care specialist, chaplain, social worker, prosthodontist and psychologist. The core team should have regular meetings where patient treatment, rehabilitation and care can be discussed and planned (BAHNO, 1998; BAOHNS, 1998).

Surgical excision of a head and neck tumour can rarely be achieved (with the exception of very small lesions which are suitable for laser vaporization, unilateral vocal cord lesions and some salivary gland tumours) without significantly altered anatomy or a substantial defect requiring reconstruction or prosthetics. The goal is to restore function and achieve acceptable cosmesis. This is sometimes achieved by the use of prostheses, which must be well fitting, secure and cosmetically acceptable in order to minimize disfigurement and dysfunction. There is a trend towards osseointegrated prosthetics for the replacement of external features, i.e. nose, ear and eye/orbit, where the prosthesis is secured by titanium screws into bone, rather than relying on prostheses that are glued on or attached to spectacles.

If it is necessary to move tissue from one area to another in order to reconstruct a defect caused by surgical excision of the tumour, several options are available depending on the site and extent of excision.

Tissue can remain attached to its blood supply by a pedicle and then be tunnelled, advanced, swung or rotated into a local defect, or can be completely detached from its site of origin and used as a 'free flap'. The advent of the microvascular free flap in the mid-1970s made a considerable impact on the surgical reconstruction of defects caused by surgical excision of a head and neck tumour, often resulting in improvements in function and appearance when compared with more traditional methods of reconstruction. The free flap (tissue based on a significant artery and vein) is completely removed from its donor site and is then attached to the recipient site by microvascular anastomosis (see Figures 11.1 and 11.2).

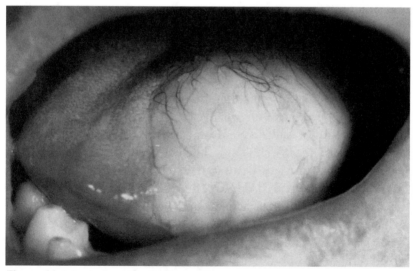

Figure 11.1 A microvascular free flap on the tongue.

Myocutaneous flaps consisting of muscle, skin and blood supply, and in some cases bone or cartilage, are especially useful when large amounts of tissue have been resected and bulk is needed to reconstruct the defect. The deltopectoral flap consisting of tissue (no

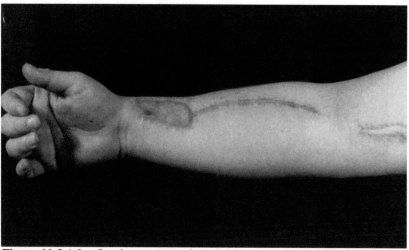

Figure 11.2 A free flap donor area on the radial forearm.

muscle) and blood supply only is a useful source of well vascularized tissue for an area that has previously been irradiated.

Management of the altered airway

Many patients undergoing surgery for head and neck cancer will have an altered airway as either a temporary or permanent feature, by the formation of a tracheostomy (temporary or permanent) or laryngectomy (permanent) (Figure 11.3). Tracheostomy is used in situations where airway obstruction or impaired pulmonary function is anticipated or already exists. For instance, elective tracheostomy is performed to relieve temporary airway obstruction anticipated as a result of oedema following resection of an oropharyngeal tumour, whilst a permanent tracheostomy may be required to prevent aspiration due to an incompetent larynx as a result of advanced disease or radionecrosis following radiotherapy.

The nursing management of tracheostomy will vary according to the reasons for performing tracheostomy and local policies and procedures. Basic principles include the necessity to provide humidification (as the normal mechanism of warming and moistening air by breathing through the nose and mouth has been bypassed) to prevent secretions becoming thick, tenacious and difficult to clear. A safe, effective suctioning technique is also necessary, as is attention to toileting of stoma and tubes, including regular cleaning of inner cannulae to

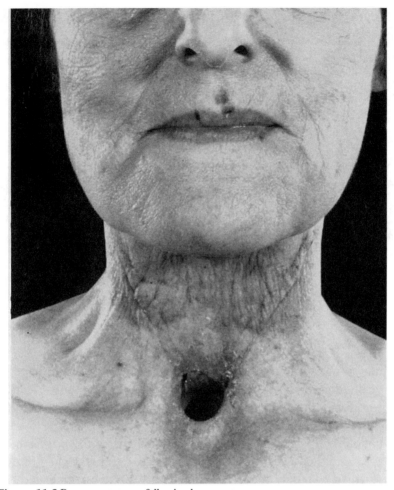

Figure 11.3 Permanent stoma following laryngectomy.

prevent occlusion, and monitoring of cuff pressures to prevent damage to the tracheal mucosa and subsequent tracheal stenosis.

It is important that patients are encouraged to perform self-care of the tracheostomy/laryngectomy both to improve confidence and to promote acceptance of altered body image. The performance of self-care in the immediate postoperative period has been highlighted as an important indicator of adjustment (Dropkin, 1989). It is important to recognize the psychological impact of altered body image; strategies for offering support in this regard will be discussed later in this chapter.

Radiotherapy

Where radiotherapy is the treatment of choice this commonly involves 30 or more daily fractions of 1.8 to 2 Gy (Levendag and Keus, 1998), although regimes will vary between centres and tumour site. A plastic shell or mask, with the radiation marks drawn on to it, is used to keep the head in the same position for each treatment and to ensure accurate beam delivery (see Chapter 2).

Interstitial or endocavitory brachytherapy by temporary iridium seeds and wires (Figure 11.4), or by permanent iodine seeds, is sometimes used because sources of irradiation within or close to the tumour have the advantage of sparing surrounding normal tissues (Levendag and Keus, 1998).

Acute effects of radiotherapy

Mucositis and skin erythema occur two weeks after treatment commences and increase in severity. Skin desquamation can occur. Xerostomia with thick ropy saliva, altered taste sensation, and mucosal oedema with pain and dysphagia mean it is necessary to monitor dietary intake, with some patients needing tube feeding or

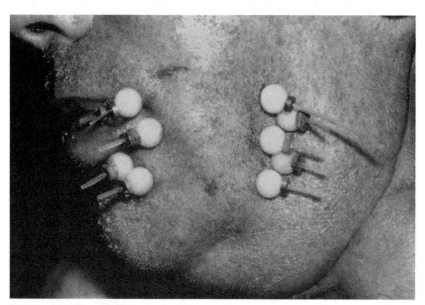

Figure 11.4 Interstitial brachytherapy.

supplements. Oral care is essential during this time to alleviate pain and prevent infection (Bildstein, 1993). Recovery from the acute side effects of radiotherapy to the head and neck begins 3–6 weeks after completion of radiotherapy (Levendag and Keus, 1998).

Late effects of radiotherapy

Permanent damage to salivary glands occurs when they receive 40 Gy or more, and this results in severe xerostomia (dry mouth). Although some improvement may occur after about a year this can be a distressing condition that is difficult to alleviate as artificial saliva sprays and lozenges tend to have a very transient benefit and many patients are unable to tolerate salivary gland stimulants (e.g. pilocarpine), due to the side effects. Any saliva that is produced tends to be thick and ropy, making chewing and swallowing difficult. The protective mechanism of saliva is lost and the patient is more prone to oral infections and dental caries, making meticulous oral hygiene and prophylactic dental care advisable (Bildstein, 1993). Osteoradionecrosis of the jaw can result from radiotherapy to the oral cavity and the importance of dental care and oral hygiene in the prevention of this needs to be emphasized (Jansma et al., 1992). Trismus can occur due to fibrosis of the temperomandibular joint and the muscles of mastication, which can further add to eating and chewing difficulties.

Radionecrosis of the larynx can sometimes necessitate laryngectomy or tracheostomy due to incompetent larynx. The eye and ocular structures may be damaged during radiation of the nasopharynx and paranasal sinus tumours. The lens is very sensitive and cataracts can result from a single dose of 2 Gy or a fractionated dose of 8 Gy. Damage to the retina and optic nerve occurs with doses in excess of 50 Gy. Radiotherapy to the lacrimal gland results in dry eye. If radiotherapy is given to the ear cartilage, necrosis of the external auditory canal can in turn result in bone necrosis. Tympanic (eardrum) fibrosis may also be a problem. Doses above 40 Gy to the skull base damage the pituitary and lead to hormonal dysfunction. Hypothyroidism can occur following radiation to the thyroid gland (Levendag and Keys, 1998).

Chemotherapy

Chemotherapy is not regarded as a curative option in head and neck cancer but may be indicated as:

- Neoadjuvant treatment followed by a definitive treatment (surgery/radiotherapy)
- Concomitant treatment given simultaneously with radiotherapy
- After surgery or radiotherapy

Trials show promising response rates with neoadjuvant chemotherapy but effects on long-term tumour control and survival are insignificant (Elwell and Tobias, 1998). However, neoadjuvant chemotherapy to improve local control prior to a definitive treatment (surgery/radiotherapy) may mean less extensive surgery or smaller radiation fields/doses, which may result in a better functional outcome, less disfigurement and improvements in quality of life.

Trials of concomitant chemoradiotherapy appear more promising, but the toxicity of treatment is considerable and intensive multiprofessional support is required (Elwell and Tobias, 1998).

Early studies on the use of chemotherapy in head and neck cancer centred on patients who had recurrent incurable disease, and although a reduction in tumour volume may have a palliative effect the side effects may make its use in palliative care inappropriate.

Support

A diagnosis of cancer presents a severe threat to an individual's physical and emotional resources (Feber, 1998) and causes great turmoil for patients and their families. The likelihood of disfigurement and dysfunction resulting from proposed treatment or the disease itself is an additional concern. Head and neck cancer is by its nature a very visible disease that impacts on many areas of an individual's life: eating, drinking, communication, breathing, body image, self-esteem and sexuality. Disfigurements and dysfunctions are often impossible to hide and a multiprofessional team approach is essential to provide the necessary help and support to enable physical and psychosocial rehabilitation.

The way a patient copes with the initial diagnosis of cancer can profoundly affect the outcome of subsequent treatment. Kumasaka and Dungan (1993) and Kalayjian (1989) identify helpful nursing behaviours as listening, providing appropriate information, availability, sensitivity, caring, empathy, respectfulness and honesty. Usual coping skills are challenged by the gravity of a cancer diagnosis and information-giving is one way of increasing decision-making ability and hence sense of control (Kumasaka and Dungan, 1993). Assessment of an individual's past coping strategies may provide a framework for offering support.

Patients studied by Edwards (1997) identified explanations and information-giving by nurses who specialize in head and neck cancer as an indicator for best practice. The support of a specialist nurse who has a sound knowledge base, counselling skills and information on that particular patient's prognosis/stage of disease means that the patient is better placed to make sense of proposed treatments, the extent of likely disfigurement and dysfunction, and is subsequently more able to make a truly informed decision about the future. In her evaluation of a support strategy for laryngectomy patients Feber (1998) found that following diagnosis a comprehensive outpatient nursing assessment, an educational and counselling session with the patient and family, provision of a comprehensive information pack and a preoperative meeting with and assessment by the community nurse at home significantly improved patient satisfaction with the whole service. The opportunity to speak to someone who has undergone similar surgery can be a source of support and encouragement to an individual awaiting surgery, and the nurse can facilitate this.

Anxiety and depression can be significant problems in head and neck cancer, sometimes predating diagnosis (Davies et al., 1986); it has been shown that in some patients this is possibly related to alcoholism and poor nutritional status, factors independently associated with depression (Vokes et al., 1993). Patients with head and neck cancers have also been identified as having a higher suicide rate than other cancer patients (Koester and Bergsma, 1990). Byrne et al. (1993) found that psychological interventions such as education and teaching of coping skills and follow-up significantly reduced the occurrence of depression in laryngectomy patients.

Health professionals have an important role to play in helping patients to develop coping strategies, and the role of surgical nurses is crucial here. Coping strategies are based on the increased use of self-care techniques leading to acceptance and social interaction with others; the optimum time for this is 4–6 days postoperatively (Dropkin, 1989). The difficulties of learning to develop coping skills are compounded by the possibility that individuals with head and neck cancer may have personality traits that lead them to develop excessive smoking habits and alcoholic tendencies, and also to have poor adaptive coping skills (Burgess, 1994).

'Rehabilitation is a process of change which may involve the patient returning to their former physical and psychosocial status, but more commonly signals successful adjustment to profound changes in body function, body image and social relationships/roles' (Whale, 1998). Social support, including that from family and self-help groups, has a positive effect on rehabilitation (Edwards, 1997; Baker, 1992), and nursing practice can be enhanced by a family focused approach to care with the provision of assistance and support in hospital and at home (Feber, 1998).

Treatment for head and neck cancer often leaves individuals with disabilities or disfigurement that marks them out as abnormal. These abnormalities or the stigma associated with them can cause unwelcome reactions from others, such as staring or comments. Immediately after surgery, patients themselves have identified the need for privacy at times (preferably a side room), but also the importance of being in an environment where other patients have similar conditions and where nurses are familiar with their care (Edwards, 1997). Peer support from individuals with the same type of cancer can play a crucial part in adjustment following surgery (Richardson et al., 1989), and patients should be given contact numbers for local self-help groups, such as the National Association of Laryngectomee Clubs (NALC), or Lets Face It. Disfigurement and dysfunction can cause major problems in social interaction, and the charity Changing Faces specializes in equipping individuals with the social skills and confidence to manage varying situations.

Individuals with head and neck cancer clearly need expert nursing, not only whilst undergoing treatment but during the period following diagnosis, through physical and psychological rehabilitation and ultimately perhaps through palliative care. If patient and family support is seen as an integral part of the treatment regime, is available from the time of diagnosis, and is seen as an essential and automatic component of care, then this may be less stigmatizing and likely to be better accepted than referral for 'counselling' once psychosocial problems become evident later in the course of the disease or treatment.

Case histories

David

David presented, aged 52 years, with a painless, hoarse voice which had been present for 3–4 months. He smoked 25 cigarettes a day, drank 30 units of beer a week, and was self-employed as a sprayer in a paint workshop. He lived with his wife. He was diagnosed with a T3 glottic (vocal cord) squamous cell carcinoma and underwent a total laryngectomy, with formation of a tracheoesophageal fistula for future placement of a voice valve. This valve allows air to be diverted from the lungs into the pharynx when David occludes his stoma, thus enabling speech.

David was discharged from hospital 12 days postoperatively and was fully self-caring. He was confident in the management of his stoma and understood the importance of humidifying inspired air by the use of a foam filter or bib. He was able to cough secretions out from his stoma and did not normally need to use suction. He received speech therapy as an outpatient and achieved good voice with his valve. Four months later he was depressed and frustrated by his inability to return to work due to the practical difficulties of working in a dusty and fume-filled environment, and both he and his wife needed considerable support form the multidisciplinary team. Three years later he is free from disease, well adjusted to his altered body

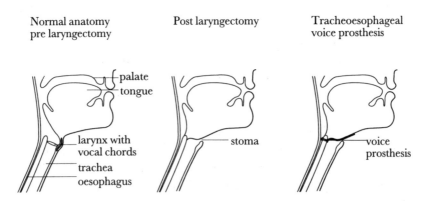

Normal anatomy
pre laryngectomy

Post laryngectomy

Tracheoesophageal
voice prosthesis

palate
tongue

larynx with
vocal chords
trachea
oesophagus

stoma

voice
prosthesis

Figure 11.5 Tracheoesophageal voice prosthesis.

image, working on a part-time basis as a decorator and still smoking and drinking.

Jim

Jim (58) presented to the head and neck oncologist as an emergency with inspiratory stridor. He was diagnosed as having a T4 N3 supraglottic squamous cell carcinoma of the larynx. He underwent urgent tracheostomy. Jim was an ex-smoker and drank about 28 units of alcohol a week. Three years previously he had undergone a left lower lobectomy for lung carcinoma and was diagnosed on this admission as having a recurrence. The recurrence of his lung tumour meant that it was inappropriate to offer radical treatment for his laryngeal cancer, and palliative care was offered. He was discharged home, where he lived with his father, once he was self-caring with his tracheostomy and was able to perform tracheal suction. He had a cuffed tracheostomy tube as he was aspirating due to the incompetence of his larynx, but he was able to obtain reasonable voice with a speaking valve. He commenced oral morphine for pain control and a steroid in an attempt to reduce oedema associated with his tumour and improve his breathlessness. Jim remained at home with the support of his district nurses, GP and Macmillan head and neck nurse for almost three months, during which time he still managed to visit his social club most lunchtimes. He was admitted two days prior to his death with haemoptysis, chest infection and breathlessness. He commenced subcutaneous diamorphine via a syringe driver and died peacefully.

Anne

Anne was a 60-year-old married woman when she presented with an early T1 N0 squamous cell carcinoma right floor of mouth. This was treated with radioactive iridium needles, and she remained tumour-free for eight years. The recurrence was treated by surgical excision, including partial mandibulectomy and reconstruction with a latissimus dorsi myocutaneous flap and mandibular plates. A percutaneous gastrostomy (PEG) tube for feeding was placed prior to surgery and Anne never managed to swallow more than a few sips of fluid. Anne was diagnosed with further recurrence two months later and had considerable pain. She was commenced on morphine, a non-steroidal anti-inflammatory, prophylactic laxative, and a tricyclic antidepressant and TENS machine for neuropathic pain. Anne developed an orocutaneous fistula and a fungating lesion on her neck which leaked copious amounts. Anne and her husband were able to manage the dressings with the support of their district nurse but she was very self-conscious and tended to remain at home. Anne died seven months later.

Conclusions

As this chapter has illustrated, head and neck cancer impacts on many areas of an individual's life. It can be a severely debilitating and disfiguring disease and often the treatment causes a great degree of dysfunction and distress. Whilst early tumours are often cured by radiotherapy or local surgery, early presentation and diagnosis remains uncommon. Many patients continue to drink and smoke, and the incidence of second primaries, either within the head and neck or lung, remains high while overall five-year survival rates remain low. Recent years, therefore, have seen increasing emphasis on maximizing quality of life and the support needs of patients and their families from the time of diagnosis, through treatment and rehabilitation and, for some, through palliative care.

Chapter 12
Childhood cancers

RUTH SADIK

Introduction

Whilst childhood cancers are rare, with 3.5 per million of the population aged 0–14 years, they still represent the second leading cause of death in this age group after accidents (Hollis, 1997). However, many malignancies once considered fatal are now curable, with the five-year survival rate for cancer in all sites improving from 26% in the 1960s (Robertson et al., 1994) to 70% in 1990 (Stiller, 1994). This means that in the near future one in 1,000 young adults will be the survivor of a childhood malignancy (Hawkins and Stevens, 1996).

Effective treatment which can improve the quality and length of children's lives is now possible, due mainly to early detection, improved and broadened treatment modalities and the concept of multidisciplinary care. The Calman-Hine Report (1995) recognized that children diagnosed as having cancer had a right to uniformly safe, effective, high quality care provided as close to their homes as possible. This has led to a rise in the number of designated paediatric specialist cancer centres, and the concept of 'shared care'. This latter concept involves staff from children's services in district general hospitals working with staff from designated cancer centres, in the provision of care and treatment protocols required by children with cancer. These initiatives appear to have had the most positive effects on both morbidity and mortality (Calman and Hine, 1995).

In the light of these recent developments, this chapter will explore the different types of childhood malignancies, predisposing

211

factors and presentation. In addition, their prevention, detection and management will be discussed, together with the support available to children and their families.

Incidence and aetiology

Whilst little is known about the cause of childhood cancers, it is known that the sites of occurrence are similar for males and females, that acute lymphoblastic leukaemia (ALL) is most common in toddlers, and that Hodgkin's disease is rarely diagnosed before 15 years of age.

Despite efforts to establish the cause of childhood cancers, no definitive answer exists. Factors known to cause malignancies in adults, such as smoking and irradiation, do not necessarily apply to infants and children, therefore current research is focused on the interaction between environmental triggers and genetic alterations (Thomson and Cohen, 1996). Despite this assertion, it has been identified that children of parents who smoke prior to conception and during the antenatal period are more at risk of developing malignancies (Golding et al., 1990).

As in the case of adult cancers, there are some common features amongst presenting malignancies in children, but also distinct characteristics that vary according to anatomical site and morphology.

Specific childhood malignancies

Leukaemias

The leukaemias are not a single disease, but a group of disorders related to an abnormal proliferation of immature, poorly differentiated white cell precursors known as blast cells. It is the replacement of normal bone marrow elements with blast cells that leads to the presenting signs and symptoms.

Leukaemia is usually classified by cell type, such as myelogenous, lymphocytic or non-lymphocytic, and by cellular differentiation such as undifferentiated or primitive. Whilst any of the white cell lines can be abnormal, in neonates the myeloid rather than the lymphoid line are usually affected (see Chapter 9).

The leukaemias are the most common form of cancer in childhood, with acute lymphoblastic leukaemia accounting for over 80%.

Most frequently affected children are white boys aged 3–4 years, with a decreasing incidence to 10 years of age.

The exact causes of leukaemia are unknown but viruses, radiation, chemical and drug exposure, familial predisposition and chromosomal abnormalities have been implicated (Toren et al., 1996). It is known to be 15 times more likely to occur in children with Trisomy 21. Whilst familial clustering has been described, as has a higher incidence in monozygotic twins, it is not clear whether this reflects genetic factors or exposure to common environmental triggers.

Immunologic studies currently suggest that 80–85% of ALL cases arise from B-cell precursors whilst 15–20% arise from T-cell lines. Few cases fall into the non-T, non-B variety which was once thought to represent the majority. B-cell has been subdivided into groups with differing prognoses. Children with mature B-cell ALL have the worst prognosis, whilst those whose cells have the common ALL antigen have the best. T-cell ALL has much in common with T-cell lymphoblastic lymphoma, and they are thought by some (Parker, 1997) to represent variants of the same disorder. Some investigators consider B-cell ALL to be a disseminated form of Burkitt's lymphoma. T-cell ALL occurs typically in older boys who present with high leucocyte counts and anterior mediastinal mass. New prognostic tests concern cytogenic factors, specifically the number of chromosomes in ALL cells. Children who have more than 50 have the best prognosis.

The presenting signs and symptoms of leukaemia are listed in Table 12.1.

Table 12.1 Common signs and symptoms in leukaemia

Local infection, typically of the respiratory tract
Pallor
Pain
Fever
Fatigue, weakness and/or malaise
Bruising
Enlarged liver and spleen (seen on X-ray as elevating the left side of the diaphragm and causing displacement of the stomach)

Whilst in many instances initial treatment with antibiotics may resolve/improve the complaints, they return once therapy has ceased.

The types of investigations carried out to ascertain a diagnosis of leukaemia may include a full blood count (FBC), which typically shows anaemia with low platelet and neutrophil counts. Radiologic assessment can demonstrate that thymic infiltration in children with T-cell leukaemia causes a mediastinal mass with possible pleural effusion, and it can also determine osteoporosis of the spine in 90% of children presenting with ALL (Parker, 1997). Aspiration of bone marrow allows differential diagnosis to be made by morphological evaluation. A specimen of cerebrospinal fluid (CSF) will also be taken to ascertain central nervous system (CNS) infiltration. At this point acute myeloid leukaemia (AML) or ALL can be determined and therapy decided upon.

Treatment includes multi-agent chemotherapy with prophylactic CNS radiation. Event-free survival of three years is considered cured, with a late relapse being extremely uncommon.

If relapse is going to happen it will manifest in the CNS, testicular tissues or occasionally the kidney. Improved survival has been as a result of CNS prophylaxis with irradiation, intrathecal chemotherapy or a combination of the two. This treatment may lead to brain atrophy, even in the absence of initial infiltration, and has led to the recommendation of baseline CT in all newly diagnosed children. The benefits of this must however be weighed against the possible long-term effects of being subjected to radiation equivalent to 40 chest X-rays.

Solid tumours of the brain and central nervous system

The second most common type of cancer, more frequently found in white males under four years old, is cancer of the brain and CNS. The World Health Organization classifies tumours by tissue of origin, and states that two-thirds arise from glial tissue in the posterior fossa. Almost half are astrocytomas and more than half of these respond poorly to treatment. The most common malignant CNS tumour in childhood is the medulloblastoma, which is highly invasive and carries a poor prognosis. According to Mason et al. (1998), survival rates for non-malignant tumours vary considerably from 90% in cerebellar astrocytoma to 20% in brainstem tumours.

CNS tumour presentation depends on the site, type of tumour and the child's age. Even though two-thirds of children present with signs of increased intracranial pressure and gait disturbances, few are diagnosed within one month of the onset of symptoms (Friedman et al., 1991). In addition to the inability of young children to describe their symptoms, Friedman et al. (1991) also recognize that doctors may mistake the symptoms for more common childhood disorders.

Referral to a paediatric neurosurgical unit maximizes surgical and medical management of the child. It provides the opportunity to define the benefits of novel surgical approaches with microsurgical techniques, allows histological examination by pathologists familiar with children's tumours, and facilitates transit to laboratories concerned with research into cranial neoplasms.

Unfortunately, at present the majority of brain tumours remain inoperable, but none the less in many cases surgical resection is the first in a series of multimodality treatments (which include radiotherapy and chemotherapy), designed to bring about a cure. The extent of tumour resection must therefore be seen in the light of the implications for the child's subsequent survival. The multidisciplinary team, including the child (if old enough) and parents, should be involved in deciding the advantages and disadvantages of surgical intervention which may leave the child with irreversible brain damage.

Hodgkin's disease

Hodgkin's disease has been reported in children under five years of age, but is rare prior to adolescence. It is a cancer of the lymphatic tissue, and usually occurs in a single lymph node or anatomic group of nodes, spreading by means of involvement of contiguous lymph node groups (see Chapter 9). There appears to be an increased risk in same-sex siblings, children with immunodeficiency syndromes, infectious mononucleosis and those with Epstein-Barr virus titre. According to Stiller (1998), children of South Asian descent born in Britain have a higher chance of suffering from Hodgkin's disease than white children.

Hodgkin's disease is commonly characterized by the presence of painless, firm, mobile cervical or supraclavicular nodes, anorexia, weight loss, malaise, lethargy and fever. It is definitively diagnosed by a lymph node biopsy, as the blood tests for alkaline phosphatase and serum copper levels, which are indicative in adults, are unreliable in childhood.

Treatment depends on the stage of the disease. Prognosis is generally good with 70–90% of stage I–II having a 90% survival rate 10 years following treatment. The Rye classification of this disease identifies four subtypes:

- Nodular sclerosis, which accounts for 40% of cases in children under 10
- Mixed cellularity, which occurs in 30% of younger and 15% of older children
- Lymphocytic predominance, which is present in 5–15% of all children
- Lymphocytic depletion type; rare in children who are not HIV positive

Non-Hodgkin's lymphoma (NHL)

These are solid tumours of the haematopoietic system presenting as diffuse lymph node enlargement, with a peak incidence between 7 and 11 years of age in white males.

In children, the disease tends to exhibit aggressive behaviour with a propensity for widespread dissemination (Kurtzberg and Graham, 1991). Despite this, the disease is responsive to chemotherapeutic treatment, leading to an overall high cure rate for children who are diagnosed early.

NHL is more common in children who have congenital immunodeficiency syndromes such as Wiskott-Aldrich or children who are chronically immunosuppressed as a result of transplantation of major organs. NHL has also been reported as being a second primary malignancy following treatment for Hodgkin's disease.

The symptoms of NHL depend upon the site of the tumour, the most common of which are the abdomen, mediastinum, head and neck. Whilst an intra-abdominal tumour will present with pain, bloatedness and vomiting, a mass in the chest would result in a persistent cough, dyspnoea and pyrexia.

Wilm's tumour

This type of tumour is also known as a nephroblastoma. It arises from the tissue of the kidney, is the most common renal malignancy and affects girls and boys equally but occurs more frequently in black populations. It is known to be associated with congenital anomalies such as hypospadias, cryptorchidism and fusion anomalies of the kidney. It is also strongly associated with chromosomal abnormalities resulting in aniridia, microcephaly, mental retardation and genito-urinary tract anomalies, whilst findings have also been made in children with Beckwith-Wiedemann syndrome and neurofibromatosis.

Diagnosis is usually made at two to three years of age, when the tumour presents as a non-tender unilateral abdominal mass. Symptoms may occasionally include abdominal pain, haematuria, fever, hypertension and malaise. As in the case of most tumours, the child's prognosis is related to the spread (or stage) of the disease. In Wilm's tumour the staging represents:

- Stage I: tumour is limited to the kidney and is completely excised
- Stage II: tumour extends beyond the kidney but is completely removed
- Stage III: residual tumour confined to the abdomen with involvement of lymph nodes which is not completely resectable
- Stage IV: metastases in lungs, liver, bone and/or brain
- Stage V: bilateral kidney involvement at diagnosis with distant metastases

Treatment for Wilm's tumour in children deemed to have stages III–V involves surgical removal of the affected kidney followed by radiation to the renal bed. Multi-agent chemotherapy has greatly increased survival rates.

Neuroblastoma

This is the most common tumour in white males under one year of age. It is a proliferation of neural crest tissue in the adrenal glands or along the craniospinal axis, therefore presenting most usually as an abdominal or pelvic mass. Occasionally, it will present in the chest where it manifests as a persistent cough, chest pain or dyspnoea. Neuroblastoma has no known pattern of congenital anomalies; however it has occasionally been seen in children with foetal hydantoin syndrome, neurofibromatosis or Beckwith-Wiedemann syndrome.

Neuroblastoma presentation depends on the site. In an abdominal mass, it is firm, irregular and crosses the midline. In the upper neck and chest it can cause Horner's syndrome; paraspinal tumours can result in spinal compression; bone marrow involvement may cause limping, pain and refusal to walk whilst retroperitoneal tumours can lead to vascular compression and oedema of the legs and feet. Diagnosis is made on bone marrow aspiration; however, elevated urinary catecholamine metabolites such as homovanillic acid and vanillyl mandelic acid are very suggestive.

Treatment modalities include multi-agent chemotherapy, surgical excision and irradiation.

Frequently, the tumours associated with neuroblastoma are large and not conducive to full resection through surgery. Despite this, children with stages I–II have been shown to go into spontaneous remission following incomplete surgical removal (Cheung, 1991). Where metastatic spread is involved the prognosis is poor, with just 10% of children in this group remaining in remission for five years (Cheung, 1991). Currently, research into increasing the longevity of children with poor prognoses is trialling adoptive immunity using antibodies and lymphocytes as vehicles. This type of therapy is, however, very much in its infancy, but results from trials using monoclonal antibodies, cytokines and gene therapy should soon become available for use with chemotherapy.

Rhabdomyosarcoma

Rhabdomyosarcoma is a rare malignancy of striated muscle and is frequently situated in the head and neck although it can be found in the bladder and vagina. Presentation is as a painless mass, although if this is large pressure symptoms may lead to pain. Symptoms are site-dependent.

Rhabdomyosarcoma can affect bone, soft tissue or connective tissue and as such presentation depends on the site affected. As it is an extremely aggressive tumour, early detection and staging is vital to both the treatment and prognosis. Staging is performed in relation to the following criteria:

- Stage I: tumour is found in the eye, head, neck, bladder or vagina
- Stage II: tumour is in one area, but not those mentioned above, is smaller than 5 cm in size and has not spread to lymph glands

- Stage III: tumour is confined to one area, is greater than 5 cm in size and has spread to local lymph nodes
- Stage IV: tumour is found in more than one site
- Stage V: recurrent tumour returns following treatment

Golding et al. (1990) have found an association between maternal exposure to carcinogens (specifically X-rays and smoking) during pregnancy and subsequent malignancy development in the newborn, especially rhabdomyosarcoma.

The treatment for all children with this type of cancer is related to surgical removal of some or all of the tumour if possible, radiation therapy either externally or internally administered in several small doses a day (hyperfractionated radiation therapy), and chemotherapy. Despite improvements in management, the prognosis remains generally poor.

Autologous bone marrow transplantation is proving valuable in recurrent cases.

Bone tumours

Bone tumours predominate in white adolescent males, with osteogenic carcinoma or osteosarcoma accounting for 60% of all tumours. Ewing's sarcoma accounts for 30%, with the other 10% comprising a variety of rare malignancies.

Generally bone tumours arise in the metaphyseal region of the long bones, with the majority of lesions occurring around the knee and the shoulder joints. Osteogenic sarcoma is positively correlated with the growth spurt of adolescence and long bone growth in particular. Ewing's is associated with skeletal or urogenital abnormalities, and both types are related to previous trauma to the involved bone.

Bone tumours present with painful swelling over the tumour site. Any activity undertaken by the child increases pain and young children may refuse to walk, whilst older ones will limp. Ewing's sarcoma is commonly found in the pelvic bones, tibia, fibula and femur. It presents with pain around the site and on X-ray can be seen as a tissue mass around the bone. Both types are managed by surgical removal and multi-agent chemotherapy. Irradiation is not used to treat osteogenic sarcoma as the tumour is radio-resistant; however it may be used palliatively. Ewing's sarcoma responds poorly to this form of treatment. The prognosis has risen from 20% in 1960 to 59% in 1990.

Investigations and treatment

Most of the tests, investigations and treatments required by children undergoing treatment for malignancies are repetitive, lasting from six months to two years, and invasive or unpleasant in nature.

To minimize the trauma experienced during these procedures, coordination and planning is required by the different teams of professionals involved in the care, to ensure that all procedures are carried out at one time.

Certain procedures such as lumbar puncture, bone marrow aspiration, venous catheter insertion or change, wound care and change of dressings, may be carried out under a short-acting general anaesthetic, which may be replaced by a local anaesthetic as the child's confidence increases (Lilley, 1990). Chest radiotherapy which requires the child to control his or her breathing for prolonged periods of time may also be undertaken whilst under general anaesthetic.

Children with malignancies require frequent venous access either for blood tests or the administration of intravenous chemotherapy. To help relieve the fear and pain of repeated cannulation, local anaesthetic creams are available that take effect within ten to 40 minutes, depending on the type used.

Long-term venous access can be accomplished by using either external tunnelled catheters, or totally implanted subcutaneous ports (Dillon and Weiner, 1997). These devices enable accurate delivery of drugs, blood and blood products and parenteral nutrition whilst allowing atraumatic blood sampling. The nurse is responsible for monitoring for complications such as infection or mechanical or thrombotic occlusion (Dillon and Weiner, 1997).

As many children may also require MRI or CT scans, the nurse should be able to recognize the implications for the child. It may involve lying still for long periods of time and the ingestion of unpalatable contrast media after being without food or drink for two hours. Some children may also find the experience of being in a scanner frightening and may require sedation.

Nuclear medicine scans involve the intravenous administration of radioactive isotopes, commonly Technetium[99] for screening tumours which metastasize to bone (Hawkins and Stevens, 1996). These are Ewing's sarcoma, rhabdomyosarcoma, neuroblastoma and osteogenic sarcoma. During administration of the drug, the child may experience a fleeting hot flushing of the skin and body. Gallium imaging of lymph nodes is performed in Hodgkin's and non-Hodgkin's lymphoma.

Table 12.2 provides a summary of the investigations required for different malignancies.

Table 12.2 Summary of investigations required for different childhood malignancies

Malignancy	Biopsy	Laboratory evaluation	Radiology
Leukaemia	Bone marrow	Full blood count, differential and platelet count	Chest X-ray
	Skin nodules	Cerebrospinal fluid Liver and renal function tests	
Brain tumours	Tumour	Cerebrospinal fluid and spine	CT scan MRI of brain
			Ultrasound
Hodgkin's disease	Lymph nodes Bone marrow	FBC	MRI CT scan Chest X-ray
Non-Hodgkin's	Lymph nodes	FBC	X-ray of site CT scan Ultrasound
Neuroblastoma	Tumour	FBC, differential and platelet count	Chest X-ray
	Metastatic lesions	Liver and renal function tests	Skeletal survey
	Bone marrow	Urinary VMA Urinary HVA	CT scan Bone scan

Common side effects of therapy

All therapy used in treating children with malignant disease involves the introduction of agents that destroy normal as well as abnormal cells, and it is this factor that leads to the extensive range of toxic effects experienced by the child. The nurse's prime responsibility is to teach the child and family about the disease and its treatment, as the more informed the family is, the better they will be able to anticipate and manage undesirable side effects (Faulkner et al., 1995).

Oral complications

Stomatitis is the inflammation and breakdown of the mucosa of the mouth, gums, tongue and lips, occurring in 90% of children receiving chemotherapy (Porter, 1994). It can be prevented by careful observation and thorough oral hygiene. Over the years different tools have been used for carrying out mouth care; however, it has been agreed that a soft-headed toothbrush remains the tool of choice used in conjunction with nationally agreed protocols (Campbell, 1994) related to mouthwash and antifungal treatment. Irradiation of the head and neck may also cause damage to the salivary glands, increasing the viscosity of saliva and precipitating dental decay. Taste alteration and difficulty in chewing, swallowing and speaking may also occur.

Poor appetite

During cytotoxic therapy children suffer readily from anorexia, which may be attributable to a sore mouth, nausea and vomiting, anxiety or constipation. Consequently the child will suffer weight loss, and a full nutritional assessment is required on admission. To ensure appropriate nutrition, it is recommended that baseline height and weight are recorded and continued weekly. If the child cannot or will not tolerate an oral bland semi-solid diet, enteral or parenteral nutrition may be considered (Sacks and Meek, 1997).

Recommended daily allowances (RDAs) (found in Table 12.3) can be used to determine normal calorific and protein needs. However, the nurse should be aware that these were devised for healthy children. To compensate for the child's previous weight loss, an increase of 15–50% may be required (Sacks and Meek, 1997).

Alopecia

Loss of hair through chemotherapy is the most difficult side effect for children to accept (Reid, 1997), as it insults the self image (Lilley, 1990). Whilst it is neither inevitable or permanent, many myths have grown up surrounding this facet of treatment. If the child opts to wear a wig, it

Table 12.3 RDA approximations for calories and protein

	Age	Calories (kcal/kg/day)	Protein (g/kg/day)
Infants	0–6 months	110	2.2
	6–12 months	100	1.5
Children	1–3 years	100	1.2
	4–6	90	1.0
	7–10	75	1.0
Adolescents	11-14	52	1.0
	15–18	47	0.8

is essential that one is provided prior to hair loss so that the stylist can match colour and texture. It may also be beneficial to encourage children to have their hair cut short in readiness for a change in appearance, and help them to develop positive coping mechanisms such as humour. Younger children tend to dismiss wigs in favour of headscarves and caps, which are presently fashionable. The nurse needs to ensure that all children and their parents understand the risk of sunburn to the scalp even in weak sun, and ensure that adequate precautions are taken (Reid, 1997). As body hair may also be affected, adolescents who may see its acquisition as a rite of passage need reassurance that regrowth is usually quite rapid on discontinuation of therapy.

Nausea and vomiting

Nausea and vomiting occur as a result of two main mechanisms (Lilley, 1990). The first is that some cytotoxic agents affect the vomiting centre situated in the medulla of the brain, and the second is the effect of irradiation on the small intestine. Psychogenic vomiting can also result if the child is anxious or has developed an aversion to the sight, sound or smell of drugs (Dolgin et al., 1989). It is this interaction between physiological and behavioural stimuli that determines each child's unique vomiting threshold.

The goal of managing drug-induced nausea and vomiting is to minimize the direct effect of treatment and facilitate the child's early recovery. In order to do this, the nurse needs to recognize the often cyclical nature of vomiting and offer interventions that help to alleviate symptoms and break the cycle (Hockenberry-Eaton and Benner, 1990).

There are several anti-emetic drugs available that are particularly useful with cytotoxic drug-induced symptoms. The most well known and effective are the group of $5HT^3$ receptor antagonists. According to the British National Formulary (BNF, 1998), a serotonin antagonist works peripherally on the vagus nerve, without causing sedation. In order to maintain serum levels the drug is commenced either intravenously immediately prior to treatment, or 1–2 hours orally before treatment. This group of anti-emetics appears to have dramatically reduced the number of children developing dehydration.

Complementary therapies such as distraction through touch, storytelling, stroking, rocking, breathing, counting or puppet play, and relaxation techniques such as guided imagery and self-hypnosis are currently finding favour in helping children cope with nausea and vomiting (Hockenberry-Eaton and Benner, 1990).

Constipation and diarrhoea

Constipation can result from the prolonged use of narcotic analgesics or cytotoxic drugs such as vincristine (BNF, 1998). The best treatment is prevention, which can be encouraged through the use of stool softening agents, a high fibre diet and appropriate fluid intake for the child's age. Whilst enemata and suppositories are avoided in the immunocompromised child, they should not be withheld when the child is suffering from painful faecal impaction.

Diarrhoea is a frequent effect of irradiation and some anti-emetic drugs (BNF, 1998). The nurse needs to monitor fluid intake and output, involve the dietitian in recommending appropriate foods and ensure that hygiene levels and skin integrity are maintained.

Bone marrow suppression can leave the child susceptible to infection, bleeding and anaemia. Nurses working with immunosuppressed children must maintain scrupulous hygiene, and ensure that staff who may be infectious do not nurse these children (see Chapter 15).

Support for the child and family

The psychological and social impact of a diagnosis of cancer is devastating for the child and family, and may result in feelings of loss of control and uncertainty about the future (Hawkins, 1996). Lewandowska (1997) has further identified that the initial impact of diagnosis can trigger shock, disbelief and denial – a concept she refers to as 'turmoil without resolution', where parents start to experience emotions of anger, despair, fear, apprehension and abandonment. These effects require all members of the multidisciplinary team to be skilled in the assessment of family dynamics and follow-up.

The acute stress and anxiety experienced by parents makes it difficult for them to absorb information. It is therefore incumbent upon the nurse to constantly reiterate information, choosing an appropriate time and place to impart it (Lewandowska, 1997). Family-centred care principles dictate that the individual needs of each family should be considered and information techniques tailored to meet them in the most beneficial manner. This may involve the use of videos, books and discussion groups.

Whilst the needs of children with cancer and their parents are well documented, the needs of siblings of children with cancer are less well recognized. Primarily through the work of Spinetta in the 1980s this is slowly being resolved. Spinetta found that siblings of children with cancer require direct information about the disease, the implications of treatment and outcome, because education and effective communication have been demonstrated to improve the ways in which siblings cope. The fear and grief suffered by parents of children with cancer cannot be hidden from siblings, and even very young children are astute observers of adult non-verbal communication cues evident in behaviour, conversation and body language (Noll et al., 1995). Doyle (1987) has reported that school-aged siblings may experience fear that the disease is something they wished on their brother or sister. She also identifies that sibling anger is common, with the unaffected child becoming an extension of the ill child with a subsequent loss of self identity. This may lead to conflicting emotions of jealousy of the attention given to the ill child, and guilt at feeling this way (Sawyer et al., 1995). One way of overcoming these difficulties and any feeling of isolation is to involve siblings in care decisions and foster an atmosphere of openness and honesty. Parents may express feelings that the siblings cannot cope and should be excluded. However, studies have demonstrated that siblings who are not involved can feel unresolved guilt and fear for years afterwards if their sibling dies (Kupst et al., 1995).

The long-term psychological effects of surviving childhood cancer affect all areas of a person's life; the main ones are listed in Table 12.4.

Table 12.4 Psychlogical effects of surviving childhood malignancy

School difficulties
Community acceptance
Employment
Dating/marriage
Conception
Transmission in offspring

Support services available to children and their families involve both statutory and voluntary sectors. These include:

- *Primary healthcare team:* GP, community children's nurse, health visitor
- *Local hospital team:* children's nurses, paediatrician, play leader, clinical psychologist, dietitian, outpatient clinic
- *Regional centre:* oncologist, surgeon, children's nurses, liaison nurses, social worker, dietitian, pathology, play specialist, clinical psychologist, cardiologist, endocrinologist, neurologist
- *School:* teachers, nurses, teaching assistants

Late effects of cancer treatment
In the past, cancer was synonymous with death and thus the psychological care of the child and his/her family was directed at preparing the family for the eventual death of their child. Recent advances in oncology care and treatment have meant that the focus has moved to include long-term effects in the child receiving treatment for cancer.

It is now estimated that before long, one in every 1,000 young adults will be the survivor of a childhood malignancy (Hawkins and Stevens, 1996), and it is therefore important that the late effects are prime considerations in total patient care.

The most devastating complication to develop in a child already cured of a malignancy is a second cancer. It has been known since the 1960s that survivors of childhood cancers have an increased risk of second cancers. However, to keep this in perspective the incidence is approximately 3.7% (Hawkins and Stevens, 1996), with the highest occurrence in children treated with chemotherapy and irradiation for Hodgkin's lymphoma.

Endocrine problems are both the most common and easily remedied in many cases, with the gonads, thyroid and pituitary being the most frequently affected glands. Children given cranial irradiation may experience early puberty, whilst those who have gonadal irradiation will suffer infertility. In males treated with MOPP (nitrogen mustard, vincristine, procarbazine and prednisolone), sterility is thought to affect 80%.

Growth hormone deficiency is most common in children who have irradiation of the pituitary field. However, it is being successfully remedied by growth hormone replacement therapy, resulting in satisfactory attainment of normal adult height.

Neurological sequelae are thought to stem from radiotherapy, particularly for brain tumours. However, recently it has been found that IQ declined following combination treatment of high-dose intravenous methotrexate and cranial irradiation, but not with either treatment alone (Waber et al., 1995). Cerebellar dysfunction or cranial nerve palsy may result from the tumour itself or from surgical intervention.

Cardiotoxicity is associated with radiotherapy and the chemotherapeutic group of anthracycline agents such as doxorubicin and duanomycin. The effects include cardiac failure and sudden death, thought to be from arrhythmias (Lipshultz et al., 1990).

Pulmonary function deviations result mainly from mediastinal or pulmonary radiation, with those children who were treated at an early age more likely to suffer than older age groups at initial treatment (Miller et al., 1986).

Case histories

Chloe

Four-year-old Chloe has been unwell for the past eight weeks. She is usually a happy, lively, independent little girl who likes playing rough and tumble with her two-year-old brother Luke and five-year-old sister Georgie. Over the past two months Chloe's parents have been worried about her inability to shake off a bout of flu which has left her with intermittent fever, some breathlessness and reluctance to walk anywhere. She is generally clingy and tired out. Various visits to the GP resulted in a possible diagnosis of pneumonia and treatment with antibiotics for ten days, during which time Chloe was back to her usual self. Three days after completing the course of antibiotics Chloe's symptoms returned and her anxious parents returned to the GP, where blood tests were taken by the practice nurse.

When the blood tests returned, they confirmed leukaemia and the family was referred to the regional centre 17 miles away for further tests and treatment. Fortunately Chloe's mother was able to stay with her, and her father went home to care for the other children.

Initially, Chloe needed further tests to establish the extent of her disease. This involved more blood tests to confirm the presence of blast cells. The hospital also tested to see whether Chloe had sufficient immunity against potentially lethal childhood illnesses such as chickenpox and measles. They also saved blood for the childhood cancer study and to check whether Chloe had any covert chromosomal abnormalities which could adversely affect her prognosis.

Under a general anaesthetic, a bone marrow aspiration was performed to help confirm the type of leukaemia, and a lumbar puncture was also done to identify whether or not Chloe had leukaemic cells in the cerebrospinal fluid around the brain.

Once it was ascertained that Chloe had acute lymphoblastic leukaemia, she was commenced on a treatment regiment consisting of four phases. The first involves inducing remission, which uses chemotherapy to kill off as many abnormal cells as possible. Once this has been achieved, and confirmed on blood test, the next phase involves intensification, where high-dose cytotoxic agents are used to eradicate any remaining cells. The third phase, called central nervous system (CNS) prophylaxis, uses drugs administered directly into the cerebrospinal fluid in combination with high-dose systemic drugs to prevent the spread of malignant cells to the brain and spinal cord. Cranial irradiation may also be considered at this time.

The final phase is maintenance therapy, which Chloe will continue for several years to keep her in remission. After a relatively uneventful remission induction, Chloe could be transferred to the local hospital to continue her treatment, where her family could have close contact.

James

James is eight years old and until six months ago when his brother Timothy was born he was developing within normal parameters and progressing well at school. During the past six months his mother has noticed that James has become disobedient and clumsy with 'selective deafness'. She has taken James to the family doctor who assured her that his behavioural problems are probably related to feeling left out by Tim's birth. Despite extra attention, James's school work is suffering. His teacher has reported that his writing has deteriorated, he is uncoordinated during games sessions and he appears to lack concentration generally.

For three mornings in a row James woke up complaining of a headache and funny vision, and vomited. His GP referred him to a consultant, who sent him for a CT scan, after confirming that James was discoordinated and unable to control a pencil smoothly. The scan revealed a brainstem glioma. His family was informed that his treatment would probably include high-dose cranial radiation to shrink the tumour, surgical removal of as much tumour as possible and chemotherapy to prevent regrowth or spread.

Conclusions

Caring for children with malignancies and their families can be physically and emotionally demanding. Whilst at one time most children died, now the outcome is much more positive with the majority of children surviving into adulthood. This brings about its own challenges for health professionals, who are now faced with the challenge of enabling children and their families to cope effectively with the long-term effects of treatment for childhood malignancies.

Chapter 13
Fungating tumours

Sylvia Hampton

Introduction

Dressing selection must be based on knowledge and experience of wound healing, although with a fungating tumour or lesion treatment objectives require different assessment criteria and treatment to that of a wound that is likely to heal. This chapter will review the types of dressings that address some of the problems experienced by patients with fungating wounds, and will supply information on when the different types should be used and their interactions.

The appearance of a wound generally leads the nurse to select a dressing based on knowledge and experience of wound healing. However, experience of wound healing is unlikely to benefit the nurse when faced with a fungating tumour. Care is often palliative, addressing uncomfortable and distressing symptoms rather than offering aggressive treatments, which may strive for an optimum healing environment. Control of pain, odour, bleeding and exudate become primary considerations and removal of necrotic tissue becomes a low priority. Unfortunately, much of the care of patients with fungating tumours is based on trial and error, rather than research (Hastings, 1993). This is unacceptable today when clinical governance and audit is becoming increasingly important and care must be based on clinical evidence. Each clinician is expected to provide a rationale for the care given in any situation and it would be difficult to rationalize why all patients' wounds are dressed with the same product when each patient's needs are different.

Care of a fungating wound requires excellent communication skills, and a knowledge of:

1. Relevant anatomy and physiology
2. The wound-healing process
3. Related microbiology
4. Dressing interactions
5. Scientific approach to treatment
6. Holistic assessment

Care of the patient with a fungating wound often requires remarkable patience as the symptoms being treated are sometimes difficult to manage.

What is a fungating lesion?

A fungating lesion is a malignant infiltration of the skin (Hastings, 1993). Cooper (1993) describes it as:

> a break in the epidermal integrity because of infiltration of malignant cells. This may be due to primary skin malignancy, including basal cell carcinoma, squamous cell carcinoma and malignant melanoma, or because of metastatic deposits or extensions of malignancy from deeper structures that may result in fungating carcinomas.

The locations of fungating wounds can vary greatly; however, the most common site is the breast (62%) (Hallett, 1993).

Treatment for control of the tumour will be dealt with elsewhere within this book and may include radiotherapy, surgery, laser, or chemotherapy; all of which will require a nurse experienced in wound healing following treatment.

Tumours can rapidly increase in size with a 'cauliflower' appearance, can quickly ulcerate and the ulceration can bring symptoms which then become the patient's primary problem. The pain, malodour, excessive exudate and the large dressings required, which show through or under clothes or wound dressings, can be distressing and embarrassing for the patient.

Cancer cells proliferate and can affect tissues within a local area, causing a hypoxic environment and necrosis. The most common emergency experienced in fungating tumours is haemorrhage due to erosion of the blood vessels by the malignancy itself, secondary necrosis or the sloughing of tissues following radiotherapy (Brunner and Suddarth, 1975). The abnormal conditions of the wound can also lead to poor drainage of interstitial fluid leading to oedema and collapse of capillaries and lymph vessels, thereby further reducing fluid drainage and supply of nutrients to the damaged area. Tissue deprived of oxygen and nutrients will eventually become non-viable and take on a black leathery appearance when exposed to air, or yellow/grey appearance when moist. The length of time this takes to occur will be different in each individual and depends largely on the underlying pathology.

The harmful influences of devitalized tissue on the body's defences are without question: moist, devitalized soft tissue acts as a culture medium promoting bacterial growth and inhibits leucocyte phagocytosis of bacteria (Haury et al., 1978). However, natural debridement is possibly the only option open in the case of fungating wounds, for obvious reasons. Surgical debridement will either cause excessive bleeding or 'seed' the malignant cells.

Management of fungating lesions

Debridement

Debridement will be difficult to achieve as poor vascularity of the wound will continually produce further necrotic tissue. If debride-ment of the wound is the overall aim then use of a dressing that promotes autolysis is the route of choice. Hydrogels, cadexomers, hydrocolloids and sugar paste all promote natural autolysis. When the wound becomes moist through the breakdown of necrotic tissue this can open it to bacterial colonization, causing increased malodour and exudate.

Malodour

Malodour can be the most distressing symptom of a fungating tumour and is most generally caused by bacterial colonization of the wound.

The hypoxic environment within the ulcerated tissue is a micro-biological heaven to anaerobic bacteria, which require an oxygen-free environment to survive. Fatty acids are released as an end product of the action of anaerobes and it is this end product that produces the characteristic odour within necrotic tissue. As blood supply to the area is likely to be poor, leucocytes are unable to attack anaerobes, thus leaving them free to proliferate and so the malodour increases.

Excessive exudate production is a byproduct of all bacteria. The colour and odour produced by the bacteria can be recognized and identified by an experienced nurse. Antibiotics are unlikely to reduce the bacterial count unless a clinical infection is present. Therefore, bacterial colonization must be addressed by the selected dressing and knowledge of the action of dressings becomes essential to the nurse.

Green exudate often signifies a pseudomonal colonisation, which has a sweet, musty smell. This is a gram-negative aerobic bacteria (requires oxygen to survive) and the colour can often be startlingly green, almost fluorescent. *Pseudomons* produces large amounts of exudate and the musty smell can be very embarrassing for the patient. Gram-negative bacteria respond very well to silver found in silver sulphadiazine cream (Flamazine) and within a charcoal, silver-impregnated dressing called Actisorb plus. Silver sulphadiazine should be used for a short period when the green discharge is first noted and discontinued when green has disappeared – probably after two or three applications. Continued use of the cream appears to lead to the *Pseudomons* remaining in the wound in small amounts. Actisorb should be used as a primary dressing, as it has two actions: (i) the charcoal filters the odour; and (ii) the silver residues in the dressing reduce the bacteria.

The author has noted an increase in pain of wounds colonized by *Pseudomons* and a reduction of pain when the bacteria are controlled. However, to date this is anecdotal and requires research.

Red/brown exudate can often be associated with staphylococcus or streptococcus colonization. This has a 'bloody' smell and is a Gram-positive bacteria that is often easily controlled by use of iodine cadexomer dressings (Iodoflex, Iodosorb). Iodine is rapidly deactivated by contact with pus and so, although it has a rapid kill rate, its value is very limited in wounds. The iodine cadexomer dressings allow slow release of iodine into the wound in exchange for exudate. This has three values:

(i) The iodine 'bathes' the wound, killing bacteria

(ii) The cadexomer dressing absorbs large quantities of exudate

(iii) The dressing is excellent for wound debridement

This makes the cadexomer dressings very useful in a malodorous, high exudate, necrotic wound.

Anaerobic bacteria create the dreadful odour associated with gangrene – often described as 'the smell of hell'! Anaerobes survive in necrotic tissue because oxygen is not found in unviable tissue. Hyperbaric oxygen may be a way forward for the future but, at present, dressings are relied on to address the problem.

Sugar paste and icing sugar create a hyperosmotic environment by forcing bacteria to give up fluid through osmosis. Bacteria cannot survive this osmotic 'pull' and malodour will decrease, along with exudate production, as bacterial count is reduced. It also has a debriding action (Topham, 1996) which makes it ideal in treatment of sloughy wounds. The problem associated with the use of sugar paste (particularly thin paste) is that it can be messy. The availability of icing sugar makes it a very simple and achievable way of reducing bacteria and exudate. However, care should be taken in painful wounds when introducing a hyperosmotic or hydrophilic dressing, as the 'pull' of these dressings can increase pain.

Metronidazole gel is effective against malodour (Newman et al., 1989), although systemic metronidazole is often given for the same reason. However, systemic administration is less likely to be effective as poor blood supply to the local tissues will prevent delivery of the treatment at the wound site, particularly as anaerobes survive in necrotic tissue. The amount that is delivered to the wound bed will have little effect on these bacteria.

Other future dressings will include homeopathic treatments, with tea tree oil controlling bacteria and aloe vera and many of the essential oils controlling the malodour and pain.

Included on the list of natural treatments will be larvae therapy. Natural myiasis (infestation of wounds) is commonly seen in hot climates but rarely in Britain, and is often greeted with horror when the dressing is removed to expose the infestation (Flanagan, 1997). Nevertheless, maggot therapy has been used for many centuries as a natural debrider of wounds. There is evidence that the benefits of maggots were noted as long ago as 1557 (Morgan, 1997). Later, in the American Civil War (Thomas et al., 1996; Morgan, 1997) there are anecdotal reports of Malay Indians using maggots to remove superficial malignancies.

The most commonly used fly in biosurgery is *Lucilia sericata* or green-bottle fly (Thomas et al., 1996). The fly is bred in the Surgical Materials Testing Laboratory in Bridgend, the only centre for larvae in Britain and one of only three centres in the world. Maggots will not pupate in the wound and so the patient and the nurse can be assured that they will not find flies in the wound when they remove the dressing. This method of debridement is increasing in popularity, particularly in difficult wounds requiring palliative management, such as fungating tumours, as a reduction of odour and exudate can be achieved by the treatment (Thomas et al., 1996). However, larvae therapy is contraindicated in bleeding wounds as it can increase the potential of haemorrhage.

Carbon dressings can filter odour and can, therefore, be very useful as primary or secondary dressings (Table 13.1)

Table 13.1 Dressings that filter odour

Carbon	
Actisorb plus	Actisorb contains silver as an antibacterial agent. Should be used as a primary dressing
Lyofoam C	Lyofoam is absorbent with a carbon centre
Carboflex	Carboflex has a unique five-layer construction, comprising a Kalto stat layer, aquacel wound contact layer, activated charcoal cloth and absorbent padding, with a charcoal dressings filter and deodorizing EMA film cover

Pain

Pain in fungating tumours may be related to size or site of the lesion, pressure from other organs (Hastings, 1993), the type of bacteria present within the wound or a psychological pain caused by the presence of the lesion. Systemic treatment for pain is addressed elsewhere in this book. This chapter will look at how pain may be dealt with through dressings.

The pain is often caused by exposed nerve endings and reduction of pain may then be achieved by 'bathing' the exposed nerves with the wound dressing. Hydrocolloids and hydrogels (Table 13.2) can soothe this pain and may be very useful. However, before they can be successfully applied, the amount of exudate and odour often requires treatment. If gels or hydrocolloids are applied to highly exuding wounds, the amount of exudate and malodour may well increase.

Hydrocolloids

These consist of a mixture of pectins, gelatines, sodium carboxymethyl-cellulose and elastomers. Hydrocolloids are available in a number of forms: as wafers, extra absorbent wafers, extra thin wafers, granules, powders, gels and pastes. On contact with wound exudate, the hydro-colloid material dissolves into a gel. This gel provides many of the conditions favourable for moist wound healing. But as it mixes with exudate it has a particular 'yellow' appearance and can give off a char-acteristic odour. Although this is normal and to be expected with these products, those handling the dressing and also the patient being treated need to be aware of it (Flanagan, 1997). Care should be taken to ensure that the correct size of dressing is applied, i.e. one large enough to cover the wound with an overlap of at least two inches. Hydrocolloids can reduce dressing change interval to around five days. Hydrocolloid paste is easily used and is an effective deslough agent, excellent for small cavity wounds. It can reduce pain by moistening the nerve endings.

Table 13.2 Hydrocolloid dressings

Hydrocolloids	
Cutinova hydro	Reduce wound pain by moistening exposed nerve ends (Flana gan, 1997)
Comfeel	Provide optimum wound healing environment (Flanagan, 1997)
Easyderm	Can be left in situ for 5 or 6 days (remove if 'strike through' is apparent
Granuflex	Patient is able to bath/shower without removing the dressing
Hydrocoll Tegasorb Duoderm extra thin	
Granuflex paste	Can be left in situ for up to 5 days Easily removable from the wound bed

NB: Easyderm does not provide a hypoxic environment but is a 'breathable' dressing

Hydrogels

Hydrogels are available in sheets or gel (Table 13.3). The sheets are made up of gelable polysaccharide agarose, cross linked with polyacry-lamide. This material provides a moist environment for fungating lesions and dry to slightly exuding wounds. The gels are suitable for cavities and are effective for desloughing and debriding wounds (Bale, 1990).

Hydrogels:

- Have a high water content.
- Are useful in rehydration of hard eschar
- Promote autolysis
- Are useful as cavity dressings

Table 13.3 Hydrogels

Hydrogels	
Aquaform	Sloughy
Geliperm	Necrotic
Granugel	Cavity
Intrasite	
Purilon	
Nugel	
Sterigel	
Hydrogel sheets	
Novogel	
Second skin	

McCaffery's (1983) work led to the belief that 'pain is what the patient says it is and exists when he/she says it does'. If the patient claims to have pain then the problem must be addressed. Use of a visual analogue scale (Hill, 1991) can be useful, particularly when assessing whether treatment is effective.

Included in the assessment of pain should be an appraisal of the dressing. Any dressing that has adhered to *any* wound and proves difficult to remove should never be used on that wound again. Certain dressings are more prone to adhere than others; impregnated tulles, (iodine, paraffin) gauze, non-adherent dressings (excluding NA Ultra) have all, at some time, adhered to wounds. This does not detract from their usefulness as dressings, but they should be reconsidered in individual cases when adherence is noted.

Exudate

Exudate is often the byproduct of bacterial colonization – reduce colonization and the exudate will also lessen in amount. Iodine cadexomers are obviously an excellent choice as they control the exudate whilst killing the bacteria and can be moulded to the wound shape. However, it is unwise to continue using iodine over long periods and, on the occasions when high exudate problems have not been addressed by cadexomers, an alternative must be selected.

Gauze is inappropriate for any wound as cotton can leave fibres in a wound which may increase the possibility of clinical infection. Gauze can also adhere to the wound bed, causing pain, bleeding and distress on removal. Therefore, a suitable alternative dressing would be a non-adherent, high absorbency dressing (Table 13.4).

Table 13.4 Moderate to high absorbency dressings

ALGINATES		
Algosteril	High exudate	The osmotic pressure caused by the
Curasorb	Cavity	alginates' hydrophilic nature may
Kaltogel		possibly increase pain in
Kaltostat		a wound that is dry (Flanagan, 1997)
Tegagen		Require a secondary dressing to
Seasorb		a) support the alginate in situ
Sorbsan		b) maintain a moist environment
Drawhex		
FOAM		
Allevyn	Moderate exudate	Foam sheets and cavity dressings are:
Allevyn		Hydrophilic
Cavity		Absorb quantities of exudate
Cavicare		Have a non-adherent surface
Flexipore		Can be used as second dressings with a
Lyofoam		desloughing agent next to the wound
Tielle		Easily applied
Spyrosorb		Highly absorbent
		Some obtainable in non-adhesive
		sheets
		Will not deslough or debride
COMBIDERM	Moderate exudate	A self adhesive dressing
		Has a central island of super-absorbent
		cellulose granules which wicks exudate
		Retains fluid
		Keeps the wound bed moist but not wet
		Will not adhere to the wound

AQUACEL	Appropriate in moderate exuding wounds Cavities	Hydrofibre sheet or ribbon dressing with high wet strength Forms a gel instantly on contact with fluid Adhesive border. Retains high amounts of water without releasing it; therefore, will not macerate peri-wound areas Will not adhere to the wound bed May assist in desloughing

Once the exudate has been controlled there are many inexpensive dressings that can be used to support the wound. The optimum dressing type would be one that can support the symptoms without misshaping the patient's clothes (Table 13.5).

Table 13.5 Dressings with low adherence for minimally exuding wounds

Multidress pad Multiaminate, non-woven pad	Non-adherent Inexpensive Easily applied Easily obtained Some absorbent properties
Multidress *Multidress compress* Folded 4-ply non-woven dressing containing gelling fibres *Multidress ribbon* Viscose ribbon with gelling fibres Knitted viscose wound contact layer containing gelling fibres *Multidress WCL* Folded 4-ply knitted viscose dressing containing gelling fibres *Multidress standard*	Retains fluid Keeps the wound bed moist but not wet Will not adhere to the wound

Range provides similar characteristics to other conventional dressings but the addition of gelling fibres gives enhanced performance, including lower adherence.

Melolin Absorbent pad bonded to a wound contact polyester perforated film	Easily applied Easily obtained Some absorbent properties Non-adherent

This dressing has limited absorbency and is most suitable for lightly exuding wounds (Bale, 1991). Can adhere to wounds (Hampton, 1997).

Multidress Extra

A cotton/acrylic viscose absorbent pad bonded to a wound contact polyester perforated film

Easily applied
Easily obtained
Some absorbent properties
Non-adherent

For primary and secondary usage.

Mepital

Silicone dressing pad

Non-adherent
Easily applied

NA Ultra

Single layer of knitted viscose with silicone

Non-adherent

Easily removed but requires secondary dressing to absorb exudate.

Telfa

A layer of cotton enclosed in a perforated film (Bale, 1991)

Easily applied
Easily obtained

Some absorbent properties.

NA Tricotex

Single layer of knitted viscose

Inexpensive
Easily applied
Easily obtained
Easily removed

Requires secondary dressing to absorb exudate
No absorbent properties

In highly exudating wounds, it would be unwise to use dressings that increase 'wetness' within the wound – i.e. hydrogels. A general rule of thumb would be, if the wound is wet, dry it and if the wound is dry, moisten it. If this rule is ignored, the problem of peri-wound skin maceration can occur, particularly as the fatty acids produced as a byproduct of metabolism of anaerobic bacteria create profuse exudate which can damage the good skin.

Although the aim is to reduce damaging exudate, some exudate can support the wound environment. Maceration continues to be a difficulty in wound healing and few studies have addressed the problem (Hampton, 1997a; 1998b). Wound exudate and 'wet' dressings such as hydrogels can exacerbate the problem. When assessment indicates that a 'wet' dressing is required to facilitate wound healing, should this decision be reversed when maceration occurs? The treatment of the wound should be appropriate and if this is changed to an inappropriate dressing to suit the peri-wound area, then deterioration in the wound could be expected.

Maceration occurs when the tissues are kept overmoist for long periods of time. The cells become 'waterlogged', softened, fragile and easily damaged. This can lead to excoriation. The tissues have the appearance of white or pink, softened skin. There are significant differences in the structure and characteristics of skin of various people of all ages. Skin will react differently to any mechanical insult applied to it depending on whether it is oily, dry, moist, papery or normal. Therefore, patients' wounds may be treated in identical ways with one having a successful outcome and another's healing delayed by complications. Maceration can be caused by a wet discharge from the wound or wound dressing which moistens the viable tissue around the wound. Tissues softened in this way become easily damaged and are vulnerable to grazing, which offers an entry for infection. There are excellent products on the market today that prevent and treat maceration. Cavilon no-sting barrier film is the first of a new type of treatment that will not cause pain on application.

Exudate, therefore, is a problem shared between nurse and patient. It is particularly problematic when the peri-wound areas deteriorate because of exudate 'over-spill'. It is important to understand exudate so that dressing selection is appropriate for the wound and treatment for the peri-wound area is relevant (see Table 13.6).

Purpose of exudate:

- Metalloproteinases break down collagens and help to remodel extracellular matrix in healing (Vickery, 1997)
- Fibroblasts grow faster in exudate (Vickery, 1997)
- Contains growth factors that promote tissue regeneration (Kreig and Eming, 1997)
- Facilitates the migration of cells involved in tissue repair
- Acts as a transport medium for white cells

Table 13.6 Factors affecting exudate production

Colonization of bacteria	Noted by the colour of exudate	*Pseudomonas*=green exudate *Staphylococcus*=brown exudate
Wound (host) infection	Noted by clinical signs (cellulitis; pain; pyrexia)	Can be any colour exudate
Temperature	Vasodilation	= increased exudate production
	Vasoconstriction	= decreased exudate
Compression	Reduction in hydrostatic pressure	Compressed dressings
Permeability of vessel walls (Thomas, 1997)	Essential part of normal inflammatory process Can be caused by large number of bacteria Can be caused by acidic extracellular fluids	Production of histamine
Type of dressing	Dry wound should have a 'wet' dressing Wet wound should have a 'dry' dressing	Hydrogels Hydrocolloids (etc.) Cadexomers Alginates Foams (etc.)

Potential damage caused by exudate:

- Can exacerbate skin damage (Cameron and Powell, 1997) through irritation
- Assists in the process of autolysis (Dealy, 1997)
- Bacteria produce proteolytic enzymes which delay healing and damage peri-wound areas
- Can require large amount of nurses' time in changing dressings
- High exudate production can equal low serum proteins. Staphylococci easily replicate in exudate (Vickery, 1997)

Therefore, dressing selection relies on reducing the bacterial count in a wound but allowing exudate to continue with support from the dressing.

Bleeding and alginates

Alginates are produced from seaweed with high calcium content. Alginates exchange sodium ions for calcium ions in the wound bed and this encourages the clotting cascade within a bleeding wound; this has led to alginates being widely used in theatres and in dental treatment. Alginates are particularly useful in bleeding fungating tumours. All alginates transform to gel in the presence of exudate, are hydrophilic and are useful in highly exuding wounds, but are best avoided in low exudate wounds (Miller and Dyson, 1996). They will not assist with reducing the bacterial count within the wound bed.

Calcium alginates were first used in the 1940s (Thomas, 1992) and are extracted from the brown seaweed harvested off the coasts of Scotland (Williams, 1994). Alginate dressings are made from different parts of the seaweed plant and can be composed of galuronic and mannuronic acid units linked together (Williams, 1994) with the proportions of these units determining the gel forming properties of the final fibre (Thomas and Loveless, 1992). The high galuronic acid alginates (e.g. Kaltostat) are slow to gel and produce firmer gels. This gives the gelled fibres strength, retains the shape in the wound bed and generally enables the dressing to be lifted out of the wound in a thick gel form. The alginates high in mannuronic acid (e.g. Sorbsan) are weaker and the gel from these can easily be rinsed out of a wound with normal saline.

Alginates are best used in moderate to highly exuding wounds (Miller and Dyson, 1996) as the fibres are hydrophilic and cause an osmotic 'pull' on the fluid within a wound. If the wound bed is dry, the fibres may 'pull' fluid from the cells, thereby drying the wound out; this goes against researched evidence that recommends a moist healing environment (Winter, 1962). When applied to a highly exuding wound, the hydrophilic fibres form a gel. When a film or hydrocolloid dressing is used as a secondary dressing, the alginate gel provides warmth, moisture, occlusion (through the secondary dressing), absorption and trauma free removal, all of which are requirements of the optimum wound environment (Torrance, 1983).

Alginates can be obtained in the following forms:

- Sheets of various sizes
- Rope
- Extra thick (Sorbsan plus or Kaltostat extra) – very useful in highly exuding fungating wounds

Many alginates are available on the drug tariff.

Considering the patient

It is important that the patient is given the opportunity to be involved in the overall management of the wound and associated problems. However, it is possible that denial will disassociate the patient from the treatment and this will require a supportive and understanding approach from the nurse.

An holistic assessment of the patient will help in making decisions for wound management; however, it is helpful to write down the patient's identified problems in priority order and then to address each problem in turn. For example, if the identified problem is malodour, then dressing treatment will rely on removing the bacteria causing the malodour. If the problem is pain, this would require a multidisciplinary approach in which the pain specialist nurse, physiotherapist, pharmacist and doctor will be involved in reducing the symptom to a level acceptable to the patient.

Chapter 14
Nutritional support

JO HUNT

Introduction

The effects of cancer on a patient's nutritional status will depend on the severity and location of the disease as well as the treatment administered to combat the disease. Some cancers (e.g. gastrointestinal and lung) are associated with an increased incidence of severe malnutrition, whereas an isolated non-spreading type of skin cancer may be removed, leaving little impact on nutritional status. Approximately 45% of adult cancer patients admitted to hospital have a weight loss exceeding 10% of their pre-illness body weight (Shills, 1979). Malnutrition in the cancer patient is associated with poor prognosis (Ottery, 1994). This chapter explores the reasons why cancer and cancer treatments necessitate nutritional support. The importance of nutritional assessment is discussed, focusing on the nurse's role in detecting those patients at risk of malnutrition. The final pages describe the variety of methods of administering nutritional support.

Cancer cachexia

The term 'cancer cachexia' describes a syndrome characterized by weakness, anorexia, weight loss, derangement in water and electrolyte metabolism and eventual impairment of vital functions (Kern and Norton, 1988). It is evident in the terminal stages of disease in a large proportion of patients with cancer, but can also be apparent at the time of diagnosis. The incidence of cancer cachexia at the time of presentation in a clinical setting varies greatly between 3% and 80% (De Blaauw et al., 1997). Cancer cachexia does not appear to be related to the size of tumour or calorie intake and can be present when the tumour represents a very small percentage of total body weight.

There have been many suggested theories regarding reduced appetite in cancer cachexia, but the exact aetiology remains unclear. Current theories include a chemical imbalance in the brain as a result of an amino acid imbalance which leads to an accumulation of tryptophan and serotonin. Coupled with reduced oral intake, patients with cancer have an increase in metabolic rate resulting in an increased energy expenditure. Some metabolic pathways are altered, leading to inefficient utilization of nutrients.

The anorexia associated with cancer cachexia may be worsened by other factors. Altered taste perception and smell will reduce oral intake. Changes in the gastrointestinal tract may result in delayed gastric emptying and therefore contribute to early satiety. Malabsorption is common in patients with cancer and can lead to excessive loss of nutrients as a result of impaired digestion, vomiting or diarrhoea. Pain, especially if aggravated by eating, will lead to an unwillingness to eat. All these physical reasons for reduced oral intake may be compounded by the psychological stress and fear of the diagnosis of cancer.

The effect of cancer treatments on nutritional status

Nutritional therapy in cancer is supportive, but not considered a treatment. The primary treatments are radiotherapy, chemotherapy and surgery. Nutritional status may be compromised by any of these treatments, which may be delivered alone or in combination.

The combination of chemotherapy and radiotherapy produces more severe side effects, which can include ulceration of the gastrointestinal tract. The immune system may be adversely affected by anti-cancer therapy, therefore increasing the risk of infection and increasing energy requirements. Quite apart from the effects of the actual treatments, hospitalization may result in reduced oral intake due to aversion to food offered in hospital and timing of meals, which may not be appropriate for the individual patient. If the patient is receiving treatment as an outpatient, journeys to and from the hospital and waiting times for treatment may affect food intake.

Radiotherapy

Nutritional complications are common in patients undergoing radiotherapy. Radiation damages all actively dividing cells. Tumour cells divide more rapidly than normal cells and are slower to recover from the effects of radiation. The cells of the gastrointestinal tract and the immune system are rapidly dividing and their cell division will also be disrupted by the irradiation.

Irradiation of the head and neck causes an altered sense of taste and a decrease in the production of saliva. This will further exacerbate any existing dysphagia and nausea. Mucositis is common, making chewing and swallowing very painful. In severe cases, patients are unable to swallow their own saliva. Symptoms can be slow to resolve, sometimes taking two to four months from the end of treatment to disappear.

Any irradiation that includes the oesophagus (e.g. chest) will result in dysphagia. Radiotherapy to the abdomen and pelvis initially causes anorexia, nausea, vomiting and diarrhoea. Malabsorption secondary to irradiation of the abdomen and pelvis occurs as a result of damage to the epithelium of the small intestine, causing malabsorption of glucose, electrolytes and protein. This is termed chronic radiation enteritis, and may occur years after the radiotherapy.

Chemotherapy

Cytotoxic drugs are used to interrupt cell division and will also affect non-malignant cells. Chemotherapy causes anorexia as a result of altered taste perception, nausea and vomiting. Patients often complain of a metallic taste in the case of some cytotoxic agents, which discourages them from eating. Ulceration of the mucosa of the lip, tongue and oesophageal cavity is also common and can lead to dysphagia. Nausea and vomiting will undoubtedly reduce oral intake. Other complications of chemotherapy can include constipation or ileus.

Surgery

Fasting prior to necessary investigations that are performed preoperatively may affect appetite and ability to eat a normal diet, especially if the tumour originates in the gastrointestinal tract. Surgery is often essential to remove the tumour, and chemotherapy or radiotherapy may be required postoperatively. Any surgery will cause the body to mount a stress response, a consequence of which is an increase in metabolism. If the surgery involves the gastrointestinal tract, effects may be more specific. Surgery to the head and neck will cause problems in swallowing and chewing. It is essential that the impact on the patient's nutritional status is kept to a minimum during the perioperative stage, as subsequent treatments (i.e. chemotherapy and radiotherapy) can compound any depletion of energy reserves and nutrients. Simple measures such as regular weighing of the patient may alert healthcare professionals to a potential problem. The importance of weighing in the outpatient setting must not be underestimated for this group of patients.

Malabsorption is common due to resection of an organ of the gastrointestinal tract. A gastrectomy will cause 'dumping syndrome', where the food rushes into the small intestine causing diarrhoea. This may result in malabsorption of iron, calcium, fat and vitamins. Resection of the terminal ileum will cause malabsorption of vitamin B and biliary salts.

Pancreatic surgery will cause general malabsorption due to insufficiency of pancreatic enzymes. A pancreatic tumour may cause obstruction of the pancreatic or bile duct resulting in malabsorption.

Nutritional assessment

Although general awareness of nutrition is improving, the detection of malnutrition remains a problem. The King's Fund Report 'A Positive Approach to Nutrition as Treatment' in 1992 recommended that simple assessment of nutritional status should be performed on all patients admitted to hospital, regardless of their age or diagnosis. This should be performed routinely on admission as part of the admission process. Nutritional assessment tools are used to determine whether a patient is suffering from, or at risk of, developing malnutrition. All cancer patients should undergo a nutritional assessment when their diagnosis is first made. This first presentation to healthcare professionals may be in hospital or in the community. Any patient regarded as at risk of developing malnutrition or who is indeed malnourished must be referred to a dietitian.

The British Association of Parenteral and Enteral Nutrition (BAPEN) promotes the use of four simple questions which should be asked to all patients on admission to hospital (Lennard-Jones et al., 1995).

- What is your normal weight in health?
- What is your normal height in health?
- Have you unintentionally lost weight recently?
- Have you been eating less than usual?

Patients should be weighed in light clothing (the same type of clothing each time if possible) using accurate scales. If weight has been lost, the percentage weight loss should be determined. Short-term fluctuations in weight loss (of more than one kilogram) are more likely to reflect changes in fluid balance. Oedema can distort weight changes.

Objective nutritional assessment is based on the following quantitative criteria:

Weight and height

An unintentional weight loss of greater than 10% in three months gives cause for concern. Besides the percentage weight change, the patient's body mass index (BMI) can be calculated. The BMI is calculated by dividing the weight in kilograms by the height (squared) in metres:

$$BMI = \frac{weight\ (kg)}{height\ (m^2)}$$

The figure obtained from the BMI calculation is used to indicate whether a patient is a healthy weight for his or her height.

<16: malnourished
16–19: underweight
20–25: normal
26–30: overweight
31–40: moderately to severely obese
>40: morbidly obese

Measurements of BMI are not accurate in children or in the elderly (whose height may be inaccurate). For the elderly, a similar calculation can be used based on the patient's demispan. For children, the centile charts should be used (Freeman et al., 1995).

Biochemical measurements

These can be used to assess nutritional status but there is no single reliable test. Certain biochemical markers may be influenced by the underlying pathology and allowances must be made for nutrition-related and disease-related abnormal parameters. Plasma proteins most commonly measured in nutritional studies (e.g. albumin and transferrin) have a long half-life and do not accurately reflect changes in food intake. Albumin falls during an inflammatory response, while the C-reactive protein increases (Pennington, 1997). Hypoalbuminaemia correlates poorly with nutritional status (Anderson and Wochers, 1982).

Anthropometric measurements

These include skin fold thickness measurements. However, these can be inaccurate if not taken in exactly the same manner each time.

Subjective nutritional assessment

An experienced clinician can accurately assess the nutritional status of a patient by taking appropriate medical history and performing appropriate physical examination. They term this 'subjective nutritional assessment'. By observing the condition of the patient's skin and hair, a prediction of nutritional status can be made. Poor wound healing may be reflected by deficiencies in vitamin C or zinc. Deficiency of the B complex vitamins can result in sore and cracked lips and other mouth disorders. Physical manifestations of weight loss include loose-fitting clothes and rings, poorly fitting dentures and sunken eyes.

Principles of nutritional support

The aim of nutritional support in the patient with cancer is to prevent any deterioration in nutritional status and restore the patient to an optimum status by the most appropriate method of nutritional support. Not all patients will have nutritional problems. This group of patients will require general healthy eating advice in order to ensure a diet well balanced in all vitamins and minerals. Nutritional assessments should be maintained and the patient must be encouraged to seek advice if any difficulties arise which compromise their nutritional status.

Pre- and postoperative nutritional support

It is inconclusive whether preoperative nutritional support reduces postoperative complications or mortality in patients with cancer (Bozzetti, 1995). There may be a reduction in wound complications, and studies of post-operative nutritional support have suggested that nutritional support does improve outcome (Yamada et al., 1983). Nevertheless, malnutrition in cancer patients does increase mortality.

Referral to the dietitian

The dietitian will normally assess the patient and calculate his or her individual nutritional requirements, taking an account of the following: dietary history; medical history (as this may affect nutrition); drug–nutrient interactions; whether the present disease is likely to change, and how it will affect nutritional status.

The dietitian will then assess whether there is likely to be an increased need for any other nutrient (e.g. there is an increased requirement for potassium when a patient is taking amphotericin).

The Schofield equations are one of the tools used in clinical situations to predict requirements for energy. There are 12 equations (based on age and sex) which are used to calculate basal metabolic rate from weight. After the basic equations are calculated, additions are made (e.g., physical activity level) in order to reach a figure of estimated energy requirements.

However, Shaffer (1998) suggests that the Schofield equations and other current methods used to calculate patients' energy and nitrogen requirements are probably a generous estimation of what patients actually require.

Meeting the nutritional requirements of cancer patients

As well as calculating the patient's requirements, a decision must be made regarding the best route of delivery of nutrients. The preferred route of feeding is always the gastrointestinal tract. The following section discusses the various ways in which nutritional support can be delivered. If nutritional support is required, the options range from simple dietary manipulation to enteral tube feeding and parenteral feeding.

Menu choice assistance

Some patients may be able to manage sufficiently with larger portions of food from the hospital menu, with additional snacks when required. Nurses are in an ideal position to advise patients on their choice of menu, taking into account special needs (e.g. diabetic diets, religious exclusions, etc.). The majority of healthy eating guidelines (e.g. low fat, high fibre, reduction in refined sugars, reduction in energy) may not be appropriate for sick patients with a poor appetite. High fibre diets increase the bulk of the food and can result in early satiety. High energy, high protein food may be rich in refined sugars and fat, but is more suitable for the patient with little appetite.

If nausea is a problem, the patient should eat small, frequent snacks and avoid the smell of foods that trigger nausea. Anti-emetics should be administered prior to meals. Fatty and greasy foods delay stomach emptying and could exacerbate nausea. Biscuits and dry toast may help control nausea, and ginger biscuits and ginger ale may be effective in some patients.

Severe mucositis may require parenteral nutrition, especially if associated with diarrhoea. If the mucositis is less severe, or if they are recovering from severe mucositis, patients should be encouraged to take analgesia before attempting to eat. Foods that are not recommended include highly spiced food, acidic and salty food, alcohol, hot food and dry or rough food. Soft food, and possibly nutritional supplements, should be encouraged.

Modification of food

Modifications can be made to hospital menu food to increase its suitability for an individual patient. Patients with chewing and/or swallowing difficulties (e.g. in the case of cancer of the oesophagus) may require liquidized or pureed diets. If pureed food requires dilution, full fat milk (not water) should be used. There are a variety of commercially available thickening agents that allow pureed food to be presented in an appetizing way. Moulds are also available to help make a pureed meal look more like a conventional meal. With some thickening solutions it is even possible to make a pureed sandwich. Hot food shaped in moulds will retain its warmth for longer, largely as a result of a decreased surface area. Traditional pureed food which is often served in hospitals tends to come in standard colours such as green, brown and cream, which rarely excite the appetite. Pureed diets should be fortified, as it is difficult for patients consuming this type of diet to achieve their nutritional requirements.

Fortification of food

Fortification of the diet may be appropriate for patients who can eat normal hospital menu food, but in insufficient quantities to meet their requirements. Foods that are low in calories and protein should be supplemented with foods of higher nutritional value. For example, jellies and soups can be supplemented with varieties which are fortified using skimmed milk powder, butter and cream. Patients and carers can be instructed how to do this easily at home. Commercially prepared products are available to boost the calorific value of food and drinks.

Nutritional supplements

Supplements are available in a variety of forms (e.g. soups, milk shakes and puddings) and can be used to boost the diet of a patient who is eating normal food from the hospital menu. A high energy liquid sip feed can be taken slowly throughout the day. Three supplements a day gives approximately 1,000 calories, which goes a long way towards achieving a patient's daily requirements. The nutritional sip feed drinks often packaged in tetrapaks are nutritionally complete and have the advantage of being lactose-free. Milk-based supplements should be used with caution, as some patients demonstrate a temporary lactose intolerance following fasting or gastrointestinal surgery.

Several studies are now showing that supplements can be given as soon as one day after elective gastrointestinal surgery. Exceptions to this include oesophagectomies, total gastrectomies and pancreatic surgery. In these cases, a nasojejunal tube can be inserted for enteral feeding. Studies suggest that the presence of food in the gastrointestinal tract may increase the blood supply to the anastamosis and possibly improve the strength of the anastamosis (Braga et al., 1998).

Tube feeding

If the patient is unable or unwilling to eat but has a functioning gastrointestinal tract, tube feeding should be considered. The method of delivery will depend on the patient's condition and preference, as well as the likely duration of feeding. The following section considers tube feeding as either a temporary or a long-term measure.

Temporary tube feeding

If tube feeding is likely to be for a short duration (i.e. 3–4 weeks), a fine-bore nasogastric tube made of silicone or polyurethane with a diameter of <3 mm is most commonly used. Ryles tubes (used for gastric drainage) are occasionally used for feeding (e.g. in intensive care units) but can cause pharyngitis, oesophagitis and gastritis, and may significantly compromise a patient's respiratory function by occluding one nostril (especially in babies and the elderly). Fine-bore nasogastric tubes are preferable.

When inserting a fine-bore tube, there is a risk of malposition and oesophageal perforation, causing a pneumothorax. They therefore need to be inserted by a suitably experienced, qualified nurse. It is essential that the patient is well informed and understands the reasons for this method of feeding. Pre-measurement of the tube is essential prior to insertion. Place the exit port of the nasogastric tube at the tip of the patient's nose. Extend the tube to the earlobe, then to the xiphoid process. The tube will have marks on it to use as a reference. Inserting excess tubing may cause the tube to become kinked and result in obstruction.

It is recommended that the position is checked by aspiration and pH testing of aspirated fluid. Low range pH reagent strips should be used, as litmus paper may not always distinguish between gastric aspirate and bronchial secretions (Methany et al., 1994). Auscultation of the epigastrium is often used to confirm tube position, but should not be used as the sole method (Rollins, 1997). The position must be checked by X-ray (both abdominal and chest) if the patient has altered consciousness, an altered gag reflex or if there are gastric anatomical abnormalities.

Nasojejunal tubes are usually placed by endoscopic guidance as only 50% will spontaneously pass though the pylorus into the duodenum. This method of tube feeding is ideal for a patient who has high nasogastric aspirates, but where the intestine is still functioning. Double lumen tubes are available, which allow gastric aspiration from a proximal lumen and feeding via a distal lumen.

Nasogastric tubes are an ideal method of supplying extra nutrition to patients who are unable to consume enough food to meet their requirements. The feed is administered overnight, leaving patients free to tempt their appetite with small, frequent meals throughout the day.

Long-term tube feeding

If it is anticipated that feeding will be required for more than four weeks, a tube may be inserted directly into the oesophagus (oesophagostomy), the stomach (a gastrostomy) or the small bowel (a jejunostomy).

An oesophagostomy may be placed after major head and neck surgery (e.g. laryngectomy). It is normally placed at the time of surgery. This route bypasses the nose, mouth and upper airway.

A gastrostomy can be placed directly into the stomach under a general anaesthetic and is sometimes performed for drainage after surgery in preference to a nasogastric tube. It can then be used for feeding at a later date if required.

A percutaneous endoscopic gastrostomy (PEG) is inserted percutaneously under endoscopic control. A mature stoma tract is formed after two weeks, but it may take longer if the patient is on steroids. If there is any risk of the patient aspirating or if there is gastric status, a conversion tube from PEG to PEJ (jejunostomy) is possible.

Complications of tube feeding

The complications associated with tube feeding are similar regardless of the method of delivery.

1. Diarrhoea

To reduce the risk of a patient developing diarrhoea whilst being tube fed, it is recommended that the patient starts with 40–50 ml an hour of full strength feed and gradually builds up to meet their fluid and nutritional requirements as quickly as tolerated (i.e. usually within 24 hours). Diarrhoea may result if the flow rate is too rapid or if certain drugs (e.g. antibiotics) are administered. It may also indicate microbial contamination, as described below. Anti-diarrhoeal agents and low fibre feeds can be used (Shankardass et al., 1990).

2. Aspiration

The position of the tube must be checked after insertion and at least daily (as described above). It is preferable for the patient to be propped up in bed with pillows or sitting in a chair, rather than lying flat. Pulmonary aspiration of gastric or small bowel contents is a potentially life-threatening complication of tube feeding. If aspiration of the feed is suspected, the feed should be discontinued immediately. An urgent chest X-ray and arterial blood gas analysis will confirm the suspicion.

3. Blockage of tube

To prevent the tube becoming blocked, it must be flushed with water regularly using a 50 ml syringe. It is recommended that the tube be flushed every six hours or after each feed is completed. If the tube does become blocked, sodium bicarbonate or a carbonated drink can be administered down the tube and it can be clamped for 15 minutes. The tube should then be flushed. Using a syringe smaller than this size may cause the tube to rupture. If the tube cannot be unblocked, it can be removed and unblocked. If the guide-wire has been kept, the tube can be washed and re-inserted. Guide wires should never be replaced if the fine-bore tube is still inside the patient (Rollins, 1997).

4. Microbial contamination

In a recent study, 29% of enteral feeds administered to patients were found to be contaminated and those patients were twice as likely to develop symptoms of diarrhoea, vomiting and abdominal pain (Navajas et al., 1992). It is therefore vital that feeds are administered in such a way that contamination is minimized as far as possible.

The person administering the feed should wash their hands before setting up or changing the feed. The tube must be flushed with water after every feed is complete to prevent bacterial colonization within the tube. Syringes used for flushing or aspirating feeding tubes should not be re-used. The risk of contamination is lower with a commercially prepared feed, especially those that require no transfer from the original container. The feed should not hang for longer than 24 hours, particularly on a warm day, as bacterial multiplication greatly increases. Giving sets must be changed every 24 hours (Cataldo et al., 1998).

PVC tubes should be resited every 14 days. Polyurethane tubes may be used for up to six months. Gastrostomies and jejunostomies should be changed as per manufacturers' and individual hospital guidelines.

5. Premature removal of tube

This is more common in a nasogastric tube, but does sometimes occur in gastrostomies. According to a study by Keoshane, Attril and Silk (1986) the reasons for premature removal of nasogastric tubes are:

50%: accidentally by the patient
5%: accidentally by staff (during turning, physio, etc.)
4%: vomited up
10%: removed following death of the patient
20%: removed on commencement of full oral diet

In addition, they may occasionally be removed due to a blockage.

Despite these complications, tube feeding can be used successfully both in hospital and in the community. The modern gastrostomy tubes are discreet and allow patients to be fed enterally overnight giving them freedom during the day.

Parenteral nutrition

Parenteral nutrition should only be used if the gut is non-functioning (i.e. intestinal failure has occurred). Causes of intestinal failure in the cancer patient include prolonged paralytic ileus, enterocutaneous fistulae and radiation enteritis. With this method of feeding, nutrients are delivered directly into the circulation via the peripheral or central route. Parenteral nutrition is not without complications arising as a result of insertion of the central line or due to metabolic consequences of intravenous feeding (Pennington, 1991).

Composition and delivery

The all-in-one system of providing intravenous nutrition was introduced in the 1970s. Standard bags can be purchased directly from
pharmaceutical companies or can be tailor-made in specially
designed sterile pharmacy compounding units. Parenteral nutrition
solutions contain glucose, a simple sugar, as the carbohydrate source.
As well as glucose, calories are also supplied in the solution from lipid.
Commercially prepared amino acid solutions are added, as well as
vitamins, trace elements and electrolytes. The volume of the
parenteral nutrition solution can be manipulated depending on the
patient's requirements. Drugs (e.g. ranitidine) can be added, although
this may affect the stability of the solution. The rate can be increased
in order to decrease the duration of feeding as the patient's condition
allows. This promotes independence and a feeling of freedom. The
parenteral nutrition should never stop abruptly or rebound hypoglycaemia may result (Cataldo et al., 1998). If the patient is receiving
parenteral nutrition over a shorter period than 24 hours, it must be
infused at half rate for the last hour of infusion. If the patient begins to
eat, he or she must reach approximately half of their requirements
enterally (or 1,000 kcal) before stopping parenteral nutrition (Dewar,
1999). For example, if the patient requires 2 litres of parenteral nutrition over 16 hours, the rate will be 125 ml per hour for 15 hours, and
62 ml per hour for the remaining hour.

To have any beneficial effect on nutritional status, parenteral
nutrition should be administered for a minimum of 7–10 days. It
should be administered via a designated lumen of a central line (or
peripherally inserted central line: PICC). An increasing number of
lines used now are tunnelled, with a cuff if the patient is likely to be
on parenteral nutrition for some time. The cuff adheres to the subcutaneous layer of skin and three weeks after insertion requires no
sutures. Patients who are to be discharged with a line should always
have a cuffed line in for security, unless a PICC is used. PICCs have
been successfully used to administer PN. Compared with the insertion of a central line, the insertion of a PICC is cheaper and simpli-
fies nursing care (Palmer and McFie, 1997).

If parenteral feeding is estimated to be required for a short
period only, commercially prepared peripheral solutions may be
administered via a peripheral cannula. To extend the life of the

cannula, a GTN patch can be applied to a site distal to the cannula (Payne-James and Khawaja, 1993). As with PICCs, peripheral cannulae avoid the risk of pneumothorax, associated with the insertion of a central venous catheter.

Nursing care of patient receiving parenteral nutrition

1. Temperature, pulse and respiration

   At least daily TPR is recommended to assess for signs of line infection. If the patient has an unexplained temperature, blood cultures should be taken aseptically from the central line. Blood pressure should be taken as the condition of the patient indicates.

2. Weight

   A weight change of greater than 1 kg is an indication of fluid gain or loss. Daily weights are a very important method of assessing fluid state.

3. Urinalysis

   A sample of urine should be tested for glucose daily as the patient receives a large amount of glucose and fat via an abnormal route. If gluscosuria is detected, a blood sugar level must be determined. Blood sugars may be elevated, especially if the patient is stressed or on steroid therapy.

4. Fluid balance

   An accurate fluid balance is required, especially if losses are high from stomas, etc. The volume of the parenteral nutrition solution can be increased to account for losses.

5. Care of central line

   The exit site dressing should be redressed according to individual hospital policies and procedures. The nurse should observe the site for signs of infection, e.g. redness, oozing from the site.

6. Psychological care

   Eating is a very social pastime, and the patient who is unable to eat may feel socially isolated. It is vital that this is not overlooked when nursing a patient dependent on parenteral nutrition.

7. Biochemical monitoring

   Daily biochemistry should be taken until the patient is stable. Large amounts of sodium may be required if the patient has a high output stoma or fistula. The sodium concentration of small bowel effluent can be as much as 100 mmol/l (Nightingale et al., 1990).

Complications of parenteral nutrition

Life-threatening complications can arise with parenteral feeding. These may be metabolic or nutritional in origin, or related to the catheter. They can include the following:

The first potential complication that can arise occurs at the time of the line insertion. Many cancer patients receiving chemotherapy may already have a double lumen central line which can be used for intravenous nutrition if required. Complications of central line insertion include pneumothorax, haemothorax and malpositioning. A chest X-ray is vital following line insertion to exclude these complications. The use of peripherally inserted central catheters (PICC) eliminates the threat of a pneumothorax or haemothorax, but an X-ray is still required to check the position of the line.

To avoid any episode of catheter-related infection, it is vital to use strict aseptic technique when dealing with any central line, especially if intravenous nutrition is being administered. The parenteral nutrition solution provides bacteria with an ideal culture medium in which to multiply. A patient who is receiving chemotherapy or radiotherapy will also be immunologically compromised, thus increasing the risk of opportunistic infection. A closed system of administration of the intravenous nutrition should be used to reduce the risk of infection.

Another catheter-related complication is catheter blockage. This can be avoided by flushing the line with sodium chloride and administering heparin into the line when not in use. Heparin and lipid from the parenteral nutrition solution should not be allowed to come into contact with each other as this causes a precipitate which can block the catheter. The line should be well flushed before and after blood sampling and drug administration, although most centres with a nutritional support team advocate the use of a lumen dedicated only for parenteral nutrition administration. Urokinase can be administered into a sluggish line assumed to be occluded by fibrin. An ethanol flush may unblock catheters that have become occluded as a result of the lipid in the PN solutions (Johnston et al., 1992).

Fracture or puncture of the catheter would cause an air leak and would be a potential site of bacterial invasion. This must be attended to immediately using commercially available repair kits.

The major cause of metabolic complications is a result of excess, rather than inadequate supply, of nutrients. Hyperglycaemia (detected by daily urinalysis) can be a result of excess infusion of glucose. Other biochemical abnormalities can be detected by regular biochemical monitoring, paying particular attention to calcium, phosphate, magnesium and zinc. Refeeding malnourished patients may precipitate deficiency of potassium, phosphate and zinc as a result of an increased requirement for tissue anabolism. Fluid overload or dehydration is possible and is the reason for careful fluid balance. Fluid balance problems are compounded by the administration of other intravenous fluids (e.g. with intravenous drugs) or by the loss of large amounts of fluid via stomas or fistulae.

Deranged liver function tests are often blamed on parenteral nutrition solutions. Hepatic dysfunction during parenteral feeding has been attributed to an excessive supply of glucose, fat or amino acids. It is often not possible to identify one single cause. Several studies suggest that a balanced mixture of glucose, fat and amino acids may be associated with a lower incidence of liver dysfunction (Tulikoura and Huikuri, 1982).

Careful monitoring of the patient receiving parenteral nutrition will enable the early detection of any catheter related or metabolic complications which do arise.

Palliative care

Not all patients suffering with cancer will be cured. The nutrition of those patients who are terminally ill is a great concern to relatives and carers as well as nurses. The aim of nutritional support in the palliative care setting is to be as simple as possible. Successful symptom control, a high standard of mouth care and meals presented in an attractive way are vital to encourage a patient to attempt small, frequent meals. There is a shift in emphasis as patients are encouraged to eat purely for pleasure and not to maintain their nutritional status. Tastes and textures become more important, especially if the patient has abnormal taste perception or dysphagia. Food and eating are associated with wellbeing and social satisfaction. Any decision to alter or withdraw nutritional support in the terminal stages of disease should be made in conjunction with a fully informed patient or relative. This will need careful and sensitive handling, especially if tube feeding or parenteral feeding is to be withdrawn (Penson and Fisher, 1991).

Case histories

Tube feeding

A 62-year-old man was admitted to a general surgical ward to undergo a routine oesophagogastrectomy for cancer of the oesophagus. At the time of operation a feeding jejunostomy was placed as it was certain that oral diet would be impossible immediately postoperatively. The patient's requirements were assessed by the dietitian whilst he was on the intensive care unit. Sterile water was first injected into the tube in bolus amounts. A standard tube feed was commenced before he left to go back to the surgical ward. This was started at a reduced rate and was slowly increased to the desired rate within 48 hours. Six days after the operation, a Gastrografin swallow was performed which revealed no leaks from the anastamosis. The patient began with sips of water orally and slowly increased to full diet. He was supported with the jejunal tube feeding until he was able to consume his total requirements. He was discharged home without requiring nutritional support 12 days postoperatively.

Parenteral nutrition

A 34-year-old man who had recently undergone a bone marrow transplantation was referred to a nutritional support team suffering from gastrointestinal graft versus host disease (GvHD). GvHD develops as the recipient's body mounts an immune system attack against the healthy donor cells which it recognizes as foreign. The patient had the following symptoms: nausea, vomiting, mucositis, severe diarrhoea and malabsorption. These symptoms made it impossible for him to receive any nutritional support via the enteral route. It was decided that parenteral nutrition should be recommenced. Based on a weight of 72 kg, the dietitian estimated his requirements as 14 g of nitrogen and 2,200 kcals per day. This would routinely be administered in 2.5 l of fluid. However, in this case, the patients was also receiving large amounts of fluid with intravenous antibiotics and blood products which could amount to 2 l per day. To avoid fluid overload, the volume of parenteral nutrition was reduced to 1.5 l per day. A double lumen cuffed line was already in situ for previous treatment.

As the mucositis and gastrointestinal symptoms resolved, the patient was encouraged to eat a lactose free, low residue, low fat diet to maximize absorption and minimize further nausea, vomiting and steatorrhoea. Solids foods were introduced gradually and the parenteral nutrition weaned. Fibre and lactose were introduced gradually to his diet with an emphasis on a high protein, high calorie diet.

Conclusions

A structured approach to nutritional support is a vital aspect of the care of the patient with cancer. During the past 20 years, many nutritional support teams have been established in hospitals in the UK. The benefits of such multidisciplinary teams are a reduction in infection rate and catheter insertion complications in parenteral feeding, reduced metabolic complications in both parenteral and enteral feeding, and reduced gastrointestinal and mechanical abnormalities in enteral feeding (Silk, 1994). In addition, the patient is assured that his nutritional needs are being met and care is explained by a group of experienced healthcare professionals. Communication is vital between the nutritional support team and healthcare professional responsible for the individual patient's care, to ensure that all involved are striving to achieve common goals.

Compared with a malnourished person, a person who is well nourished feels and functions better, is are more active, stronger and actually eats more. It is hard to quantify these benefits, but to the individual with cancer they are undoubtedly of great importance.

Chapter 15
Infection control issues

SARAH BALCHIN

Introduction

Hospital-acquired infections (HAI) affect approximately 10% of all inpatients who receive treatment and care in the NHS in the UK (Meers et al., 1994). These infections have a dramatic impact in terms of both human and financial costs. The individual patient may suffer pain and discomfort, require additional treatment and may even die. The organization that has provided the care will incur financial costs associated with additional drugs, equipment, supplies, dressings and extended length of stay. It has been reported that over 30% of these infections would be directly preventable if healthcare professionals complied fully with good infection control practice recommendations (Haley, 1985).

Risk factors associated with HAI include immunocompromise, prior treatment with antibiotics, increased hospitalization with long length of stay and exposure to invasive devices such as indwelling urinary catheters or intravenous devices (Craven et al., 1996). It is apparent, therefore, that patients with cancer have an increased risk of acquiring infection and greater difficulty obtaining successful treatment.

This chapter will identify the effects of disease and treatment on the patient's immune system, describe the types of infections to which oncology patients are susceptible, and clarify prophylactic measures to minimize the risk of infection to the patient.

The immune system

The human body has a variety of mechanisms that enable the body to: a) prevent micro-organisms and other foreign bodies entering; and b) limit their spread if they are successful in doing so.

If one or both of these systems are damaged in any way the ability of the host to minimize or fight infection is reduced. This is known as immunocompromise.

The immune system itself can be divided into two separate parts: the non-specific or innate immune system and the specific immune system.

Non-specific immunity

This system comprises non-specific physical, chemical and cellular barriers that act unselectively against most micro-organisms. These include the skin, saliva and acid and bile in the gastrointestinal tract (see Figure 15.1).

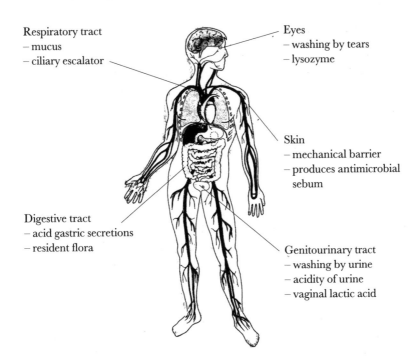

Respiratory tract
– mucus
– ciliary escalator

Eyes
– washing by tears
– lysozyme

Skin
– mechanical barrier
– produces antimicrobial
  sebum

Digestive tract
– acid gastric secretions
– resident flora

Genitourinary tract
– washing by urine
– acidity of urine
– vaginal lactic acid

Figure 15.1 Physical, cellular and chemical barriers to infection.

The skin

The skin provides a mechanical barrier against penetration by micro-organisms. It also secretes sebum, which has an antimicrobial action that inhibits the multiplication of micro-organisms. The skin has micro-organisms as permanent residents, known as resident flora, which may produce metabolic products which inhibit the multiplication of non-resident micro-organisms.

Mucosal defences

Mucosal defences provide protection against infection by a variety of natural defences. These include:

1. Mechanical washing by tears (tears contain lysozyme, which breaks down bacterial cell walls) or urine
2. The ciliary escalator system which moves mucus and debris
3. Surface phagocytes which consume and destroy micro-organisms.

Gastrointestinal defence systems

The chemical action, i.e. acidity, of gastric secretions effectively destroys a large number of bacteria, and bile produced in the small intestine also inhibits bacterial growth. The large intestine has resident flora which effectively minimize the growth of non-resident flora.

The inflammatory response

If a micro-organism or other foreign body is successful in entering the body, the normal response is one of inflammation, i.e. signs of heat, redness, tenderness or pain and swelling around the affected site. These signs will be the same for many micro-organisms and foreign bodies: that is the response will be non-specific.

The inflammatory response is divided in to four stages (see Table 15.1).

As a result of the inflammatory response a large amount of fluid, comprising white cells and a few red blood cells, enters the tissues. The damaged tissues produce chemicals which attract phagocytes which engulf foreign bodies (including micro-organisms). These foreign bodies are recognised quite easily but the process is more effective when the cells are marked with complement proteins (see below) to aid identification of host cells.

Table 15.1 The inflammatory response

Response	Mediator	Effect	Visible sign
Dilation of blood vessels	Histamine from mast cells	Increase blood flow to area	Redness and heat
Blood vessel become more permeable	Prostaglandins	Plasma and white blood cells migrate into tissue	Swelling
Pressure on nerve endings	Swollen tissue	Discourages movement of affected part	Pain

The complement system

The system comprises nine enzymes and proteins which interact with each other to aid in the destruction of invading micro-organisms. They circulate in the bloodstream in an inactive form and are activated as a result of contact with some organisms. This process is essential for phagocytosis to take place.

Two complement activation pathways have been described: the classical pathway and the alternative pathway (see Figure 15.2).

The classical pathway responds in the presence of antibody and is rapid-acting. The alternative pathway is slower acting, but can act in the absence of antibody and provides a defence against serious infection including meningococcal septicaemia.

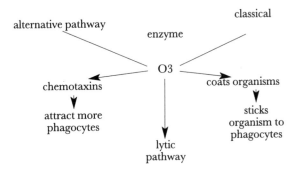

Figure 15.2 Activation of the complement system.

The specific immune response

The specific immune response supports the action of the non-specific immune response in destroying micro-organisms that are not affected by phagocytes. The specific immune response is based on recognition of antigens present in the pathogen.

This immune response is induced when the body identifies an organism which appears *foreign* (see Figure 15.3). This is achieved as the invading organisms have a unique combination of enzymes, toxins and cytoplasms (known as antigens), and they appear totally different from the host's cells. The antigens from the invading organism circulate through the lymphoid system and come into contact with lymphocytes. The lymphocytes have receptors on their surface that which enable them to identify an antigen. If this particular antigen contacts the appropriate receptor, a large number of the lymphocytes able to recognize this antigen are produced. In turn, these additional lymphocytes enter the bloodstream and move to the site of infection and support the body's fight against infection in a variety of ways. A very brief outline of these methods follows.

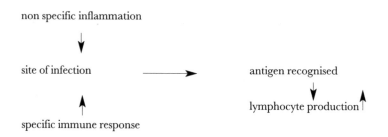

Figure 15.3 Induction of the immune response.

Humoral immunity

There are two types of lymphocytes:

1. B-lymphocytes (B-cells)   – produced by stem cells in the bone marrow
                             – responsible for production of antibodies

2. T-lymphocytes (T-cells)   – produced also in the bone marrow but requiring the thymus gland for development
– responsible for
a) providing a defence against micro-organisms which enter and survive in host cells
b) coordinating the immune response.

B-lymphocytes

The B-lymphocytes provide the basis for humoral immunity and precede antibody-producing *plasma cells*.
The effects of antibody are:

1. Neutralization of toxins
2. Neutralization of virus
3. Agglutination
4. Killing of organisms: activation of complement system
5. Opsonization (enhancement of phagocytosis).

Cell-mediated immunity

T-lymphocytes

The T-lymphocytes protect against:

1. Intracellular bacterial infections
2. Viral infections
3. Some fungal infections.

They are not present in children with a rare congenital absence of the thymus and who hence have a very low resistance to infection.

The T-lymphocytes interact with the antigen and assist in localizing infection by attacking cells and interrupting the virus replication cycle. As the T-cells increase in number they divide into two different groups: *helper T-cells*, which encourage B-cell production; and *suppresser T-cells*, which prevent over-reaction and tissue damage.

Natural killer cells

These lymphocytes are neither B- nor T-cells and it appears they may have a role in helping to prevent cancers (Wilson, 1995).

Immune deficiencies

Immune deficiencies can be can be broadly divided into two categories: primary or congenital immunodeficiency – including B- or T-cell defects and secondary or acquired immunodeficiency – resulting from malignancy or immunosuppressive therapy.

They can be further divided in to seven main groups:

1. Disorders of the non-specific immune system
2. Neutropenia and neutrophil dysfunction
3. T-cell deficit
4. Hypogammaglobulinaemia
5. Complement deficiencies
6. Splenectomy
7. Immunodeficiency associated related to haematological or other malignancy, intensive chemotherapy or after transplant

The host defences of a patient with cancer are undermined by the underlying disease, the therapy required to treat that disease and the interventions (iatrogenic manipulation) that take place. The severity of immunocompromise means that the patient is more susceptible to micro-organisms that would not cause infections in individuals with an adequate immune system.

The effects of cancer on the immune system

It is very rare that immunodeficiency can be classified as having a singular cause. As previously stated, patients with cancer are affected not only by the cancer but by their treatment and even by the care they receive. The type and severity of immunocompromise will indicate which infection they are particularly susceptible to (see Table 15.2).

It must also be noted that less easily recognizable stresses on the patient's immune systems, such as poor nutritional status, will have an impact on his or her ability to fight an infection.

Table 15. 2 Common deficits in immune function and the infections with which they are associated

Immune deficit	Caused by	Bacterial infections	Other infections
Complement	Congenital	Neisserie spp Streptococcus pneumoniae	
Spleen	Surgery, trauma, sickle cell anaemia	S. pneumoniae Haemophilus influenzae (type B)	Plasmodium spp Babesia spp
Gammaglobulin	Congenital, multiple myeloma, CLL, AIDS	S. pneumoniae H. influenzae	Pneumocystis carinii Giardia intestinalis Cryptosporidium parvum
Neutrophils	Chemotherapy, bone marrow transplantation	Enterobacteriaceae Oral streptococci Pseudomonas aeroginosa Enterococcus spp	Candida spp Aspergillus spp
T-cells	Marrow and other transplants, AIDS, cancer chemotherapy	Listeria monocytogenes Mycobacterium tuberculosis M. avium-intracellulare Salmonella spp Rhodococcus equi	P. carinii Toxoplasma gondi Cryptosporidium parvum Leishmania spp Herpes virus spp Histoplasma spp

In addition, the patient with cancer is now more likely to receive intensive care than ever before. Due to the severity of their illness and the level of iatrogenic manipulation, intensive care patients have always reported a higher level of nosocomial (hospital-acquired) infection (Inglis et al., 1992). In a medical–surgical ITU in the USA, a two-year study identified an acquired infection rate of 50% in oncology patients (Velasco et al., 1997). They identified a positive correlation rate between the use of devices (ventilator, indwelling urinary catheter and central venous catheter, etc.) and the incidence of nosocomial infection.

Immune suppression can be very specific and cause depression of the cellular immune response limiting T-cell responses. It can also be totally non-specific and impair the whole system's function. Haematological diseases that affect the bone marrow, for example, also affect the production of cells. For example, in leukaemia, immature or abnormal white blood cells are produced, while normal cell production is suppressed.

The organs of the immune system are vital in fighting disease; see Table 15.3 for a list of these organs and their functions.

Table 15.3 Organs of the immune system

Organ	Function
Bone marrow	Production of cells
Spleen	Filter and destroy foreign matter
Liver	Filter and destroy foreign matter
Lymphoid tissue	Filter and destroy foreign matter
Lymph nodes	Contain macrophages and lymphocytes

The system is connected and the nodes closest to the site of infection will provide the greatest number of lymphocytes and macrophages in the early stages of infection. This is why they appear swollen.

It is clear, therefore, that any cancer which affects the lymphatic system or one of the aforementioned organs of the immune system has the capacity to induce a state of immunodeficiency.

The effects of treatment on the immune system

Many immunosuppressive therapies are used in the course of modern medical care and they are on the increase. This has led to a comparative increase in the incidence of acquired or secondary immunodeficiency. This is often related to the use of drug therapies such as corticosteroids and cyclosporin (Pryor et al., 1996). The anti-rejection attributes of these drugs reduce the effects of host cytotoxic and natural killer cells – an essential part of the body's response to infection. In addition, the anti-inflammatory nature of these drugs also inhibits the body's inflammatory response, which will delay the onset of signs indicating an infection (attenuated clinical signs) (Antrum, 1996). This leads to difficulty diagnosing infection, as often the traditionally perceived signs of infection, e.g. raised temperature, inflammation and pain are not present until very much later in the infection process (Ringden et al., 1991).

Cytotoxic treatments currently used in cancer care have highly toxic effects (see Table 15.4) and serious consideration must be given to the risk of infection to this group of patients. The combination of the effects on the immune system of the disease process compounded by the effects of the treatment increase the risk of infection considerably. The precautions required to protect patients are described below.

Table 15.4 The effects on the immune system of drug treatment for cancer

Effect/side effect	Result
Bone marrow suppression	Reduction in production of cells
Nausea and vomiting	Potential dehydration and poor nutritional status
Extravasation of intravenous fluid (escape from of fluid into surrounding tissue)	Necrosis of surrounding tissue with increased risk of localized infection
Renal impairment	Reduced production of urine and subsequent mechanical flushing of genitourinary system
Hepatic impairment	Reduced efficiency in filtering as part of lymphatic system

Common infections in oncology patients

Individuals with fully functioning immune systems are still susceptible, at times, to infection. People with cancer, whose immunity has been affected by both the disease process and the treatment, can be affected by the organisms that cause disease in a host with normal immunity. They can also, however, develop infections as a result of micro-organisms with low virulence (infectiousness) which are incapable of causing infection in a host with a non-compromised immune system. In one study, persistent infection combined with other complications was found to be the primary cause of death in a group of immunocompromised patients (Ringden et al., 1991). This caused a greater number of deaths than progression of the underlying disease, which preceded bacterial and fungal infection alone as a cause of death.

Often these organisms are part of the normal bacterial flora of a person and it requires considerable skill to interpret the implications of the presence of such micro-organisms. Differences between carrying an organism (colonization) and infection by an organism need to be clarified as the implications are very different for each case (see Table 15.5)

Table 15.5 Colonization and infection

Colonization:	When a microbe establishes itself in a particular environment such as a body surface without producing disease. These organisms are known as commensal organisms. However, they are capable of causing disease if virulent or if the host is compromised.
Infection:	When a harmful micro-organism enters the body and multiplies in the tissue.
	In the host with a normal immune system the commensal organisms pose no threat day to day. If the immune system becomes depressed these commensal organisms have the potential to take advantage and become able to cause disease in the host: the organism develops pathogenic capabilities. This is known as *opportunistic* infection.

When caring for patients with cancer, therefore, infection control measures extend not only to the prevention of entry of *normally* harmful micro-organisms to the body, but they also aim to reduce the risk of colonization by organisms that may potentially be harmful to the immunocompromised host. A smaller number of micro-organisms may be able to cause infection in a patient who is immunocompromised in comparison to a host with normal defences.

Problem organisms for cancer patients

Fungal infections

Candida

Candida infections have been increasing in incidence over the last 20 years and are often associated with patients with compromised immune systems. Candida septicaemia, preceded by oral candida, has been reported as a cause of death in immunocompromised patients

(Mills et al., 1994). A variety of types of candida are reported: *Candida albicans* accounts for 46% of those identified (Wingard, 1995).

It is resident in or on the normal flora of the mucous membranes of mouth, intestinal tract and vagina. It causes local infections of mouth, e.g. thrush, or less frequently reported widespread systemic disease, for example a rare occurrence that predominantly affects the lungs and more rarely the heart, kidneys and meninges. Predisposing factors for infection by candida include immunocompromise and pregnancy.

Aspergillus

Aspergillus infection is caused by a variety of types of aspergillus with *A. fumigatus* being the main pathogen. It is resident in soil and dust particles. The infection may come about as a result of superficial infections in the ears, burns and surgical wounds, and pulmonary aspergillosis may arise after the patient has inhaled fungal spores. The patient may be affected by:

1. The growth of a fungal ball in an existing tuberculous cavity
2. The development of an allergic form of hypersensitivity
3. Invasive aspergillosis when the lung infection spreads to other organs.

Predisposing factors to such an infection include severe immunosuppression, and exposure to building work.

Bacterial infections

Enterobacter

This group of organisms comprises a large number of Gram-negative bacilli. Many are normal residents of the gastrointestinal tract of human and animals but some are pathogenic. *Escherichia coli* (E. coli) is a normal resident of the gut.

Enterobacters are the commonest cause of urinary tract infections, but they also cause wound infections, septicaemia and biliary tract infection. Specific types can cause neonatal meningitis, traveller's diarrhoea and infantile gastroenteritis. In the immunocompromised patient, chest infections have been reported associated with altered respiratory tract flora as a result of extended antibiotic therapy.

Predisposing factors include hospital admissions (E. coli has been reported as responsible for approximately one-quarter of HAI), immunocompromise.

Klebsiella

This is a normal resident of the gut. It causes urinary tract infection, wound and respiratory tract infections, and predisposing factors include hospital admission (particularly intensive care admission), antibiotic therapy and immunocompromise.

Salmonellae

Salmonellae are normal residents of the gut in man and animals. They cause 'food poisoning' and enteric fever (the latter caused by S. typhi and S. paratyphi). Sufferers can go on to develop bacteraemia and associated bone, joint or meningitic infection. Immunocompromise is a predisposing factor.

Shigellae

This is another normal resident of the gut in man and other animals which causes dysentery (diarrhoea with blood). The tropical type of this disease produces severe symptoms but in the UK symptoms are less severe. Some outbreaks have been associated with hospitals for people with learning difficulties who may have some congenital immunocompromise.

Streptococcus

These oval-shaped organisms form pairs or chains and are a very complex group which can be harmless commensals or devastating pathogens. They can be resident on mucous membrane and cause a wide variety of infection problems (see Table 15.6). The organism has the potential to cause outbreaks of infection in the hospital and is therefore treated quite aggressively in the inpatient setting.

Table 15.6 Streptococcal infections

TYPE	ILLNESS CAUSED
Beta-haemolytic streptococcus group A	Tonsillitis, scarlet fever, wound infections, impetigo
Beta-haemolytic streptococcus group B	Septicaemia and meningitis in neonates
Streptococcus pneumoniae	Exacerbation of chronic chest disease, pneumonia, sinusitis, otitis media and conjunctivitis
Viridans-type streptococcus	Infective endocarditis after entry to bloodstream

Staphylococcus aureus

Staphylococcus aureus is carried by approximately 40% of the population. In normal circumstances the micro-organism is a commensal of the skin, but it readily becomes a pathogen. It is responsible for a large number of hospital-acquired wound infections and septicaemias.

It is resident on the anterior nares (front of the nose), and less frequently the axilla, vagina and mucous membranes.

Staphylococcus aureus causes superficial abscesses, carbuncles and impetigo, as well as more serious infections such as wound infections, osteomyelitis and septicaemia.

Predisposing factors include immunocompromise and iatrogenic manipulation

Pseudomonas

This organism is found predominantly in moist areas in the hospital setting and poses a risk to patients with cancer, particularly as many reported cases are opportunistic. Pseudomonas can be found in stale flower water and is the cause of rot in some fruit and vegetables. In the past transplant wards have barred fruit or flowers from being brought in by friends and relatives, and some still do so. There remains a debate on whether these sources provide a true risk. Pseudomonas infection is usually easily recognizable by the presence of a very distinctive sweet odour and green pus which has been coloured by pyocyanin, a blue–green pigment.

Pseudomonas is found in water and soil and in the gut. Patients in hospital who have had antibiotic therapy are more likely to be colonized. Equipment including ventilator humidifiers, ice machines and contaminated antiseptic solutions have been reported as the source of outbreaks.

Pseudomonas causes respiratory tract infections and wound infections, but it most often colonizes chronic ulcers and pressure sores.

Predisposing factors: previous antibiotic therapy, chronic wounds, chronic chest disease, immunocompromise.

Listeria

This infection can exhibit very mild symptoms, such as headache and nausea, or none at all in individuals with normal immune systems. In the immunocompromised host symptoms appear subacute and can lead to collapse and delirium. Lesions that affect the liver and other organs may occur with external abscesses.

Listeria is resident in soil, water, unpasteurized soft cheeses and milk. It causes meningoencephalitis and/or septicaemia, and abortion in pregnant women. Predisposing factors include immunocompromise, and it tends to affect the very young and the elderly.

Tuberculosis

This infection remains the biggest killer worldwide as a result of infectious disease. Mycobacterium tuberculosis predominantly affects the lungs (pulmonary tuberculosis), causing development of lesions, but it can also affect other organs and tissues (extrapulmonary tuberculosis). If untreated, approximately half of patients will die within five years. Adequate and appropriate chemotherapy almost always results in eradication of the infection. The immunocompromised patient also responds well to therapy. There has, however, been an increased incidence of tuberculosis which is resistant to the drugs commonly used to treat the infection. Drug resistance is discussed below.

Mycobacterium tuberculosis is resident in infected humans (primarily pulmonary), and it causes lung lesions, lymph node calcifications, meningitis, involvement of the pleura, kidneys, bones and joints, skin and the gut.

Predisposing factors to infection include immunocompromise, poor nutritional state and socio-economic group (reported incidence is greater in social classes IV and V).

Viral infections

Viruses are responsible for the majority of infections affecting humans. In most cases the infection is mild and self limiting, but some have the ability to cause latent infection and others, such as the rabies virus, are almost always fatal. Viruses are not effectively treated with antibiotics but there are developments in the field of antiviral therapy. Many viruses may result in secondary bacterial infection, which *can* be treated effectively with antibiotics. Patients who are severely immunocompromised are particularly susceptible to a variety of common viral infections, and normally innocuous infections have the potential of being life threatening in a person whose defences are damaged.

Varicella (chickenpox)

Chickenpox is an infection common in children and causes a maculopapular rash developing into vesicles. These vesicles appear on the trunk or face and can spread to the limbs. It causes a rash with irritation, and complications include encephalitis and pneumonia. Disseminated lesions are common in the immunocompromised. Secondary bacterial infection of the lesions can occur if they are scratched or contaminated.

Zoster (shingles)

Shingles is the reactivation of infection that has been latent. Immunocompromised patients may develop another infection as their immune system becomes further depressed as a result of anti-cancer therapy. It is not a result of contact with a person with shingles or chickenpox but *is* capable of causing varicella in a person who has not had it.

It is characterized by painful lesions corresponding to particular dermatomes. Patients are often left with a severe neuralgia.

Immunocompromised patients are very susceptible to varicella–zoster infection and morbidity is relatively high. Patients on chemotherapy are at particular risk and are advised to contact their oncologist if a rash develops. Affected patients may be treated successfully with acyclovir.

Cytomegalovirus (CMV)

The presence of antibody to cytomegalovirus in a large proportion of the population indicates that CMV infection is prevalent but causes very little serious infection in the host with a normal immune system.

Cytomegalovirus causes a glandular fever-like illness and very rarely, hepatic disease, retinitis and pneumonitis.

Epstein-Barr virus (EBV)

This causes many symptomless infections and glandular fever, which is characterized by sore throat, lymphadenopathy, pyrexia and general malaise.

Drug-resistant organisms

Antibiotics have been used to treat infections for over 40 years and during this time the bacteria that cause the infections have developed a variety of mechanisms to reduce the effectiveness of the therapy. Acquired resistance occurs with excessive, and sometimes inappropriate, use of antibiotics. A clear example of this acquired resistance is MRSA (methicillin-resistant Staphylococcus aureus). S. aureus was initially always sensitive, i.e. treatable with penicillin, but with the increased use of antibiotics in the 1950s the organism developed resistance. Now, it is estimated that only 10% of all S. aureus are sensitive to penicillin. A number of different types of MRSA have been identified and a total of 16 types of epidemic strain MRSA (EMRSA). The EMRSA have been reported as being more easily transmissible and in the hospital situation the rapid movement between patients has led to problems with outbreaks of EMRSA. Methods of reducing and preventing the transmission of drug-resistant organisms are discussed below.

Minimizing the risk of infection

Acquired infections affect approximately 10% of all hospital inpatients, and patients with suppressed immune systems account for a large proportion of these cases. It is impossible to prevent all acquired infections in patients affected by cancer, but good practice will reduce the risks and improve the quality of care a patient receives.

If a patient with cancer does develop an infection it may be difficult to treat as previously described. It is essential that a proactive approach of preventative practice rather than curative practice is adopted. Individual clinicians and cancer centres/units have their own policies for prophylactic antibiotic cover for patients undergoing some chemotherapy regimes.

Key principles of infection control practice

All healthcare professionals are responsible for working in a way that affords protection to patients. Infection control practice has the additional benefit of protecting the staff providing the care as well. There is very little new about infection control practice and new national initiatives are focusing on the need to promote the fundamental aspects of nursing care.

Hand hygiene

Hand washing is the simplest, most cost effective way of preventing the transmission of infection in any setting (Wilson, 1995; Philpott-Howard and Casewell, 1994; Ayliffe et al., 1992). It is an issue that has been emphasized by infection control practitioners for many years but there is much evidence that many staff do not comply with recommended practices. This has been attributed to lack of knowledge, lack of motivation and very often lack of time as well. Consideration must be given, therefore, to ensuring that individuals' knowledge bases are such that they realize the implications of failing to wash their hands appropriately. Many of the organisms described previously are transmitted by contact and adequate hand hygiene will reduce this risk.

There are three main types of hand washing, which will provide different levels of hand decontamination. An assessment of the task to be undertaken must be performed to establish what method and products must be used.

How to wash your hands

Much hand washing is inadequate and does not effectively reduce the number of potentially harmful organisms from the hands. The following simple five-point exercise will ensure hand hygiene is effective:

1. Thoroughly wet hands under warm running water
2. Apply one dose of cleansing agent (this may be soap or antiseptic hand wash, according to which level of decontamination is required – see following section)
3. Using rubbing motion, cover hands with cleansing agent ensuring all surfaces are covered. Pay particular attention to thumbs, fingertips and between the fingers.
4. Rinse hands thoroughly under warm, running water ensuring all traces of cleansing agent are removed
5. Dry hands thoroughly.

Social hand wash

Product to use: soap (liquid soap is preferable).

This method will reduce the number of micro-organisms on the hands by physical means. It should be used before and after patient contact, before serving meals and after using the toilet.

Antiseptic hand wash

Product to use: antiseptic hand wash.

This method reduces by physical and chemical means the number of micro-organisms on the hand. It should be used prior to undertaking clean procedures such as wound dressing or catheter care, or after undertaking dirty procedures, or when there is a risk that hands have become contaminated with body fluids. Consideration may need to be given to using this method with immunosuppressed patients.

Surgical hand scrub

Product to use: surgical hand scrub.
This method again reduces the number of viable micro-organisms on the hand and should be performed prior to any surgical or invasive procedure such as insertion of central vascular devices. It must be noted that this method is always used in conjunction with additional protective equipment such as sterile gloves.

Use of protective clothing

Since the introduction of universal precautions in the late 1980s it has been accepted that additional precautions are needed to protect staff and patients from the risk of infection. A simple assessment of that risk will enable practitioners to identify what additional protective clothing is required for what task.

Protective clothing will also provide protection to a patient who is immunosuppressed, and consideration must be given to using gloves and aprons when caring for a patient in protective isolation. Isolation precautions will be discussed below.

Patient personal hygiene

When a patient's immune system is suppressed, they have increased risk of acquiring infection not only from external sources as described earlier, but also from themselves. All humans have a large number of micro-organisms living on them as part of the norm. Poor hygiene will enable these micro-organisms to move from their normal area of residence, for example the gut, to an area where they are not normally present; for example, the vagina in a woman, or possibly an open lesion. This enables the micro-organism to change from being a commensal, i.e. not causing disease, to a pathogen which does. It is important therefore, that patients are given guidance and support on how best to minimize the risk.

Hand hygiene

The importance of hand hygiene by staff was described in the previous section, but is also vitally important that patients be advised of the importance of their own standard of hand hygiene. Patients will only ever have to use the social hand wash method as they are unlikely to have the large number of organisms on their hands that healthcare workers do (patients who are performing their own intravenous therapy will be advised on additional measures to be taken). They should be advised to use the same five-point exercise, and also advised when to wash their hands. That is, before eating, after using the toilet and after blowing their nose or using tissues. The increase in washing and drying of hands may lead to some dryness, and a simple hand cream for both male and female patients will help alleviate this problem. It is important to prevent drying and cracking of the skin on the hands, as this provides an ideal portal of entry for micro-organisms.

Washing and bathing

It is important to ensure that each individual patient keeps as clean as possible within the limits of their illness and their own personal practices. The emphasis should be on a regular, but not onerous, routine of washing to ensure there is no buildup of organisms that may increase the risk of infection to themselves. The type of organism that will be present should not pose a risk to others, but will pose a risk to the patient as previously described. Ideally, a patient should shower on a daily basis. A shower is the method of choice as the running water supports the physical removal of resident organisms. Particular attention should be paid to thorough drying and checking of all skin creases to ensure there are no excoriated or broken areas. A perfume-free cleansing agent will assist in the maintenance of skin integrity as will a gentle, perfume-free emollient. Clothing and towels should also ideally be changed daily. This will prevent the collection of skin scales which harbour organisms.

Mouth care

Patients with cancer have an increased risk of developing mouth problems associated with their radiotherapy and chemotherapy particularly. This may be compounded by a reduced fluid intake and poor nutritional status. As a result, the incidence of Candida albicans (thrush) is considerably higher in this group of patients. In a patient with a normal immune system a topical infection of candida is not a major problem. However, in this group of patients candida has the potential of causing a gross systemic infection. Mortality rates from systemic fungal infection are high in cancer patients (Antrum, 1996). It is essential that a regular review of at-risk patients is undertaken by clinically skilled nurses. Twice-daily checks will ensure rapid identification of early onset fungal disease and antifungal therapy commenced immediately systemic infection is suspected.

Cleansing agents

There are many different types of products available for mouth care. In the main, patient preference is probably the best guide when choosing which one to use along with an adequate nursing assessment of the oral cavity (Pritchard and Mallett, 1995). For product types and their action see Table 15.7.

Table 15.7 Oral cleansing agents

Type	Action
Chlorhexidine 0.1–0.2%	Disinfectant action. Prevents accumulation of plaque and gingivitis. Tastes unpleasant but can be used for soaking dentures.
Hydrogen peroxide	Mechanical action of bubbles which loosens crusting and debris. Foaming effect can cause problems if cough reflex impaired – do not use unless suction available.
Sodium bicarbonate 1%	Loosens debris and cleansing action. If too concentrated causes damage to mucus.
Commercial mouthwashes	Useful for freshening mouth. Can have high alcohol content and cause discomfort.
Commercial toothpastes	Very useful if patient is able to brush teeth on his/her own or with minimal support. Foaming action can cause problems if cough reflex inhibited – see hydrogen peroxide.

Method

The best way to remove any debris or plaque that will provide a focus for infection is by using a small headed brush and the 'Bass' method (see Figure 15.4). Dental floss may aid patient comfort by removing debris from between the teeth. Oncology patients undergoing chemotherapy should be encouraged to keep routine appointments with their own dentist. They should not, however, embark upon treatment, including polishing and descaling, before the dentist has discussed the proposed treatment with the oncologist responsible for the patient's care.

Frequency

The type and frequency of mouth care will depend on the needs of the patient. Some factors, such as mouth breathing and oxygen therapy, will exacerbate dryness and therefore care aimed at moistening the mouth will be required more frequently, as often as hourly.

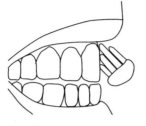

Place toothbrush at 45° angle at gingival margin.

Move brush in very small circular movements around teeth and gums.

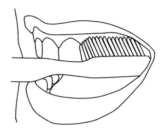

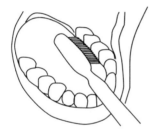

The brush will work subgingivally and collect plaque.

Figure 15.4 The Bass method of teeth cleaning.

Wounds, lesions and indwelling devices

Many patient will, as a result of treatment or disease, have a number of wounds, lesions or indwelling devices. It is essential that patients, as well as healthcare staff, are aware of what they are able to do to reduce the risk of infection from any one of these.

Wound management

When developing a plan of wound care patients can and should be involved in the decisions regarding their care. They should be advised of the importance of ensuring wound dressings remain intact and given information about what to do if the dressing becomes loose or falls off. It is also good practice to ask patients to leave dressings alone and not to attempt to loosen and remove them without a nurse being present, unless it has been previously agreed. This is to reduce the risk of the dressing becoming contaminated and then replaced on the wound. If a patient is able to replace a simple dressing, he or she should be given adequate instruction on technique and adequate supplies provided. Patients must be informed of the risks associated with touching and moving dressing on infected sites. This raises the risk of transferring infection from one site to another.

Lesions

The importance of lesions, even very small ones, as an infection risk is frequently underestimated. A lesion provides a portal of entry for infection and must be considered as important as a major wound. Care must be taken to minimize the risk of lesions, such as excoriation and pressure sores developing, in line with all good nursing practice (see washing and bathing). If a lesion does develop then regular – at least daily – checks of the site must be made. These checks must be documented to ensure that progress or deterioration is recognised. It may be useful to protect the lesion with a dressing but appropriate assessment of the lesion and other risks, such as other sites of infection, must be made.

Indwelling devices

Intravascular and central vascular devices

The majority of patients who require hospital care will at some time during their stay receive intravenous therapy for treatment or support (Angeles and Barbone, 1994). Most devices in cancer care are inserted in a planned manner and are used for chemotherapy. Many lines stay in situ for weeks and sometimes months, depending on the duration of the treatment. It is essential that all lines that provide access to the bloodstream are treated as a potential portal of entry for micro-organisms (Maki, 1987; Dennis et al., 1991). Because it leads directly into the bloodstream, the intravascular device has the potential of introducing a number of organisms into an ideal breeding ground. Septicaemia, or blood poisoning, is serious enough in patients with fully functioning immune systems, but in cancer patients it will be life threatening. The emphasis must therefore be on exemplary practice to reduce to an absolute minimum the risk of infection (Campbell, 1998; Vost, 1997; Clark, 1997).

The following key points must be addressed:

1. Assessment of the patient is undertaken to ensure the most appropriate venous access device (VAD) is used.
2. Full aseptic technique is adhered to when preparing the patient for insertion of the line. This includes hand decontamination for the operator, skin preparation of the patient and method used to insert the line.
3. Once inserted the line must be firmly secured with a sterile dressing.
4. Handling of the line must be kept to a minimum once inserted and any dressings changed using aseptic technique.
5. Patients must be advised about care of the line, even if they are inpatients who are not undertaking any of the care. This will ensure they can alert staff if a problem arises.
6. When the line is removed, aseptic technique must be used.
7. All aspects of intravascular device care must be documented in patients' notes.

Urinary catheters

Urinary catheters are used for a variety of reasons, including incontinence and obstruction. It is essential that prior to planning care the practitioner is aware of the reason for a patient being catheterized. Urinary tract infections account for approximately 30% of all hospital-acquired infections, and the majority are associated with urinary catheterization (Emmerson et al., 1996). It can be expected that within 72 hours of being catheterized a patient's bladder will become colonized with organisms that have the potential of becoming pathogenic (Ward et al., 1997). Careful consideration must be given to whether a patient needs a catheter or whether an alternative method may be used.

As with venous access device management, the emphasis must be on prevention of infection. The key points that must be addressed are as follows:

1. Consider whether the patient's problem may be better managed by an alternative method
2. When choosing a catheter, choose the smallest one that will do the job. Contrary to popular belief, the bigger the catheter the more likely it is to leak as it will cause intense mucosal irritation. It may also cause substantial trauma on insertion
3. Use aseptic technique for insertion
4. Use closed system of drainage to minimize risk of introduction of organisms
5. Ensure appropriate bag is used and when emptied use clean technique
6. Manipulate as little as possible. This applies to patient as well as staff.
7. Advise patient about care
8. Remove catheter at earliest opportunity.

Support for the patient and the family

Infection control is an issue that many patients will not have thought about at all until they are diagnosed with cancer, when they are forced to contend with a variety of practical and emotional issues. It is important, therefore, that practitioners are confident of their ability to support the patient and family by providing them with sensible, realistic advice about how to reduce the risk of infection. Some examples of effective methods are:

- Involving the patient and carers/relatives in the care planning process
- Patient information leaflets
- Accessing specialist nurses for advice
- Involving the patient and carers/relatives in the care planning process

This provides an opportunity for patients and relatives to ask questions at the outset of the care process. Notes should be made of questions asked, answers given and questions requiring further information or investigation. Encouraging integration of infection control recommendations in the core plan ensures this issue is not seen as a separate entity but as an integral part of the patient's care.

Patient information leaflets

Locally prepared information leaflets containing guidance on infection control practice for patients will provide the written information that patients often need. Written information allows time for an individual to read and decide what additional information they may require. Combining leaflets with other methods provides opportunities for relatives who are not with the patient at the time to find out what is expected of them.

Accessing specialist nurses

Many areas have infection control specialist nurses who, as part of their role, provide advice and information on reducing the risk of infection to staff and patients. They should be involved in the preparation of information leaflets and may visit patients with specific problems or queries.

Management of patients with infection problems

Caring for a patient with cancer and infection problems provides a challenge for the most experienced practitioner. Isolation precautions may be the only method by which other patients can be protected from the infection affecting this patient. It is important to emphasize that the patient remains the focus and the precautions taken are to isolate the organism not the patient. The aim is to prevent transmission of infection to other patients who may also be compromised.

In addition to the basic principles of infection control practice, some infections require additional measures to be taken to reduce the risk of transmission of infection to other patients and staff.

The commonest method used is source isolation. Attempts must be made to identify what type of infection the patient has and how that organism is transmitted. The precautions required will be dictated by whether the infection is contact spread or airborne spread. If this information is not available, precautions for airborne transmission should be implemented.

Precautions required for contact spread infection

A risk assessment must be undertaken prior to implementation of precautions and documented in the patient's notes. The following precautions are required:

- Single room, preferably with en suite facilities. If a patient is not suitable for caring for in a single room, the patient should be placed by a wash hand basin in the ward and all other precautions implemented.
- Staff to wash hands and don gloves and aprons prior to entering room. On completing care, gloves and aprons should be removed and disposed of in the room and hands thoroughly washed and dried with antiseptic hand wash.
- Bed linen should be changed daily as a minimum, more often if required. Linen should be treated as contaminated and local policy followed for disposal.
- Disposable crockery and cutlery are not required.
- Equipment for patient use should be dedicated to the patient for the duration of the treatment. Once treatment is completed all equipment must be removed and thoroughly cleaned.
- The room should be cleaned after all other areas on a daily basis. The equipment should then be thoroughly decontaminated. Once the room is vacated or the patient's infection problem resolved, the room should be given a full terminal clean which includes changing curtains. The room can then be re-used.

Precautions required for airborne (aerosol) spread infection

Precautions required are as for contact spread infection with the following additions:

- A single room is essential, with the door kept closed. The room must be well ventilated.
- A mask may be required in addition to gloves and aprons. This should be put on outside the room and removed and disposed of in the room on leaving.

Psychological aspects of isolation

Many patients do not respond well to entering isolation for an infection problem. It is essential that they are given a full explanation of why isolation is required, the type of precautions others will be taking and how long they are likely to be isolated for. As far as possible, the patient's routine should not be changed and normal activities such as watching television, listening to the radio or reading should be actively encouraged.

A confused patient or someone with communication difficulties will experience problems in isolation due to the loss of contact with the general hustle and bustle of the ward area. In some circumstances it may be inappropriate to isolate such a patient despite the risk of infection. It is essential that when this occurs a full risk assessment is made and alternative precautions taken to limit the risk to others.

Case history

Angela

Angela Jones is the 27-year-old mother of Jack, who is two years old. She is married and lives 40 miles from the hospital. She has been admitted after a course of chemotherapy and prior to a bone marrow transplant. On admission she is accompanied by her husband and appears very anxious. This is her first time away from her family for any length of time and she expresses concern about Jack, who is going to be looked after by his grandmother.

The infection control precautions instituted for Angela are listed below, together with the rationale for each.

Aims

To minimize the risk of transmission of infection to the patient.
To reduce potential psychological and physical problems associated with isolation.

Infection control precautions	**Rationale**
Single room with wash hand basin and en suite facilities.	To encourage high standard of personal hygiene and staff hand hygiene.
Single-use disposable aprons and gloves, alcohol hand rub for staff use and adequate supply of liquid soap and paper hand towels must be available in the room.	To encourage greater compliance with precautions required to reduce risk of infection.

Equipment to be used by the patient should be cleaned prior to use and placed in room for duration of stay if possible.	To facilitate ease of access to clean equipment for use by patient.
Written and verbal information should be made available to patient on additional measures required to reduce the risk of infection.	To ensure patient has adequate information about hygiene issues related to her care and to enable her to revisit information at her convenience.
Full body screen of patient to identify commensal organisms.	To establish whether prophylactic antibiotic therapy is required to reduce microbial load.
Advice should be given about limiting visitors to reduce risk of exposure to unknown risks of infection. Consideration must be given to the adverse psychological effects of limiting Jack's visits and care planned accordingly.	Visitors may unknowingly have an infection which is a risk to the patient. Children are exposed to a large number of potentially pathogenic organisms and Jack may be a risk to his mother.

Conclusions

Good infection control practice ensures that patients and staff are not put unnecessarily at risk from infection. Methods that afford protection to both staff and patients are simple, cost effective and promote high quality patient care. Infection control has been seen as uninteresting in the past and there is still little new. However, with the focus on the patient, working in such a way that reduces the risk of pain and discomfort, unnecessary interventions and possibly untimely death, should be every healthcare worker's aim. The implementation of simple precautions such as hand washing will increase the quality of care a patient receives and will ensure that they continue to have confidence in the individuals providing that care.

Chapter 16
Body image and sexuality

JANIE WHITTAKER
CARMEL SHEPPARD

Introduction

This chapter begins to explore the concepts of body image and sexuality relating to patients with cancer. Society places a heavy influence on the formation of self-concepts, and the expectations of body image and sexuality. It is therefore important for nurses to explore their own attitudes in relation to this subject when attempting to support the cancer patient, and thereby avoid the danger of hindering the therapeutic relationship.

Body image and sexuality

The concepts of body image and sexuality are closely entwined and difficult to separate, as they are interwoven with every aspect of daily life. This chapter will attempt to explore the possible effects of cancer treatments on both body image and sexuality within the biological and the psychological domains.

'Volumes are now written and spoken upon the effects of the mind on the body. Much of it is true. But I wish a little more was thought of the effect of the body on the mind' (Florence Nightingale, 1859 cited in Price, 1990, p.xii).

Despite Florence Nightingale's words, and the notion of holistic care mentioned in many nursing models, it is easy to forget the importance of body image and the effects that altered body image may have on the physical and mental wellbeing of the patients; particularly within the environment of a busy surgical ward. Cancer is often a prolonged illness with acute and chronic phases. Patients with cancer have prolonged contact with their health professionals, which makes it easier to address their holistic needs.

Traditional medicine has paid little attention overall to the effects of the body on the mind, yet one assumes both of these are intrinsically linked.

Plato suggested that 'I am a mind which just happens to be associated with a body; I am chained to my body, until death unchains me from it' (cited in Hospers, 1990, p.266). Descartes argued that 'it would be possible for you to exist without any body at all. Bodies happen to be the means whereby we are enabled to identify other persons; we can perceive their bodies and thus know that they exist' (cited in Hospers, 1990, p.267). Both of these quotations leave little more than an overall suggestion that the body is merely something to which we are chained and serves little relevance other than to let others recognize our existence; that it is the mind which represents the real 'I'. Assuming, then, that the mind is the person, what is the mind? Hospers (1990) suggests that the word 'mind' is a collective name for all your experiences, just as society is a collective name for a large group of individual persons. Thus, we are all unique and our experiences will differ. Nelson-Jones describes individuals' self-concepts as 'unique complexes of many different conceptions which constitute their way of describing and distinguishing themselves' (Nelson-Jones, 1995, p.32).

Dryden (1990, p.125) suggests that the 'self-concept develops over time and is heavily dependent on the attitudes of those who constitute the individual's significant others'. Similar views regarding individual sexuality were reported by Masters and Johnston, 1982, p.3:

> every person has sexual feeling, attitudes and beliefs but everyone's experience of sexuality is unique because it is processed through an intensely personal perspective. This perspective comes from both private and personal experience and public social sources. It is impossible to understand human sexuality without recognizing its multidimensional nature.

This indicates that self-concepts and sexuality may be influenced not only by significant others, but also by society in general. The media heavily influence how we look, how we act, our political beliefs, what class and social status we hold, women's and men's role in society, body image, sexual beliefs, etc. There is evidence that society depicts attractive people as more intelligent, attractive children are more likely to do well at school, and attractive adults are more likely to gain employment (Adams and Cohen, 1976, cited in Price, 1990, p.4). Another example of society's influence on attitudes can be seen in the change of attitude from the Victorian preference for well-rounded bodies to the modern preference for the thin, shapeless waiflike bodies of current supermodels.

All this suggests that people are likely to make judgements according to how a person looks. We are all guilty of making judgements of others; however, it is important to remember that our judgements may not always be correct. It is often incorrectly assumed, for example, that the elderly are not sexually active, and that body image and sexuality is less important to them than to younger people.

Irrespective of age, race, appearance, gender, etc., many forms of cancer may have a devastating effect on both the physical and psychological domains – including organic impotence in the male following low anterior resection for rectal cancer or cystectomy. During radical cystectomy for male bladder tumour, it is necessary to cut the nerves that are essential for erection (Joels, 1989). Many of the men who undergo this procedure are aged from the late sixties upwards. Ageist theorists might conclude that at this age sexual intercourse should not be a relevant issue for consideration. However, sexual activity should not be regarded as a pursuit for the younger age group only; sexuality and its effect upon our lives often only ends upon our death. Borwell (1997) explains that 'sexual expression is not simply sexual intercourse but encompasses human contact, comfort security and self worth, which provides cohesion within a relationship'.

The male patient who has had a cystectomy will have to deal with an alteration in both body image and sexual function. It is important to recognize that an inability to achieve an erection does not exclude the need for physical intimacy. As William Shakespeare concluded: 'is it not strange that desire should so many years outlive performance?'

For these groups of patients cancer and its treatment have affected not only their physical domain but also their psychological domain. Every day, these patients have visible evidence of the effect the cancer has had upon their body. For example, patients with urostomy will have to empty and change their urostomy pouches every day, reinforcing this constant reminder. This does not offer much of an opportunity to explore the phase of denial that many patients experience within the process of grieving, as described by Kubler-Ross (1970). Equally, there may be a tendency for society to assume that a less attractive person would be less likely to suffer psychological problems as a result of an altered body image than someone who might be considered attractive.

People may also assume that a male patient would care less than a female about an alteration in body image, but care more about an alteration in his sexuality. Women may be affected by the loss of a breast, hysterectomy, and/or removal of the vagina. These limited examples by no mean encompass the total arena of bodily cancers and their effects. Simple skin cancers, although easily treated and not life-threatening, can leave significant scarring.

Nurses may make assumptions and judgements about patients based on their own personal beliefs. Consequently, there is a danger that unless nurses are aware of their own beliefs, judgements and prejudices, the care of the patient will be far from holistic, and that the patient's psychological needs may not be addressed. Fallowfield (1991, p.23) suggests that 'Healthy psychological functioning, that is freedom from anxiety or depression and the ability to adapt and adjust to different illness states, is crucial for the maintenance of a good quality of life. It may even sustain life.' Maslow (1943, cited in Burns, 1980, p.110) describes each of us having a core pyramid of hierarchical needs in order to become fully functioning. Any interruption of this pyramid prevents us from achieving our full potential thus leading to dysfunction. Included in self-esteem needs is the need for self confidence, self respect, recognition and respect.

Maslow suggests that satisfying these needs leads to feelings of self worth. However, an inability to satisfy these needs can lead to feelings of weakness, loss of confidence, and helplessness (see Figure 16.1).

In helping the patient to achieve healthy psychological functioning, it is essential that the nurse has an understanding of the meaning of altered body image, and the ways in which altered body image might affect the patient's self-concept. If they can master this, nurses can begin to understand their patients better and focus on helping them adjust to their diagnosis and altered body image.

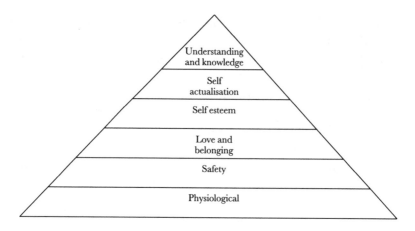

Figure 16.1 A hierarchy of need based on Maslow, 1943.

Dryden (1990, p.125) suggests that 'the need for positive regard or approval from others is overwhelming and is present from earliest infancy', Price (1990, p.4) suggests that body image is made up from three factors:

- Body reality – 'the way in which we perceive and feel about our body' (i.e. fat, thin, tall, small)
- Body presentation – 'how it responds to our command' (to include not only dress but also actions and pose)
- Body ideal – how we would like to look and be seen by others; a touchstone by which we judge ourselves.

The diagnosis of cancer may engender many fears and assumptions in relation to a patient's personal beliefs about cancer, all of which may affect body image. These may include fear of isolation from others, which may have come from a belief or stigma that cancer might be contagious. Thus, they may consider themselves unclean, or dirty and in turn avoid others for fear of rejection. A study in 1982 by Peters-Golden (cited in Fallowfield, 1990) found that of 100 healthy individuals, 61% suggested they would avoid physical contact with a friend suffering from cancer; 50% of patients diagnosed with breast cancer felt that others avoided them. It is also not uncommon to hear of patients visualizing an alien, or something with tentacles, invading and taking over their bodies. Thus the patient may come to avoid touching, and rejecting the affected part of their body, and may also avoid or push away others whom they have intimate contact with. Nurses too may adopt avoidance, or use blocking techniques to escape difficult situations with cancer patients. As well as the stigma and associated body image feelings resulting from the diagnosis of cancer, treatments equally can have devastating effects as demonstrated in Table 16.1.

It is important to understand that the side effects listed are by no means universal to all patients. However, it is vital that the information given to patients is reflective of their specific illness and treatments.

Breast cancer

Historically the importance of the breast has been represented in a number of different ways. Within the art world the breast is often representative of beauty, femininity and female sexuality. Images of a young infant attached to its mother's breast remind us of the importance of the breast in bonding, nurturing and expressing love and affection. The importance of the breast in terms of power has also been suggested (Richardson and Robertson, 1993). The women's liberation movement in the 1960s burned bras in protest against men's ideological control and stereotyping. It might, however, be argued that some women emphasize and use their breasts in order to gain control. A further almost unavoidable representation of the breast is the seductive and sexually arousing nature of breasts as portrayed by various media and advertising channels.

With constant exposure to the 'body ideal' in the media it is not surprising that any alteration or threat of loss of the breast can have devastating effects on the patient's self-concept and psychological wellbeing. The importance of the breast will vary in each individual. For some women the breast is significant part of their persona, femininity, sexual attractiveness, and sexual relationship. As well as having an effect on their body ideal, it may also have an effect on their body presentation. It is not uncommon to see women alter their posture after a mastectomy, becoming far more round shouldered in an attempt to conceal their chests. The way in which a woman dresses post-mastectomy may also alter, resulting in a complete change of wardrobe. Low-plunging necklines, sleeveless dresses and figure hugging clothes may no longer be acceptable to the patient.

Table 16.1 The effect of cancer treatments

Treatment	Effect	Outcome
Chemotherapy	Alopecia	Loss of their 'crowning glory' (head hair). Loss of pubic hair, and other bodily hair – leading to feelings of being child-like, regression and loss of sexual identity
	Weakness/lethargy/apathy	Feeling of weakness from being unable to fight infection/bone marrow suppression and anaemia
		Loss of libido, motivation and feelings of depression sometimes leading to a distortion of reality
	Loss of fertility	Altered perception of sexuality, and the ability to be a fully functioning human being
	Nausea and vomiting	Loss of weight, physical appearance of wasting
Radiotherapy	Skin dryness	Burning skin may interfere with intimacy. Patients are unable to use deodorants on the treated area which may lead to feelings of being dirty or unclean
	Lymphoedema	Further evidence of disease, and alteration of body image due to limb swelling
	Alopecia	If cranial contents or scalp are treated (this can be permanent)
Endocrine treatments	Weight gain/loss menopausal symptoms, hirsutism, amenorrhoea, hair thinning	Decline in sexual interest and activity due to vaginal dryness, loss of femininity/masculinity, alteration in body image
Surgery	Scars/loss of limb/ or alteration of anatomy	Sense of grief. Loss of identity or self. Feelings of mutilation. Loss of femininity/masculinity. Sexual dysfunction – organic or psychogenic

The patient may visualize the cancer invading her body, or regard the cancer as something alien or dirty. Many patients still fear that cancer may be contagious, and it is important not to dismiss this fear out of hand without giving the patient the opportunity to express her fears.

The patient's altered view of her body may make her feel overwhelming disgust, and she may even be unable to look at or touch the breast. Patients may continue these thoughts after surgery, regardless of the type of surgery. For this reason, some women may, if given the option, choose to have a mastectomy rather than a local excision of the cancer, as for them it may be easier to visualize that the cancer has gone along with their breast. Fallowfield et al. (1986) demonstrated no differences in psychological outcome amongst women undergoing wide local excision compared with those undergoing mastectomy. It is essential, therefore, that all women be given a choice of surgery. Equally, some women may insist on both breasts being removed, not only for fear that the other may be affected but also because they feel let down by their body, or that they cannot cope with the idea of an asymmetric bodily shape. Other women may not feel that they can cope with the loss of a breast and therefore may seek advice on breast reconstruction. Advice may also be given regarding the availability of adhesive prostheses.

Fortunately, the presentation of a patient with a fungating breast neoplasm is relatively rare; nevertheless, constant denial of the presence of a lump may eventually lead to fungation. In this regard Doyle (1980) says:

> Can we begin to imagine what it must feel like for a patient to see part of his/her body rotting and to have to live with the offensive smell from it, see the reaction of his visitors (including doctors and nurses) and to know that it signifies lingering death?

A sensitive approach to dealing with such patients is essential. Often the patient may feel guilt for having not addressed the problem earlier. Many of the patients will continue in denial, and may never wish to uncover or discuss their feelings in relation to the cancer. However, non-judgemental acceptance of the patient's condition and opportunities for counselling can be offered if the patient chooses to explore those issues. Practical solutions, such as odour-reducing dressings containing charcoal, may help to reduce the impact of the odour.

In caring for a woman with altered body image the nurse's primary role lies in offering time, support, acceptance, and the opportunity to discuss her fear; all of which are extremely valuable to the patient at this time. Whether or not the patient's breasts have previously been particularly important to her, an overwhelming feeling of loss and sadness may still be present. Practical help should be given on clothing and prostheses.

Many women feel that after a mastectomy they will no longer be able to wear lacy, attractive underwear, so it might be helpful to provide samples and picture of bras, prostheses and swimwear. Looking at the scar for the first time might be quite difficult, and some women may fear rejection from their partner. The breast plays an important part in many women's sexual relationships and patients may have concerns about this. Sheppard and Markby (1995) identify the experience many partners have in the sharing of altered body image. In their research one partner reveals his fears about looking at the scar: 'I would just like to know what I am going to be looking at ... I am a bit apprehensive at how I am going to look, if you like. I don't want to appear shocked to her ... I am not going to be horrified ... well I might.'

This suggests that both the patient and her partner need equal support in the discussion and exploration of their feelings in relation to future sexual intimacy.

Bowel cancer

Another area of possible significant altered body image for the patient is centred on the area of stoma formation for the treatment of bowel or bladder cancers. A stoma is an artificial opening on the body from which bodily fluids, usually urine or faeces, excrete. The patient has no control over defecation or urination and is technically now incontinent.

In Western society faecal and urinary incontinence are primarily associated with children or, at the other end of the spectrum, the very old. These conditions are considered to be dirty and unacceptable (Reeves, 1984). When children are able to control elimination they are rewarded positively with love and support from their parents (Morrow, 1976) and are taught that defecation is undertaken in private in a locked room or cubicle. Stoma formation and its function often leads to a negative alteration in body image and an alteration in body presentation as described by Price (1990). Body presentation concerns itself with how 'we are able to consciously review not only how our body looks but how it functions as an expression of our will, our intentions and our feelings' (Price, 1990, p.10).

Stoma patients are now unable to control how their body looks or how it functions, thus influencing how they feel about their altered body image. This in turn will affect the other domains of self-concept or body reality, as the stoma will have changed how the patient now sees his or her body. There will be scarring and the stoma itself protruding from the abdomen.

Body ideal is related to body function and how reliably it serves us. Stoma patients are now faced with an alteration in body function over which they can have no control. With the realization that their body has failed them and has developed cancer, it is not surprising that a number of patients experience difficulties adapting to their altered body image. Kelly writes (1985, p.7)

> what really alarmed me were the physiological consequences, especially the incontinence and the smell. These I believed would become the defining characteristics of my social identity and everything about me, my relationships and the way others viewed me would be conditioned by these.

It is important that such patients are supported by nurses and other healthcare professionals who have experience in discussing these issues. Failure to recognize the importance of this aspect of their care can have a devastating effect on the patient's life. The first time a patient visualizes his or her stoma, the nurse can support the patient by allowing them to express their feelings. By showing their acceptance of the patient and the stoma, the nurse will be giving the patient a basis to develop a positive response to their altered body image. Tschudin (1987, cited in Salter, 1988) illustrates this process of unconditional support:

> do you understand this grief of mine, my despair and my fear? I cannot stop thinking what is happening to me, I am not what I was a few weeks ago and I don't know who I am any more. How reassuring if we can say in reply 'yes, to me you are still you'.

Other patients may react in a different way and withdraw from intimacy and ultimately society, as fear of rejection by partners may override their need for an intimate relationship. This belief can be supported by the development of a pen-pal page in ostomate magazines published by the various manufacturing companies or delivery companies, in which patients with stomas seek out partners with stomas. Some of the readers of, and responders to, these pages reason that prospective partners from these adverts will be able to identify with their altered body image. In addition, these prospective partners will already have an understanding of an altered body image, and so it will not be so traumatic for them to have to explain their condition. Although these pen-pal pages are a help to their users, a more long-term solution for these patients would be integration into mainstream society and the opportunity to regain their self-esteem and a more positive body image. Some patients, acknowledging their fear of rejection and embarrassment, decide to withdraw from any intimacy, often rejecting their partners before their partners have an opportunity to even decide how they feel about their altered body image. White (1997) recognizes this response and concludes that:

> sometimes worries about rejection from a partner can be a reflection of thoughts you are feeling, such as 'I feel unattractive'; these thoughts are not usually what other people are actually thinking about you.

Practical advice from the stoma care nurse may be given, such as the wearing of a more discreet appliance during intimacy called a stoma cap (which is a small round device approximately 3 inches in circumference). Also, use of the drug Imodium as a method of reducing ileostomy output during sexual activity may help to allay a common fear among ostomates of appliance leakage during sex.

Colostomists may consider the use of a colostomy plug (a tampon shaped device that is inserted into the colostomy). This prevents faeces from being a discharged from the colostomy during intercourse and also stops embarrassing noise from the colostomy. It is, however, not suitable for all ostomates, only colostomists, and requires a period of training in its use.

Another option is the wearing of selected types of underwear, such as a teddy or camisole with an opening underneath, so that the appliance is hidden during intercourse. It can also be suggested to the patient and their partner that they try experimenting with alternative sexual positions for intercourse (Price, 1990).

Conclusions

Patients with cancer often experience alteration in both their perception of their body image and their sexuality. In recognizing this, nurses can assist patients by acknowledging that every patient will have an experience that is unique and individual. In addition, through reflective practice and clinical supervision, nurses can explore their own prejudices and inhibitions, and thus be able to offer the patient unconditional positive regard, and non-judgemental support. In this way the relationship can become one of trust and empathy in which the client feels understood and equal.

In attempting to explore the patient's world, the nurse should become aware of the emerging family dynamics, and the need to include the patient's social/external world in relation to his or her adjustment to an altered body image. Discussion, advice and support to both the patient and their partner can be undertaken separately or together. As with all relationships, often a lack of communication can cause barriers and misunderstandings. Often a simple open discussion in a supporting environment can help to bring down those barriers, enabling patients to develop a more positive body image and regain their previous sexual intimacy with their partners.

Support and advice from well informed nurses on the issues surrounding alteration in body image and sexuality can help to reduce anxiety on the part of both patients and their partners. It may also help reduce the feeling of isolation and fear of rejection. If patients are unable to adjust, intense counselling may be necessary. At this point it is essential that the nurse reassesses his/her ability to provide safe ongoing psychological care. Referral to a more appropriate agency, such as psycho-sexual therapist or qualified counsellor, should be considered.

Chapter 17
Complementary therapies

DEREK JOHN ACE

Introduction

Writing a chapter about complementary therapies is not easy. 'Complementary therapies' is a term that embraces strategies of intervention which are not controlled or readily recognized by the British Medical Association and generally not available through the National Health Service. However there is nothing sacred about modern medicine and we are only in the early stages of scientific discovery and control, but many doctors and nurses still condemn any suggestion that complementary health provision serves any useful purpose. Others show cautious optimism but are restricted by financial limits and considerations. In the field of palliative and cancer care there is a greater emphasis on holistic health and quality of life, and the use of supportive complementary strategies is increasingly valued. An enquiring mind and positive attitude by professionals, patients and in some instances relatives and significant others, can enhance feelings of worth and create feelings of wellbeing.

Medical techniques, including pharmaceutical, surgical and technological advances, are sophisticated and often effective, treating and maintaining optimum ability and capability for the majority of patients. Any painful or unpleasant side effects of treatment, irrespective of severity, are often disparaged and the patient rapidly learns that fortitude is an essential part of progress. Courageous coping therefore becomes admired and respected. But pain can lead to gloomy and depressing thought processes which may leave the patient and carers with little or no hope and even less control.

Orthodox, compassionate, holistic professional healthcare, including control of pain and other distressing symptoms, may be the only support necessary to nurture a change in philosophical outlook and improve ability to cope. The individual needs of cancer patients in the light of personal attitudes, beliefs and values, must be explored in order to build a supportive network of empathic understanding. Physical, social, psychological and spiritual dimensions often need sensitive exploration with multidisciplinary professional information and explanation.

Whether these options should include complementary therapies is debatable, however. There is a paucity of comprehensive and evidence-based research into such therapies, and hence a lack of scientific validation needed to prove their effectiveness beyond reasonable doubt. Couple this with unlegislated training, disparate and divisive leadership, and a vast range of strategies under the umbrella of complementary therapies, and you have the potential for non-recognition and limited control. This opens the door to charlatanism and the ultimate exploitation of vulnerable people. It is essential to protect patients from such exploitation if we are to meet the needs of an increasingly informed general public who are now prepared to share responsibility for their own health, welfare and wellbeing, and additionally satisfy the high professional standards demanded by doctors and other healthcare professionals.

Patients may welcome the opportunity to examine and explore complementary health supporting and health promoting strategies that offer effective control of distressing symptomology, and it is becoming almost impossible to ignore the increasing interest and demand for information and access to complementary therapies. This chapter will attempt to describe some of the better known and increasingly valued therapies, which are subdivided into the following categories:

Therapies that require physical touch and body manipulation
    Chiropractic and Osteopathy
    Massage (including reflexology)
Therapies that use naturally occurring organic substances
    Herbalism
    Aromatherapy
    Homeopathy

Therapies that rely on alternative philosophies and concepts
    Acupuncture
    Hypnosis

Chiropractic and osteopathy

The word 'chiropractic', from the Greek *cheiro* and *practikos* meaning 'done by hands', was used in 1895 by a Canadian doctor, Daniel Palmer, to describe a strategy of spinal manipulation to influence and relieve clinical symptoms of specific medical problems, especially where the problem is linked to poor posture and spinal misalignments. The theory underpinning the spinal manipulative strategy was based on the knowledge that all tissues and organs of the body are supplied with both motor and sensory nerves. Messages and instructions are interpreted and activated at a conscious and unconscious level to maintain a healthy balance in the body. The theory was that physical interference by spinal problems and misalignment could be corrected by skilled manipulation and pressure.

Historically some form of spinal manipulation has existed since Hippocrates and possibly much earlier, and has been evident in different forms in different cultures, for example the American practice of backwalking (Olsen, cited in Booth, 1993), and European 'bone setters' (Inglis, cited in Booth, 1993).

Currently chiropractic is one of the complementary therapies most accepted by the British Medical Council, which states:

> In the clinical practices of osteopathy and chiropractic, the basic training is largely grounded in the orthodox medical sciences and, as such, practitioners of these disciplines are able to have a close dialogue with their medical colleagues which is based upon a common language (BMA, 1993, p.6).

Although research is limited, a study carried out by Medical Research Council epidemiologists and rheumatologists concluded:

> For patients with low back pain in whom manipulation is not contraindicated, chiropractic almost certainly confers worthwhile long term benefit in comparison with hospital outpatient management. The benefit is mainly seen in those with chronic and severe pain. Introducing chiropractic into NHS practice should be considered (Meade et al., cited in Booth, 1993, p.54).

There are obvious similarities between treatment by an osteopath and a chiropractic in that each uses massage and manipulation to a greater or lesser degree. However, osteopathy has tended to place a greater emphasis on the circulation of blood and uses massage to stimulate blood flow and manipulation to correct misalignment. As a discipline it preceded chiropractic by 21 years (1874) when its founder Dr Andrew Taylor Still laid down the philosophy and principles of treatment. He developed the therapy in response to what he saw as the limits of medicine. Still was a deeply religious man who 'saw the body as a machine made in God's likeness and therefore perfect in design' (Trevelyan and Booth, 1994). The tragic death of three of his children with cerebrospinal meningitis alerted him to the limitations of medicine and motivated him to look for alternatives. Clearly the spiritual and scientific aspect of Still's theories are now dated and disputed, but the legacy of what appears to be an effective antidote to a variety of ailments and their symptoms still persists. A survey by Which (1986) cited in Trevelyan and Booth (1994) reported that 82% of patients using osteopathy said their problem was cured or improved by the treatment. As with chiropractors, the British Medical Association is beginning to accept and often recommend the use of an osteopath, but it still refuses to endorse the osteopath's right to diagnose, reserving that clinical responsibility for the medical profession.

Massage and reflexology

Massage can be described as the extension, standardization and normalization of touch arising from a primitive and instinctive means of communicating compassion, care and concern about another individual. Being touched and massaged where intent and consent are mutually acknowledged and agreed appears to provide a sense of security, comfort and healing. The need for touch extends from the cradle to the grave and is especially welcome in times of illness and crisis.

The history of massage can be traced back to 3,000 years before the birth of Christ when the Chinese produced a medical treatise called *Nei Ching*, which contains references to massage. The Indian books of the *Ayurveda*, written about 1800 BC, refer to massage as rubbing and shampooing, which they recommend as a means of helping the body to heal itself. Egyptians, Persians, Japanese, Greeks and Romans firmly believed in the benefits of massage. Homer in *The Odyssey* spoke of the restorative powers for exhausted war heroes of rubdowns with oil, and Hippocrates wrote in the fifth century BC: 'the physician should be experienced in many things but assuredly in rubbing, for rubbing can bind a joint that is too loose and loosen a joint that is too tight' (Fromant, 1991).

Massage strategies and techniques also have their variations. Some of the different methods available include aromatherapy, reflexology, Reichian therapy, rolfing, shiatsu, and Swedish massage. It is important to inform the client about the varieties available and what they entail. For example, reflexology is a sophisticated massage of the feet, or to a lesser degree the hands, having its origins in China and India. In addition to producing deep relaxation and a sense of wellbeing, reflexologists claim it can be used as a diagnostic aid and treat problems in other parts of the body.

Massage is therefore not just a form of healthy behaviour that can both stimulate and relax, but a potent form of interpersonal communication which crosses the boundaries of colour, culture, class and mental agility and ability. Obviously consideration must be given to the recipient's attitude to being touched, as fear and suspicion arising from bad experiences would need to be respected and the professional responsibility of always acting in the best interests of the patient must prevail.

The comedian Bob Hope once said 'If you don't cuddle you curdle' (Jackson, p.43). Perhaps uncurdling people with cancer should be an objective worth pursuing in the quest for improved management of the disease.

Therapies that use natural organic substances

Herbalism

'The Lord hath created medicines out of the earth: and he that is wise will not abhor them' (Ecclesiastes 38:4). Stanway (1986) points out that 'there are at least 350,000 known species of plants ... yet we have only looked at 10,000 plants from a medicinal point of view'. From earliest times man has used and later cultivated plants for food and to improve the taste of food. It is difficult to identify at what precise moment and in which culture various plants were found to have additional properties of pain relief and other health promoting and life enhancing effects.

The earliest evidence of the use of wheat and barley dates back to 6750 BC and was found during excavations in Iraq. By 3500 BC Egyptians were increasingly using herbs and relying less on magic to cure ailments and disease, but it is in China in 2600 BC that the Emperor Huang-Ti is credited with writing a herbal treatise on medicine. In India too the *Rig Veda* (one of the sacred books of the Brahmins) mentions the use of medicinal plants. However, it is generally accepted that the Egyptian Ebers Papyrus written about 1550 BC, which listed 800 botanical prescriptions, laid the foundation stones for Greek and Roman medicine and later developments in Europe and other regions.

The advent of the industrial revolution heralded a medical move away from the use of natural remedies, first by isolating and then extracting the specific substance that affected the outcome of an illness or disease, and then later chemically and biomedically changing and refining more remedies – thereby giving greater control over life-threatening and debilitating conditions. The drugs produced, for example antibiotics, allowed doctors to manage and control the disease process in a way that had never previously been possible. Dosages could be measured accurately and prescribed specifically to give optimum effect with minimum side effects. Unwanted side effects were inevitable, but often considered too minor to cause concern or, alternatively, controlled by other drugs as the need arose. By contrast herbal remedies appear to take longer to achieve the desired effect, there is limited control and legislation over standards and quality, doubtful accuracy of a measured dose and some doubt as to whether they work at all. Irrespective of these criticisms, herbal remedies are increasingly available and often used in preference to synthetic preparations. In some cases they are effective where orthodox treatment is unsuccessful. The knowledge gained and passed on by many generations cannot be ignored and, as Weiss (1998, p.10) says, 'It is one of the functions of modern science to unearth the treasure now partly buried under superstitious mystical concepts and learn to give it its rightful value'.

The British Medical Association (BMA 1993, p.107) states:

> It [was] unfortunate that there is such a gulf between the medical herbalists
> and the orthodox physicians ... It may be that the formulary of the medical
> herbalist has something to offer; and, indeed, many of our potent orthodox
> medicines were originally herbals.

Carefully chosen herbal remedies may not appear to be as effective as conventional cures but they may make a meaningful contribution to the quality of life of patients.

Aromatherapy

Aromatherapy, as the name implies, involves using substances that are scented and inhaled. Oils, classed as essential oils, are extracted by distillation and other processes, from trees, herbs, and other plants or parts of plants. For example, the orange plant produces the essential oil of orange from the fruit, pettigrain from the leaves, and neroli from the flower. The oils come from many countries and some, like herbs, have been used by the indigenous populations for generations.

They are administered in a variety of ways, including inhalation (burners and ionizers are often used to enhance this process); baths; where both inhalation and absorption through the skin can take place, and massage, using diluted oils.

The modern usage of essential oils for medicinal purposes is attributed to Rene Gattefose, who is reputed to have thrust his badly burned arm into a vat of lavender oil. The wound healed exceptionally fast and left no scar (Lawless, 1992 p.16). Gattefose also coined the word *Aromatherapie* in a scientific paper, and published a book of the same name in 1928. Although aromatherapy in its present form is a relatively new concept, the use of perfumes as antidotes, antiseptics, aphrodisiacs, cosmetics and even embalming fluids appear in the history of China, Egypt, Greece and Rome as far back as 3000 BC. The preservative properties of scented embalming fluid used in the mummification process have been a source of wonder and amazement to anthropologists and scientists. In England in the Middle Ages pine wood and perfumed candles were burned in homes to relieve symptoms and combat disease.

The medicinal, therapeutic and aphrodisiac properties of oils, including inhaled and absorbed concentrations, are open to debate. The dilutions used for massage are also low, adding to the controversy on effectiveness but supporting the safety aspects of the therapy. Additionally there has been little research into the claimed antiseptic, antibacterial and antiviral effects of essential oils, including their use for skin disorders and wound care. Other terminology associated with essential oils include 'aromatology' (oils used orally), aroma care, and even 'aromafun' (oils used for fun and pleasure).

Currently the preferred method of using oils is administration by massage. Not only do the oils get absorbed through the skin and inhaled but the time, touch and trusting relationship can result in feelings of relaxation and positive reinforcement of worth, rarely found in conventional medicine. The only problem is trying to isolate the relative contribution of the oils, the time, the touch and the skill and charisma of the masseur. Table 17.1 lists seven oils (the 'magnificent seven') chosen not only for their ability to enhance health and healing but also for their aromatic properties including blending compatibilities.

Table 17.1 Seven essential oils

Chamomile (Matricaria chamomilla)
A heavy, musty smelling oil with analgesic and sedative properties. Effective in many skin conditions including dermatitis, eczema, psoriasis, nappy rash and other rashes.
Eucalyptus (Eucalyptus globulus)
A strong camphoraceous oil with powerful antiseptic properties. Additionally has antirheumatic and analgesic properties and is useful for virtually all respiratory disorders.
Lavender (Lavandula augustifolia/officinalis)
Known as the king of essential oils, unsurpassed as an all-purpose oil.
Lemon (Citrus limon)
A fruity and fresh oil with antiseptic, fungicidal and mentally stimulating effects.
Rosemary (Rosemarinus officinalis)
A fresh, sweet and camphoraceous oil with many attributes including the ability to enhance concentration and memory.
Ti-Tree (tea tree) (Melaleuca alternifolia)
An extremely versatile oil with antiseptic and antiviral properties. A highly acclaimed oil with a spicy camphoraceous smell.
Ylang-Ylang (Cananga odorata)
A heavy, sweet, floral oil with sedative and aphrodisiac properties. Also effective against insomnia, anxiety, depression and stress.

Homeopathy

In the fifth century BC Hippocrates wrote there were two methods of healing: 'by contraries' and 'by similaris'. In the 18th century Samuel Hahnermann wrote: 'If I mistake not, practical medicine has devised three ways of applying remedies for the relief of disorders of the human body. The first

method is that of removing or destroying the cause of the malady ... the
second and most common, contrara contraris, that is healing by opposites ...
and the third similia similibus, that is, to cure disease, we must seek medicines that can excite similar symptoms in the healthy body.' (Hahnermann,
cited in Castro, 1990).

Hahnermann then developed a new method of dilution which he
called 'succusion' and which he claimed potentiated the remedy. The
method involved taking a substance and dissolving it in 100 ml of a
solvent (usually water or alcohol). Further dilutions were made by
taking one drop of the new solution and diluting it in another 100 ml
of water. This process was repeated up to another 29 times, by which
time it was called a 30th potency. The resulting submolecular level of
the original substance militates against any scientific effect, and as yet
the treatment cannot be explained by the laws of science as we understand them. One possible explanation is that the imprinted memory
of the original substance lives on in the prescribed homeopathic
medicine and it is this that acts as a catalyst stimulating a curative
body reaction.

There are obvious similarities to being vaccinated by a weak-
ened and attenuated substance that also stimulates the immune
system to develop antibodies and therefore prevent disease.
However, homeopathy uses much greater dilutions and can trigger
a response during, as well as prior to, the disease process. Other
theories of how it works explore the exploitation of human
suggestibility by a charismatic professional. However, Christopher
Day (an homeopathic vet) conducted an experiment to prevent
mastitis in cows. A herd of 80 cows was divided into two groups of
40. One group had an homeopathic remedy added to the drinking
water and the other had only water. The experiment lasted six
months and in the treated herd only 2 out of 40 cows developed
mastitis, compared to 18 out of 40 in the untreated herd (Horizon
television programme, 1991).

Homeopathy provides a safe strategy with no unwanted or
distressing side effects, providing for some a cure way beyond their
wildest expectations. Can we professionally justify not considering
the use of homeopathy, even for a short period, before embarking on
more damaging conventional treatments?

Therapies that rely on alternative explanations

Acupuncture

Acupuncture is a method of healing that originated in China and is thought to be over 5,000 years old. According to Chinese folklore, acupuncture was developed accidentally through observation and linking unconnected healing following a puncture wound. This was then followed by many years of investigation and development to produce an effective remedy for sickness, which is used in conjunction with health advice and guidance.

The philosophy underpinning acupuncture is based on the ancient Chinese belief that the material world is part of a cyclical movement of forces throughout the universe. People are affected both by changes in extrinsic energy (the elements and nature), and imbalances in intrinsic energy, which cause disease. Acupuncture provides a strategy for correcting destructive energy imbalances by the insertion of needles at specific points on the body, restoring balance by reducing or increasing energy to target organs or systems. The points lie on energy channels called meridians, which were often linked to and named for the internal organs they were associated with.

The links with the natural world could be seen by the fact that there were 365 points on 12 meridians, and each point was given a name corresponding to phenomena in the natural environment.

The Chinese called energy in the body the *Chi*, and this was divided equally between the meridians into Yin (negative) and Yang (positive). Since the Chinese see every illness as a result of energy imbalance, cures must aim at correcting that imbalance, but can only be effective if the degenerative process has not caused damage beyond natural repair.

The Chinese also stress the importance of treating the person, not the disease, which means the treatment strategy can only be implemented following an holistic examination which uses diagnostic strategies unfamiliar and often unacceptable to Western medicine.

The effectiveness of acupuncture in symptom control is evident by its increased popularity, often based on recommendations by satisfied customers. One day science may be able to categorically confirm or deny the theoretical concepts underpinning acupuncture;

until then adequately funded and professionally administered trials and research into effectiveness need to be conducted and the results distributed to professionals and patients.

Hypnotherapy

Hypnotherapy is the use of hypnosis in a wide variety of medical and psychological disorders. Integral to the successful use of hypnosis is a sound professional knowledge of psychotherapeutic theory and practice. Hypnosis can access and explore subconscious mechanisms, controls and functions, revive, relive and resolve previously unconscious and unacknowledged significant events and nuances and improve coping strategies. Hypnosis can be used as an independent therapy but its effectiveness may be enhanced when combined with other compatible psychological interventions. Hypnosis is undoubtedly an authentic phenomenon, and arguably the most effective method of relieving distressing mental symptomology including fear and anxiety. It can anaesthetize and reduce to an acceptable level the experience of pain, induce a state of imagined virtual reality, and redefine and reinforce the coping mechanisms for cancer patients. Indeed, one could argue that the influence of the mind on the central nervous system and subsequently the physical body could not only relieve distressing symptomology but inhibit the degenerative pathology of the disease process.

A possible explanation for the reluctance to use hypnosis lies in the fact that such a powerful tool could easily lead to the exploitation of vulnerable, desperate cancer patients. Apart from this, hypnotherapy suffers from poor self-governance and professional control, and the fact that it is the only complementary therapy that has a stage equivalent where the hypnotist creates an illusion and is given licence to fool people for the entertainment of others. All in all, it is not surprising that the discipline has credibility problems. Finally, there may be a professional fear that other psychological interventions may be undermined or made redundant by the use of hypnotherapy. This professional anxiety can undoubtedly cloud meaningful debate and research.

Ethically, good hypnotherapists should only treat problems that they are qualified and experienced to treat, but until hypnotherapy is officially recognised, accepted and respected the opportunity to practise and receive hypnotherapy will remain limited and its potential benefits sadly unexplored.

Conclusions

The debate on the value and effectiveness of complementary therapies seems set to continue, with the British Medical Association holding the key to acceptance. This clinical and ethical guardian of the nation's health carries an awesome professional responsibility for not only monitoring and disciplining its own members, but also for protecting gullible and poorly informed patients from dangerous and unproven complementary practices detrimental to health.

Deontological codes of conduct based on the categorical imperative offer guidelines for good practice and emphasize acting in the best interests of the patient. Beauchamp and Childress (1983, p.7) identified the principles of medical ethics as those that maximize beneficence, minimize maleficence, demonstrate respect for patients' autonomy, and furthermore are just. Emphasis must be placed on autonomy, which entails respecting the right of patients to think and act for themselves and to make decisions about their own lives. This includes self-care taught by experienced practitioners, and is already an option for many conditions: for example self-administration of insulin by diabetics or administration by nominated and educated significant others. Patients may choose to waive that option and place their faith totally in the integrity and skill of healthcare professionals, who are duty bound to use their expertise and continue to act in the best interests of the patients, performing their duties to the level of a reasonable practitioner. Any violation of that duty by act or omission leaves the practitioner vulnerable to professional misconduct, and this should be extended to monitor and control complementary therapies. Additionally, if research is considered to be the only acceptable way to evaluate the effectiveness of complementary therapies, then the responsibility and funding of research lies with the British Medical Association and healthcare professional bodies.

Gibran (1987) wrote in 1923: 'Work is love made visible. And if you cannot work with love but only with distaste, it is better that you should leave your work and sit at the gate of the temple and take alms of those who work with joy.' Competent healthcare professionals and complementary therapists who appear to actually enjoy treating, supporting and demonstrating their professional skills with cheerful optimism and enthusiasm, may be an important contributory factor to the success of the therapy. This concept is often devalued and difficult to promote where success is measured by financial goals, statistics and a market mentality. However, the contribution and potential of such an attitude should be realistically researched in an impartial and exploratory manner.

Complementary therapies performed by competent and experienced practitioners can offer comfort and relief of painful and distressing symptomology. 'Mixing and matching' complementary and orthodox medicine to provide advantageous caring and treatment strategies requires true professional collaboration. Palliative and cancer patients deserve the best of both disciplines and delays in investigating, monitoring and legislating the use of complementary therapies could arguably be tantamount to professional negligence.

Chapter 18
Pain control in palliative care

WENDY YOUNG

Introduction

People with serious illnesses are being referred earlier for treatment and are living for long periods with cancer and the possible side effects of treatment. Patients therefore require a plan of care that takes into account all facets of their potential requirements. Effective pain control is of paramount importance within this plan.

Palliative care

- Is the active total care of patients and their families, usually when their disease is no longer responsive to potentially curative treatment, although it may be applicable earlier in the illness
- Provides relief from pain and other symptoms
- Aims to achieve the highest possible quality of life for patients and their families
- Responds to physical, psychological, social and spiritual needs
- Extends as necessary to support in bereavement
  (Earl Mountbatten Hospice Guidelines, 1998)
  in association with the Wessex Specialist Palliative Care units.

This chapter proposes to consider pain management in the context of nursing today, and suggests an inventory that may be used as a framework in order to determine the education and practice needs of nurses who give palliative care within a wide range of settings.

Each person's pain is unique and needs individual nursing management. There is a dearth of valid research on all aspects of pain control in palliative care. Despite this, pain is a subject that is often surrounded by confusion and fear. Sadly and unforgivably, pain is often unrelieved.

It must be remembered that not all pain is caused by a patient's cancer. People can be made extremely uncomfortable by the pain of toothache and many other problems which we all experience from time to time. According to McCaffery (1972), 'pain is what the patient says it is, not what we think it ought to be', i.e. pain is an individual, subjective experience.

Pain in the context of nursing today

According to Hancock (1994), the three '*Es*' driving the health service today are *economy*, *effectiveness* and *efficiency*. These can sometimes undermine knowledge, care and understanding. If we consider that reflective practice underpins the essence of caring today, it may be considered that through practising reflection nurses will learn a skill that is not only useful in today's health systems, but an essential aspect of enabling nurses to rise to future challenges (Glen, 1995; Schank, 1990).

The advocacy role of nurses is an increasingly important element in order to promote caring within a marketplace ideology. There is no stronger way to defend this than in the context of nursing the patient who is in pain.

Schon (1987) proposes that practitioners use theories which are generated from their experience, education, values and beliefs, whilst Walsh and Ford (1989) note that 'there may be a place for intuition in the art of nursing', but the emphasis is on the rational, technical and scientific. Benner and Wrubel (1989) also see experience, as well as intuition, as central to nursing action and nursing care. In many ways this is the opposite of what Schon (1987) proposes that reflection aims to achieve.

Emphasis on competent performance defines more clearly the components of nursing within the context of the delivery of patient care. Perhaps it may be considered that in the context of today's marketplace ideology a competency-based method of pain control from a nursing perspective could help nurses enhance their proficiency in caring for a person in pain. It is most definitely not enough for nurses to verbalize a given situation (Alspach, 1984); as professionals they must be able to demonstrate enquiry-based practice.

The pain control inventory in palliative care

The pain control inventory (Table 18.1) is designed to determine nurses' education and practice needs, and also to promote enquiry-based practice.

Each factor is followed by a choice of responses for your consideration, i.e. 1, 2, 3 and 4. Please consider each factor and decide which is most appropriate to you. Tick the box that corresponds with the choice that you have made. It is very important that you give each factor due consideration. It will help you to make the appropriate response if you use the following key:

1. No knowledge or practical experience in this area
2. Have some theoretical knowledge but no practical experience
3. No theoretical knowledge, limited practical experience
4. Theoretical knowledge – have been able to put into practice.

Table 18.1 The pain control inventory

	1	2	3	4
1. Methods of pain assessment (please identify, e.g. pain thermometer)				
2. Professional care plans				
3. Pharmacological ladder				
4. Decision-making regarding analgesic administration				
5. Standards for administration of medicines				
6. Knowledge of drugs administration				
7. Nursing care, e.g. positioning physical aids emotional support distraction empathic communication				
8. Current nursing research information				

All the factors identified are vital elements in palliative care from the nursing perspective. If any of your responses are in the 1–3 inclusive range, *please take appropriate action*. This will vary according to your requirements. It may be any, or all, of the following, depending on your individual circumstances:

- personal study
- literature review
- tutorial support
- supervised practice
- peer group discussion.

Caring for people in pain

According to Brykczynska (1992), professional empathy is:

> Not so much a personal projection of effective and cognitive modes of being concerning another, but rather an ability to enter the world of a stranger and identify with the preferences, loves and hurts of the other so as to be able effectively to help the other towards the restoration of health and wellbeing.

Whilst Darbyshire (1991) discusses the fact that the theme of caring should be a golden thread running through the curriculum, Manley (1991) observes that 'theory' should not curtail practice. Manley also points out the very important relationship between knowledge and accountability.

When nursing a patient in pain, empathy, caring and accountability must be the prime considerations and the sound foundation on which further theoretical knowledge will be built. Professional competence will only be gained if nurses take responsibility for their professional self-development and reflect on their current practice.

Why may a patient's pain not be relieved?

There are two major underlying reasons for this: (i) patient expectation and (ii) nursing factors.

Patient expectation

- The patient may feel that 'pain is inevitable' – 'Everyone who has cancer has pain'
- The patient may fear the outcome if he/she admits to pain – fear of injections, further treatment, delay in returning home from hospice or hospital

- Cultural factors may affect patients' response to pain – putting on a brave face, not making a fuss and maintaining a 'stiff upper lip' may be important to them
- The patient may feel unable to approach nurses, who always seem so busy
- The patient may have a lack of understanding of the meaning of pain
- The patient may be unable to communicate the problem effectively – perhaps because of an inability to think of certain words, or aphasia, mental confusion, emotional stress, etc.

Nursing factors

- Lack of assessment – due to lack of knowledge, perceived lack of time
- Lack of knowledge (both theoretical and practical) – needs urgent attention
- Inability to manage workload – that is, not inability on the nurse's part, but due to a variety of other factors such as shortage of nursing staff
- Lack of understanding of the meaning of pain – this needs urgent attention; the professional team has a responsibility to address any shortcomings of this nature
- Lack of communication
- Not involving the patient in care
- Judgemental attitude – 'pain does not exist'/ 'pain should be accepted or endured'
- Inadequate monitoring
- Poor communication with doctors/other healthcare professionals
- Inability to advocate for the patient.

Nursing management of pain: the principles

1. Show empathy and understanding
2. Assess and re-assess regularly (include onset, duration and nature)
3. Set goals that are realistic
4. Don't wait for a patient to complain about pain – monitor repeatedly. A simple pain thermometer can help a person to express the degree of pain.
5. Ensure that the whole team has adequate skills and knowledge,

and appropriate attitudes towards the patients

6. Monitor communication within the team frequently
7. Ensure that analgesia is given regularly and monitored frequently
8. Ensure that the site(s) of pain is determined. Pain charts can play a very valuable part here, and can be devised by individual teams to best meet the needs of the appropriate client group. A simple body chart can be helpful, particularly if a patient has difficulty in communicating
9. Observe the body language of the person
10. Ensure that essential needs are met for each individual person, for e.g.:
    • environment appropriately and well ventilated
    • position comfortable and physiologically appropriate
    • fluid/dietary needs appropriately met
    • bed linen loose and wrinkle-free
    • receptors protected, if appropriate (e.g. dark glasses)
    • offer diversion if relevant – reading, hobbies, listening to music
    • drugs given as prescribed and the effects monitored
    • attention given to bowel care – a must for anyone taking analgesics
    • monitor any associated symptoms, e.g. vomiting
    • consider alternative therapies, for example aromatherapy
    • radiotherapy may be considered
    • application of heat/cold pads.

Analgesics and co-analgesics

The World Health Organization analgesia ladder (see Figure 18.1) emphasizes how important it is that the analgesia used is appropriate for the severity of the patient's pain. Alternative methods of pain relief must always be considered in *all* patients. The following must be considered:

• psychological problems
• social problems
• radiotherapy
• surgery
• chemotherapy
• complementary therapy

- use of co-analgesics, e.g. nerve blocks, TENS machine (see below), relaxation, acupuncture, drugs.

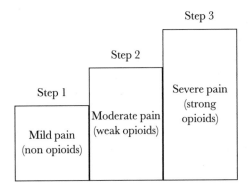

Figure 18.2 Analgesia ladder.

The TENS machine

The TENS (transcutaneous electrical nerve stimulation) machine produces a current that causes the body to release endorphins, natural painkilling substances that help block pain messages to the brain. TENS can be used on its own or in conjunction with prescribed medication. Electrodes are placed around the pain site on self-adhesive pads. They allow mild electrical impulses to stimulate the nerves in the area.

Case study

George

George, a 70-year-old retired man, was admitted to a hospice for pain assessment. He was diagnosed as having prostatic cancer 18 months earlier, for which he underwent a prostatectomy.

George was known to have bony metastases. He had suffered from osteoarthritis for many years in various parts of his body. Although he readily admitted to being in constant pain, he refused all prescribed medication. His only daughter had died of a drug overdose at the age of 16, and the healthcare team wondered if this had an influence on his refusal to take any medication.

George was seen by a consultant from the radiotherapy department, but palliative radiotherapy was not recommended. Osteoarthritis was thought to be the main cause of his pain.

The multidisciplinary team caring for George believed that he was suffering as much from spiritual pain as from physical pain. However, despite, constant encouragement he would not communicate his anxieties to anyone, either in his family or the professional team. Regular case conferences were held to discuss the case and plan accordingly.

The highest possible quality of nursing was given to George, with his total comfort being the main consideration. Careful positioning of heat pads applied to his hips and scapula seemed to have most effect and was acceptable to George.

George gradually became weaker over a period of five days and died peacefully in his sleep, with his wife present.

Conclusions

Realistic goals must be set for people who have pain. Any failure to meet targets, however unrealistic, increases both patients' and nurses' feelings of despair. It is essential that pain is patient-controlled, i.e. the patient is the person who makes the final decisions about his or her pain and any methods used to control it. Nurses must ensure that they have the appropriate knowledge, attitude and skills to provide pain control in palliative care.

Chapter 19
Breaking bad news

WENDY YOUNG

Introduction

This chapter seeks to explore some of the issues involved in the breaking of bad news and to consider how healthcare professionals need to consider possible factors that may potentially cause hurt to patients, their relatives and significant others.

If we consider that bad news is any information that drastically and negatively alters a person's view of their future (Kaye, 1996; Buckman, 1992), and that the people we meet as patients are perhaps some of the most vulnerable in society today, the necessity of ensuring that bad news is given as sensitively and gently as possible becomes apparent. According to Twycross and Lack (1990, p.212) 'truth has a broad spectrum with gentleness at one end and harshness at the other'. People can often cope with gentle truth, but not with harsh reality.

All human beings experience losses throughout their lives, with all the implications that are attached to loss. When bad news is given to an individual, where, how, why and when that news is communicated can assist or prevent that individual in working through their grieving process. This indicates how important it is for healthcare professionals to have, and to apply, the knowledge that underpins the giving of bad news. Also, it underlines the responsibility of each professional person to understand the necessity for humanity and empathy in all our communications.

In the first half of this chapter an attempt will be made to look at the nature of the factors involved in loss and the subsequent role of the healthcare professional. The second part looks at the factors involved in good practice when breaking bad news, and concludes with further suggestions for consideration and a short case study.

As we progressed through the twentieth century it was accepted, and understood, that we live in a complex, changing and challenging world. Technological development, higher expectations of life and increased longevity are just a few of the factors with which the people who make up the cultures in a rapidly changing Britain are faced. People also have to make sense of a wide range of attitudes and behaviour, of which most are acceptable and permissible within our society. People from ethnic minority groups have their lack of understanding exacerbated when English is not their first language.

Bad news is not acceptable for most people and brings to the fore social stigmata; people feel marginalized and fearful. Their expectations of life, of technological innovation and of health are put into question. People want definite and positive answers. If the bad news carries with it the threat of dying, many people will find the situation overtly distressing. Cancer itself conjures up fear, yet some cancers can be easily treated. Nevertheless, the word 'cancer' has been used when imparting a diagnosis to a patient. The healthcare professional must not be dismissive of the patient's potential distress at such a diagnosis, but explain what 'cancer' actually is.

In order for healthcare professionals to conceptualize, recognize and validate a person's distress, they need to understand the factors that are necessary in order for that person to work through their grief. We need to be aware that our initial approach may influence how someone progresses through their grieving process.

How people react depends upon their experience of managing change and also their personal circumstances. For some people the process of grief starts before they actually receive the news. They may have been receiving active treatment for a while, but fear that it will not be successful. For other people, their grief may start when they are formally given the information i.e. the bad news.

Working with grieving people

The following is intended as an outline framework to the process:

- Acknowledge the person's pain, e.g. say 'This must be very difficult for you...'
- Help the person to talk, e.g. say 'How can I help you at the moment?'
- Clarify their understanding/fill in any gaps as appropriate
- Be comfortable with silences – they are important
- Give information at the rate that an individual requires it. Written information can be helpful, particularly if the subject matter is presented professionally, and clearly written in terms that the individual can understand. It is helpful for reference when required. Written information should never be given without providing an opportunity for the recipient to receive an explanation regarding content, and the opportunity for questions to be asked, and for discussion to take place.

The main pitfalls of written information are that

   i) it may not be written at an appropriate level, e.g. too complex, too simple or too patronizing
   ii) it may contain information that the recipient is not ready to receive.

- Find out who the person has to support him/her
- Acknowledge behaviour that is demonstrated, e.g. anger, by saying 'I understand your need to be _____ '
- Allow time for emotions to be expressed
- Acknowledge sadness and concern for the future
- Realistically reassure, ensuring that false hope is not given.

We can never know how someone is going to react. There are, however, certain factors that can make the situation more difficult:

- Financial worries
- Living alone
- Concurrent losses such as divorce, job loss
- Other medical problems
- Disabled patients/partners – this can influence concerns not only for the future, but regarding consent to treatment. It may present difficulties in a situation where, for example, a patient

has to receive daily radiotherapy for up to six weeks and must travel to and from hospital
- Drug or alcohol-related problems
- Family worries, for example
financial
emotional
psychological
physical
spiritual
sexual

Preparation and practice are the key points to giving bad news sensitively and objectively, clearly and empathetically. Please remember that responsibility for successful communication rests with each individual.

Essential factors when breaking bad news

The following outline information can be used as a checklist or as a basis for monitoring professional standards.

Preparation

- Do you have time?
- Where is the news to be given?
- Who gives the news?
- Is the environment private and quiet? (avoid telephones, bleepers or interruptions)
- Is the environment suitably arranged? (chairs comfortable, barriers, such as desks, movable)
- Can you sit squarely to the person?
- What does the person already know?
- Do you know the necessary facts?
- Who else needs to be present?
- Who is available to support the individual afterwards?

Breaking the bad news

- Always introduce yourself
- Ensure empathetic communication
- Determine what the person knows, e.g. ask 'Tell me what happened to you ...'

- Start from the person's starting point
- Find out what is appropriate for the individual, e.g. ask 'Would you like more detail?
- Always warn the person that you are going to give serious information
- Pause frequently to allow for reflection and responses
- Give explanation as required, narrowing the information gap, i.e. try to get the person from where they think they are to where they actually are, in a sensitive manner
- Convey empathy throughout
- Consider the posture of the individually, i.e. never give news to someone who is lying on an examination couch, or is partly dressed. The person will be concentrating on maintaining some degree of modesty, not on what is being said.

Ending off

- Discuss any concerns
- Plan the next step
- Refer appropriately
- Foster realistic hope
- End the meeting appropriately
- Ensure that documentation is clear and concise
- Ensure that professional communication takes place, e.g. letters to other departments, as appropriate.

Throughout the whole process it is important to take into account the person's coping mechanisms.

- Allow for denial
- Allow for anger
- Do not get involved in apportioning blame.

Points to remember

- Grieving people retain only 30–40% of the information given them. What is communicated must be relevant and in a language that the individual understands.
- Our interpretation of what is causing the person anxiety may not be accurate. Always ascertain what individuals see as their main problem; do not make assumptions.

- Avoid false reassurance; the person can be left feeling that there is not a problem.
- Anger is a common reaction when someone is given bad news. The anger may be focused or unfocused.
- Maintain realistic hope.
- Avoid misleading euphemisms where possible. Use the word 'cancer' if appropriate.
- Try to include all the family in the sharing of information, but please remember it is technically breaching confidentiality to tell relatives anything without the patient's consent.

Case history

Megan

Megan, a middle-aged woman, had taken early retirement to look after her husband, who had a serious heart problem. Her husband died suddenly in her presence. A few weeks after the death Megan developed vague symptoms that seemed stress-related. Her doctor prescribed a mild sedative, but Megan believed that she had cancer. The symptoms continued – the nausea which had been the main problem developed into vomiting. Following gastroscopy an adeno-carcinoma of the stomach was diagnosed. When the consultant saw Megan in outpatients to give her the gastroscopy results she said, 'I was right, wasn't I? It is cancer, isn't it?' The consultant confirmed that it was. Megan became extremely angry and said that she was going to complain about the delay in diagnosis.

Conclusions

It is the professional responsibility of all healthcare professionals to understand the factors involved in giving bad news. This role never becomes easy, and it continues to be stressful. Not only do we need to consider the welfare of the patient, relatives and significant other people, but also our own welfare and that of our colleagues. Support and supervision is not an optional extra but is an essential component of the process. The simple strategies and skills will enable healthcare professionals to positively assist people who have serious illnesses.

References

Abdulla A, Daneshmend T (1995) Management of nausea in various conditions. Prescriber September: 40–46.

Ablin AR (Ed) (1997) Supportive Care of Children with Cancer: Current Therapy and Guidelines from the Children's Cancer Group (2nd edition). London: Johns Hopkins University Press.

Allwood M, Wright P (1993) The Cytotoxic Handbook. Oxford: Radcliffe Medical Press.

Alspach J (1984) Designing a competency-based orientation for critical care nurses. Heart & Lung 13: 655–62.

Anderson CF, Wochers DN (1982) The utility of serum albumin values in the nutritional assessment of hospitalised patients. Mayo Clinic Proceedings 57:181.

Angeles T, Barbone M (1994) Infiltration and phlebitis: assessment, management and documentation. Journal of Home Healthcare Practitioners 7(1): 16–21.

Antrum J (1996) Meeting the challenge of systemic fungal infections in cancer: nursing implications. European Journal of Haematology (Suppl.) 57: 7–11.

Armstrong B, Doll R (1975) Environmental factors and cancer incidence and mortality in different countries, with special references to dietary practices. Internal Journal of Cancer 15: 617–31.

Assikis V, Neven P, Jordan V, Vergote I (1996) A realistic clinical perspective of tamoxifen and endometrial carcinogenesis. European Journal of Cancer 32A(9): 1464–76.

Ayliffe GAJ, Lowbury EJL, Geddes AM, Williams JD (1992) Control of Hospital Infection: a practical handbook (3rd edition). London: Chapman and Hall.

BAHNO (1988) Provision and quality assurance for head and neck cancer care in the UK. London: British Association of Head and Neck Oncologists.

Baker C (1992) Factors associated with rehabilitation in head and neck cancer. Cancer Nursing 15(6): 395–400.

Balch CM, Houghton A, Peters L. Cutaneous melanoma. In: De Vita V, HellPan S, Rosenberg SA (Eds) (1989) Cancer: Principles and Practice of Oncology (3rd edition). Philadelphia: Lippincott.

Bale S, Harding KG (1990) Using modern dressings to effect debridement. Professional Nurse (Feb.) 5(5): 244–5.

BAOHNS (1998) Effective head and neck cancer management – consensus document. London: British Association of Otorhinolaryngologists Head and Neck Surgeons.

Barnes J, Chamberlain G (1988) Lecture notes on gynaecology (6th edition). London: Blackwell Scientific Publications.

Bass EM, Del Pino A, Tan A, Pearl RK, Orsay CP, Abcarian H (1997) Does pre-operative stoma marking and education by the enterstomal therapists affect outcome? Diseases of the Colon and Rectum April: 440–42.

Baum M (1995) Screening for breast cancer, time to think and stop? Lancet 346: 436.

Beauchamp T, Childress J (1983) Principles of Biomedical Ethics. New York: Oxford University Press.

Ben-Joseph E, Shamsa F, Forman JD (1998) Predicting the outcome of radiotherapy for prostate cancer. Cancer 82(7): 1334–41.

Benner P, Wrubel J (1989) The Primacy of Care. Menlo Park: Addison-Wesley.

Bennett RS (1976) The place of the pull through operations in treatment of carcinoma of the rectum. Diseases of the Colon and Rectum 19: 420–24.

Berrino F, Sant M, Verdecchia A et al. (Eds) Survival in Cancer Patients in Europe: the Eurocare Study. Lyon: International Agency for Research on Cancer.

Bertero C, Ek A (1993) Quality of life with acute leukaemia. Journal of Advanced Nursing 18: 1346–53.

Bildstein CY (1993) Head and neck malignancies. In: Groenwald S, Frogge M, Goodman M, Yarbo C (Eds) Cancer Nursing: Principles and Practice. London, Boston: Jones and Bartlett.

Black P (1997) Practical stoma care. Nursing Standard 11(47): 49–55.

Bleehen NM, Glatstein E, Haybittle JL (1983) Radiation Therapy Planning. New York: Marcel Dekker.

Blot WJ, McLaughlin JK, Winn DM, Austin DF, Greenberg RS, Preston-Martin S, Bernstein L, Schoenberg JB, Stemhagen A, Fraumeni JF jnr (1988) Smoking and drinking in relation to oral and pharyngeal cancer. Cancer Research 48: 3282–7.

Bomford CK, Hunkler IH, Sherriff SB (1993) Textbook of Radiotherapy: Radiation Physics, Therapy and Oncology (5th edition). Edinburgh: Churchill Livingstone.

Bonner J (1995) Recent Advances in Obstetrics and Gynaecology. London: Churchill Livingstone.

Booth (1993) Chiropractic. Nursing Times 89(22): 52–4.

Borwell B (1997) Psychological considerations of stoma care nursing. Nursing Standard 11(48): 49–52.

Bowers KS (1976) Hypnosis for the seriously curious. New York and London: W Norton & Co.

Boyle P, Maisonneuve P, Dore J (1995) British Medical Bulletin 51(3): 523–47.

Boyle P, Marshall JR, Maisonneuve P, Cattaruzza MS, Nickolas TJ, Zheng T, Tedescos B, Chiesa F, Scully C (1998) Epidemiology of head and neck tumours. In: Jones AS, Phillips DE, Hilgers FJ Diseases of the Head & Neck, Nose and Throat. London: Edward Arnold.

Bozzetti (1995) Nutrition Support in Patients with Cancer. In: Payne-James J et al. (1995) Artificial Nutrition Support in Clinical Practice. London: Edward Arnold.

Braga M, Gianotti L, Vignali A (1998) Artificial nutrition after major abdominal surgery. Impact on the route of administration and composition of the diet. Critical Care Medicine 26: 24–30.

Brambille EC (Ed) (1998) Lung Tumours: Fundamental Biology and Clinical Management. New York: Marcel Dekker.

Brandt B (1994) Nursing protocol for the patient with neutropenia. Oncology Nursing Forum 17(1) (Suppl.): 9–15.

British Medical Association (BMA) (1993) Complementary medicine: new approaches to good practice. New York: Oxford University Press.

British Medical Association (BMA) (1997) Family Health Encyclopaedia.

British National Formulary (BNF) (1998) (British Medical Association/Royal Pharmaceutical Society of Great Britain). London: BMA & Pharmaceutical Press.

Brunner L, Suddarth D (1975) Textbook of Medical–Surgical Nursing (3rd edition) p.242. Oxford: Blackwell Scientific Publications.

Buckman R (1992) How to Break Bad News. London: Papermac.

Bullock N, Sibley G, Whitaker R (1995) Essential Urology (2nd edition) pp.311–12. Edinburgh: Churchill Livingstone.

Bundred N, Morgan D, Dixon J (1994) Management of regional nodes in breast cancer. BMJ 6961(309): 1222–25.

Burgess L (1994) Facing the reality of head and neck cancer. Nursing Standard 8(32): 30–34.

Burns R (1980) Essential Psychology. Lancaster: MTP Press Ltd.

Buzdar A, Jonat, W, Howell A, Jones SE, Blomqvist C, Vogel CL et al. (1996) Anastrozole, a potent and selective aromatase inhibitor, versus megestrol acetate in postmenopausal women with advanced breast cancer: results of overview analysis of two phase 111 trials. Journal of Clinical Oncology 14: 2000–2011.

Byrne A, Walsh M, O'Driscoll K (1993) Depression following laryngectomy. British Journal of Psychiatry 163: 173–6.

Calman K, Hine D (1995) A policy framework for commissioning cancer services. London: Department of Health (DoH).

Calvert H, McElwain T (1978) Principles of chemotherapy. In: Tiffany R (Ed) Oncology for Nurses and Health Care Professionals. Cambridge: Harper and Row.

Campbell K (1996) Lymphocytic leukaemia: classification and treatment. Nursing Times 93(5): 31–2.

Campbell L (1998) Intravenous related phlebitis: complications and length of stay. British Journal of Nursing 7(21): 1304–12.

Campbell ST (1994) Guidelines for Mouth Care. London: Royal College of Nursing.

Cancer Research Campaign (CRC) (1993). Factsheet 18.1. London: Imperial Cancer Research.

Cancer Research Campaign (CRC) (1996a) Breast Cancer Factsheet 6.1. London: CRC.

Cancer Research Campaign (CRC) (1996b) Breast Cancer Factsheet 6.4. London: CRC.

Cancer Research Campaign (CRC) (1996c) Breast Cancer Factsheet 6.5. London: CRC.

Cancer Research Campaign (CRC) (1996d) Lung Cancer and Smoking Factsheet 11.1. London: CRC.

Cancer Guidance subgroup of the Clinical Outcomes Group (Cancer guidance) (1997) Improving the Outcome of Colorectal Cancer: The Manual. Leeds: NHS Executive Department of Health.

Carter LW (1994) Bacterial translocation: Nursing implications in the care of patients with neutropenia. Oncology Nursing Forum 21(5): 857–65.

Cartmel B, Reid M (1993) Cancer control and epidemiology. In: Groenwald S,

Frogge M, Goodman M, Yarbo C (Eds) Cancer Nursing: Principles and Practice. London, Boston: Jones and Bartlett.

Castro M (1990) The complete homeopathy handbook. London: Macmillan.

Cataldo CB, Rolfes SR, Whitney EN (1998) Understanding Clinical Nutrition (2nd edition). West Wadsworth.

Chamberlain G (1995) Gynaecology by Ten Teachers (16th edition). London: Edward Arnold.

Chamberlain J (1978) Screening for early detection of cancer. In: Pritchard P (Ed) Oncology for Nurses and Health Care Professionals Vol. 1 (Pathology Diagnosis and Treatment). London: Harper and Row.

Chamberlain J (1998) Cited in Cancer of the Prostate 3: Men's Health Care Needs. British Journal Nursing 7(5): 262–79.

Cheung N (1991) Immunotherapy: Neuroblastoma as a model. In: Horowitz M, Pizzo P (Eds) The Pediatric Clinics of North America: Solid Tumors in Children 38 (2): 425–441.

Clark A (1997) The nursing management of IV drug therapy. British Journal of Nursing 6(4): 201–6.

Cooper D (1993) Managing malignant ulcers effectively. Nursing Standard 8(2): 24–8.

Corner J, Plant A, A'Hern R et al. (1996) Non pharmacological intervention for breathlessness in lung cancer. Palliative Medicine. 10: 299–305.

Cooper D (1993) Nursing Standard 8(2): 24–8.

Corner J et al. (1997) The Palliation of Breathlessness in Patients with Lung Cancer. Conclusions from a consensus workshop at the European Congress for Palliative care. London.

Cornwell J (1997) Cancer: the war against it. Sunday Times 1 June pp.14–19.

Corriere JD (Ed) (1986) Essentials of Urology pp.205–7. Edinburgh: Churchill Livingstone.

Corydon-Hammond D (Ed) (1990) Hypnotic suggestions and metaphors. New York, London: WW Norton & Co.

Coultas DB, Samet JM (1992) Occupational Lung Cancer. Clin. Chest. Med. 13: 341–54.

Craven D, Steger K, Hirschen L (1996) Nosocomial colonisation and infection in persons infected with human immunodeficiency virus. Infection control and hospital epidemiology 17(5): 304–18.

Croner (1996). Control of Substances Hazardous to Health (COSHH). London: Croner's Health and Safety at Work.

Cummings J, Bingham S (1998) Diet and the prevention of cancer 1. BMJ 317: 1636–40.

Darby S, Whikley E, Silcocks P et al. (1998) Risk of lung cancer associated with residential radon exposure in South-West England: a Case Control. Br. J. Cancer 78.

Darbyshire P (1991) The American Revolution. Nursing Times 87(6): 57–8.

David J (1995) Cancer Care Prevention, Treatment and Palliation. London: Chapman and Hall.

Davies T (1978) The biology of cancer. In: Pritchard P (Ed) Oncology for Nurses and Health Care Professionals Vol. 1 (Pathology, Diagnosis and Treatment). London: Harper and Row.

Davies AD, Davies C, Delpo MC (1986) Depression and anxiety in patients undergoing diagnostic investigations for head and neck cancers. British Journal of Psychiatry 149: 491–3.

Dawson C, Whitfield M (1996) BMJ 312: 1090–94.

De Blaauw I, Deutz NEP, von Meyenfeldt MF (1997) Metabolic changes in cancer cachexia. Clinical Nutrition 16: 169–76.

Dennis G, Maki MD, Ringer M (1991) Risk factors for infusion related phlebitis with small peripheral venous catheters. Annals of Internal Medicine 114: 845–54.

Department of Health (1991) Breast Awareness. London. Department of Health (Professional Letter: PL/CMO(91)15).

Department of Health (DoH) (1994) Consultative Document: A Policy Framework for Commissioning Cancer Services. London: HMSO.

Department of Health (DoH) (1998) Clinical examination of the breast. London: Department of Health (Professional Letter: PL/CMO/98/1, PL/CNO/98/1).

Department of Public Health (1993) Strategy for Cancer of Cervix: The health of Portsmouth and South East Hampshire. London: DoH.

Dewar H (2000) Dietetic management. In: TPN: A Practical Guide for Nurses London: Harcourt Brace.

Dillon P, Weiner E (1997) Venous access devices in children. In: Ablin AR (Ed) Supportive Care of Children with Cancer: Current Therapy and Guidelines from the Children's Cancer Group pp.217–28. London: Johns Hopkins University Press.

Ditroia JF (1972) Nodal metastases and prognosis in carcinoma of the oral cavity. Otolaryngological Clinics of North America 5: 333–42.

Doherty AP, Christmas TS (1996) British Journal of Medical Medicine 55(3): 104–6.

Dolgin MJ, Katz ER, Zelter LK, Landverk J (1989). Behavioral distress in pediatric patients with cancer receiving radiotherapy. Pediatrics 84(1): 103–10.

Doll, Peto (1981) The causes of cancer: quantitative estimates of avoidable risks of cancer in the United States today. J. Natl. Cancer Institute 66: 1191–1308.

Donohoe G (1992) Sensitivity can break the taboo. Professional Nurse (Feb.): 304–8.

Doyle B (1987) I wish you were dead! Nursing Times 83(45): 44–6.

Doyle D (1980) Domiciliary terminal care. The Practitioner 224(1344): 575–82.

Dreicer R, Williams RE (1992) Cited in Tanagho E, McAninch JW, Smith's General Urology p.361. London: Prentice Hall.

Dropkin MJ (1989) Coping with disfigurement and dysfunction after head and neck cancer surgery: a conceptual framework. Seminars in Oncology Nursing 5(3): 213–19.

Dryden W (1990) Handbook of Individual Therapy. London: Sage.

Dryden H, Whyte F (1997) Comparison of cutaneous malignant melanoma in two European countries. Journal of Cancer Nursing 1(4): 208–14.

Dufour DT (1990) Information for teachers of children with central venous catheters. Journal of Pediatric and Oncologic Nursing 7(1): 37–8.

Dukes CE (1932) The classification of cancer of the rectum. Journal Pathol. Bacteriol. 35: 323–32.

Earl H (1995) Gynaecological Tumours. Medicine (UK edition) 23: 11 November.

Earl Mountbatten Hospice, in association with all the Wessex Specialist Palliative Care Units (1998) Guidelines in Clinical Management.

Edwards D (1997) Face to Face: Patient, family and professional perspectives of head and neck cancer care. London: Kings Fund Publishing.

Edwards L, Levine N (1986) Skin cancer: The best route to early diagnosis. Modern Medicine 54(42): 54.

Ekman P, Li C, Pan Y, Dich J (1997) Environmental factors: A possible link with prostate cancer. British Journal Urology 79 (Suppl. 2): 35–41.

Elcoat C (1986) Stoma Care Nursing. East Sussex: Baillière Tindall.

Elwell CM, Tobias JS (1998) Chemotherapy in head and neck oncology. In: Jones AS, Phillips DE, Hilgers FJ (1998) Diseases of the Head & Neck, Nose and Throat. London: Arnold.

Emmerson AM, Enstone JE, Griffin M, Kelsey MC and Smyth ETM (1996) The second national prevalence study of infection in hospitals – overview of the results. Journal of Hospital Infection 32: 175–90.

Facchino F, Spiro SG (1998) Chemotherapy in Small Cell Lung Cancer – is more better?

Fallowfield L, Baum M, Maguire GP (1986) Effects of breast conservation on psychological morbidity associated with diagnosis and treatment of early breast cancer. BMJ 293: 1331–4.

Fallowfield L (1990) The Quality of Life. London: Souvenir Press.

Fallowfield L, Hall A, Maguire P, Baum M (1990) Psychological outcomes of different treatment policies in women with early breast cancer outside a clinical trial. BMJ 305: 575–80.

Fallowfield L (1991) Breast Cancer. London: Routledge.

Farmer A, Payne S, Royle G (1995) A comparative study of psychological morbidity in women with screen detected and symptomatic breast cancer. In: Richardson A, Macleod Clarke J (Eds) Nursing Research in Cancer Care. London: Scutari Press.

Faulkner A, Peace G, O'Keefe C (1995) When a Child has Cancer. London: Chapman and Hall.

Faulkner A, Maguire P (1996) Talking to Cancer Patients and their Relatives. Oxford: Oxford University Press.

Feber P (1998) Design and evaluation of a strategy to provide support and information for people with cancer of the larynx. European Journal of Oncology Nursing 2(2): 106–114.

Fenlon LE (1995) Protective isolation: Who needs it? Journal of Hospital Infection 30 June (Suppl.): 218–31.

Fielding JE, Phenow KJ (1988) Health effects of involuntary smoking. New England Journal of Medicine 319: 1452–60.

Fillingham S, Douglas (1994) Urological Nursing (2nd edition). London: Baillière Tindall.

Fisher B, Redmond C, Poisson R et al. (1989) Eight-year results for a randomized clinical trial comparing total mastectomy and lumpectomy with or without irradiation in the treatment of breast cancer. New England Journal of Medicine 320(8): 22–8.

Fitzgerald V, Sims R (1987) A positive approach. Community Nurse (Nov.): 16–21.

Flanagan M (1997) Wound Management. Edinburgh: Churchill Livingstone.

Forrest APM (1986) Breast Cancer Screening: Report to the Health Ministers of England, Scotland and Northern Ireland. London.

Frank-Stromborg M, Cohen RF (1993) Assessment and interventions for cancer prevention and detection. In: Groenwald S, Frogge M, Goodman M, Yarbo C (Eds) Cancer Nursing: Principles and Practice. London, Boston: Jones and Bartlett.

Freeman JV, Cole TJ, Chinn S, Jones PRM, White EM, Preece MA (1995) Cross-sectional stature weight reference curves for the UK (1990). Archives of Disease in Childhood 73: 17–24.

Friedman H, Horowitz M, Oakes J (1991) Tumors of the central nervous system. In: Horowitz M, Pizzo P (Eds) The Pediatric Clinics of North America: Solid Tumors in Children 38(2): 381–91.

Fromant P (1991) Let me rub it better. Nursing 4(46): 18–19.

Gabriel J (1999) Central venous access devices. In: Dougherty L, Lamb J (Eds) Intravenous Therapy in Nursing Practice. London: Harcourt Brace.

Gibran K (1987) The Prophet. London: William Heinemann Ltd.

Gibson J (1975) Modern Physiology and Anatomy for Nurses. Oxford: Blackwell Scientific.

Gillis C (1978) The epidemiology of human cancers. In: Pritchard P (Ed) Oncology for Nurses and Health Care Professionals Vol. 1 (Pathology, Diagnosis and Treatment). London: Harper and Row.

Gillis C, Holes D (1996) Survival outcome of care by specialist surgeons in breast cancer. BMJ 312(7024): 145–8.

Golding J, Paterson M, Kinlen L (1990) Factors associated with childhood cancer in a national cohort study. British Journal of Cancer 62(2): 304–8.

Goodman M, Ladd L, Purl S (1993) Integumentary and mucous membrane alterations. In: Groenwald S, Frogge M, Goodman M, Yarbo C (Eds) Cancer Nursing: Principles and Practice. London, Boston: Jones and Bartlett.

Greening JR (1985) Fundamentals of Radiation Dosimetry. Bristol: Adam Hilger Ltd.

Haley RW (1985) Surveillance by objectives: a new priority directed approach to the control of nosocomial infection. American Journal of Infection Control 13: 78–89.

Hallett A (1993) Fungating Wounds. Wound Care Society Education Leaflet. Huntingdon: Wound Care Society.

Hampton S (1997a) Germ warfare. Nursing Times 93(40): 74–9.

Hampton S (1997b) The Treatment of Macerated and Excoriated Peri-Wound Areas. Paper presented at the Seventh European Conference on Wound Management, Harrogate.

Hampton S (1998) Film subjects win the day. Nursing Times 94(24): 80–82.

Hancock C (1994) Paper presented at the Conference of the National Association for Staff Support.

Hancock B (1996a) Cancer Care in the Hospital. Oxford: Radcliffe Medical Press.

Hancock B (1996b) Cancer Care in the Community. Oxford: Radcliffe Medical Press.

Harrocopus CM, Myers C (Eds) (1996) Stoma Care Nursing. London: Edward Arnold.

Hastings D (1993) Basing care on research. Nursing Times 89(13): 70–76.

Haury B, Rodheaver G, Vensko J, Edgerton MT, Edlich RF (1978) Debridement: an essential component of traumatic wound care. American Journal of Surgery 135(2): 238–42.

Hausen L (1991) Viruses in human cancers. Science 254: 1167–73.

Hawkins MM, Stevens MCG (1996) The long term survivors. British Medical Bulletin 52(4): 898–923.

The Health of the Nation (1992) A Strategy for Health in England. London: HMSO.

Henson DE (1988) The histological grading of neoplasms. Archives of Pathology and Laboratory Medicine 112: 1091–6.

Hernandez E, Rosenhein N (1989) Manual of Gynaecological Oncology. Edinburgh: Churchill Livingstone.

Hill J (1991) Assessing rheumatic disease. Nursing Times 87(4): 33–5.

Hin K (1988) Chinese massage and acupressure. New York: Bergh Publishing.

Hockenberry-Eaton M, Benner A (1990) Patterns of nausea and vomiting in children: nursing assessment and intervention. Oncology Nurses Forum 17(4): 575–83.

Hoffbrand AV, Pettit JE (1993) Clinical Haematology (2nd edition). London: Mosby-Wolfe.

Hoffbrand AV, Pettit JE (1994) Essential Haematology (3rd edition). Oxford: Blackwell Science.

Hollis R (1997) Childhood malignancy into the 21st century. Paediatric Nursing 9(3): 12–15.

Holt PJ (1988) Cryotherapy for skin cancer: Results over a 5 year period using liquid nitrogen spray and cryosurgery. British Journal of Dermatology 119: 231–40.

Holy Bible

Hopwood P, Swindell R, Burr P et al. (1997) Clinically relevant quality of life outcomes in the first randomised trial of endobronchial radiotherapy patients with inoperable non-small cell lung cancer. Lung Cancer 18 (Suppl. 1): S130.

Horizon (1991) Homeopathy: myth or magic? London: BBC Television.

Hospers J (1990) An Introduction to Philosophical Analysis (3rd edition). London: Routledge.

Hunter M (1994) Counselling in Obstectrics & Gynaecology. British Psychological Society (BPS Books).

Independent Review Group (1998) Silicone Gel Breast Implants. Report to the Department of Health.

Inglis TJJ, Sproat RJ, Hawkey PM, Knappett P (1992) Infection control in Intensive Care Units: UK National Survey.

Ionising Radiations Regulations (IRR) (1999), Statutory Instrument No. 3232, HMSO, London.

Ionising Radiations (Medical Exposure) Regulations (IR(ME)R) (2000), Statutory Instruments No. 1059, HMSO, London.

Irizarry L, Merlin T, Rupp J, Griffith J (1996) Reduced Susceptibility of Methicillin-resistant Staphylococcus aureus to Cetylpyridinium chloride and Chlorhexidine. Chemotherapy 42: 248–52.

Jackson S (1985) The touching process in rehabilitation. Australian Nursing Journal 14(11): 43–5.

James N, Field D (1992) The routinization of hospice: charisma and bureaucratization. Social Science & Medicine 34: 1363–75.

Jansma J, Vissink A, Spijkervet FKL, Roodenbury JLN, Panders AK, Vermey A, Szabo BG, 's-Gravenmade EJ (1992) Protocol for prevention and treatment of oral sequlae resulting from head and neck radiotherapy. Cancer 70: 2171–80.

Jarvinen HJ (1992) Epidemiology of familial adenomatous polyposis in Finland. Gut 33: 357–60.

Joels J (1989) Psychological implications of having a stoma. Surgical Nurse 2(6) (Suppl.): x–xii.

Johnston DA, Walker K, Richards J, Pennington CR (1992) Ethanol flush for the prevention of catheter occlusion. Clinical Nutrition 11: 97–100.

Jolley M, Brykczynska G (1992) Nursing care: the challenge to change. London: Edward Arnold.

Jones AS (1998) General introduction. In: Jones AS, Phillips DE, Hilgers FJ Diseases of the Head & Neck, Nose and Throat. London: Arnold.

Jones DJ, James RD (1993) Anal cancer. ABC of Colorectal Disease. British Medical Journal.

Kalayjian AS (1989) Coping with cancer: the spouse's perspective. Archives of Psychiatric Nursing 3: 166–72.

Kalnins IK, Leonard AG, Sako K, Razack MS, Shedd DP (1977) Correlations between signals and degree of lymph node involvement in carcinoma of the oral cavity. American Journal of Surgery 134: 450–54.

Kaye P (1996) Breaking Bad News. Northampton: EPL Publications.

Kelly MP (1985) Loss and grief as responses to surgery. Journal of Advanced Nursing 10: 517–25.

Keoshane PP, Attril H, Silk DBA (1986) Clinical effectiveness of weighted and unweighted 'fine bore' nasogastric tubes in enteral nutrition: a controlled clinical trial. Journal of Clinical Nutrition and Gastroenterology 1: 189–93.

Kern KA, Norton JA (1988) Cancer cachexia. Journal of Parenteral and Enteral Nutrition 12: 286–98.

Ketcham M, Loescher, LJ (1993) Skin cancers. In: Groenwald SL, Frogge MH Goodman M, Yarbo C (Eds) Cancer Nursing: Principles and Practice. London, Boston: Jones and Bartlett.

Kirby RS (Ed) (1995) Prostatic Disease and Treatments. Health Press Page.

Knapman J (1993) Controlling emesis after chemotherapy. Nursing Standard 7(1): 38–9.

Knobf MT, Durivage HJ (1983)Therapy. In: Groenwald S, Frogge M, Goodman M, Yarbo C (Eds) Cancer Nursing: Principles and Practice. London, Boston: Jones and Bartlett.

Koester M, Bergsma J (1990) Problems and coping behaviour of facial cancer patients. Social Science and Medicine 30: 569–78.

Krebs L (1993) Sexual and reproductive dysfunction. In: Groenwald S, Frogge M, Goodman M, Yarbo C (Eds) Cancer Nursing: Principles and Practice. London, Boston: Jones and Bartlett.

Kreig T, Eming AS (1997) Is Exudate a clinical problem? A dermatologist's perspective. In: Cherry C, Harding K (Eds) Management of Wound Exudate. Proceedings of Joint meeting of EWMA and ETRS. London: Churchill Communications.

Krishnasamy M, Wilkie M (1997) Lung Cancer Patients' Families and Professionals' Perceptions of Health Care Need. A National Needs Assessment Study. Preliminary Report to Macmillan Cancer Relief.

Kubler-Ross E (1970) On Death and Dying. London: Tavistock.

Kumasaka LMKB, Dungan JM (1993) Nursing strategy for initial emotional response to cancer diagnosis. Cancer Nursing 16(4): 296–303.

Kupst MJ, Natta MB, Richardson CC, Shulman JL, Lavigne JV, Das L (1995). Family coping with pediatric leukemia: ten years after treatment. Journal of Pediatric Psychology 20(5): 601–17.

Kurtzberg J, Graham M (1991) Non-Hodgkin's Lymphoma: Biologic classification and implications for therapy. In: Horowitz M, Pizzo P (Eds) The Pediatric Clinics of North America: Solid Tumors in Children 38(2): 443–56

Laker C (Ed) (1994) Urological Nursing (Chapter 10). London: Scutari Press.

Lawless J (1992) The encyclopaedia of essential oils. Element Books Ltd.

Lederle FA, Niewoehner DE (1994) Lung Cancer Surgery: A critical review of the evidence. Arch. Intern. Med. 154: 2397–2400.

Lennard-Jones JE, Arrowsmith H, Davidson C, Denham AF, Micklewright A (1995) Screening by nurses and junior doctors to detect malnutrition when patients are first admitted to hospital. Clinical Nutrition 14: 336–40

Levendag PC, Keus RB (1998). Radiotherapy in head and neck oncology. In: Groenwald S, Frogge M, Goodman M, Yarbo C (Eds) Cancer Nursing: Principles and Practice. London, Boston: Jones and Bartlett.

Levi F, Franceschi S, Negri E, La Vecchia C (1993) Dietary Factors and the risk of Endometrial Cancer. Cancer (June) 71(11): 3575–81.

Lewandowska S (1997) A model for parent education. Paediatric Nursing 9(7): 21–3.

Lilley L (1990) Side effects associated with pediatric chemotherapy: management and patient education issues. Paediatric Nursing 16(3): 252–6.

Lipshultz SE, Colan SD, Walsh EP (1990) Ventricular tachycardia and sudden unexplained death in late survivors of childhood malignancy treated with doxorubicin (abstract). Pediatric Research 27: 853a.

Loevinger R, Budinger TF, Watson EE (1989) MIRD Primer for Absorbed Dose Calculations. New York: Society of Nuclear Medicine.

Lowden B (1998) The care and treatment of lung cancer. Nursing Times 94(9): 61–2.

Luesley DM (1997) Common Conditions in Gyneacology: A problem-solving approach. London: Chapman and Hall.

MacFarlane MT(1988) Urology for the House Officer (Chapter 26).

Maguire P, Lee E, Bevington D et al. (1978) Psychiatric problems in the first year after mastectomy. BMJ (i):963–5.

Maguire P (1994) Psychological Aspects. BMJ 6969(309):1649–52.

Maier H (1998) Staging and prognosis of head and neck oncology. In: Groenwald S, Frogge M, Goodman M, Yarbo C (Eds) Cancer Nursing: Principles and Practice. London, Boston: Jones and Bartlett.

Maki MD (1987) Prospective study of replacing administration sets for IV therapy at 48 hours vs 72 hours intervals. JAMA 258(13): 1777–81.

Manni JJ (1998) Diagnostic methods in head and neck oncology. In: Groenwald S, Frogge M, Goodman M, Yarbo C (Eds) Cancer Nursing: Principles and Practice. London, Boston: Jones and Bartlett.

Maran AGD (Ed) (1988) Logan Turner's Diseases of the Nose Throat and Ear (10th edition). Oxford: Butterworth-Heinemann.

Maran AGD, Gaze M, Wilson JA (1993) Stell and Maran's Head and Neck Surgery (3rd edition). Oxford: Butterworth-Heinemann.

Mason P (1992) Beware the sun. Nursing Times 88(12): 19.

Mason WP, Grovas A, Halpern S, Dunkel IJ, Garvin J, Heller G, Rosenblum M, Gardner S, Lyden D, Sands S, Puccetti D, Lindsley K, Merchant TE, O'Malley B, Bayer L, Petriccione MM, Allen J, Finlay JL (1998) Intensive chemotherapy and bone marrow rescue for young children with newly diagnosed malignant brain tumors. Journal of Clinical Oncology 16(1): 210–21.

Masters and Johnston (1982) On Sex and Human Loving. London: Macmillan.

Mathe et al. (1959) Cited in Trelevan J, Barrett J (1994) Bone Marrow Transplant in Practice. Edinburgh: Churchill Livingstone.

McCaffery M (1983) Nursing the Patient in Pain. London: Harper & Row.

McIndoe W, Maclean M, Jones R, Mullins P (1984) The invasive Ppotential of carcinoma in situ of the cervix. Obstetrics and Gynecology 64(4): 451–8.

McKie L (1993) Women's views of the cervical smear test: Implications for nursing practice – women who have not had a smear test. Journal of Advanced Nursing 18: 972–79.

McLaughlin J, Thompson D (1995) Drugs for the treatment of nausea and vertigo. Prescriber September: 31–8.

McPherson A (1994) Women's Problems in General Practice (3rd edition). Oxford: Oxford University Press.

McPherson A, Waller D (1997) Women's Health (4th edition). Oxford: Oxford University Press.

Meadows AT, Baum E, Fossati-Bellani F (1985) Second malignant neoplasms in children: an update from the Late Effects Study Group. Journal of Clinical Oncology 3: 532.

Meers P, Jacobsen W, McPherson M (1994) Hospital Infection Control for Nurses. London: Chapman and Hall.

Mehta AC, Marty JJ, Lee FYW (1993) Sputum cytology. Clin. Chest. Med. 14: 69–85.

Melville and Eastwood (1998) A wider role in managing patients with lung cancer. Nursing Times 19(94): 33.

Meredith WJ (Ed) (1967) Radium Dosage – The Manchester System (2nd edition). Edinburgh: E&S Livingstone Press.

Methany N, Clouse RE, Clark JM (1994) pH testing of feeding tube aspirates to determine placement. Nutrition in Clinical Practice 9: 185–90.

Miller RW, Fusner JE, Fink RJ (1986) Pulmonary function abnormalities in long-term survivors of childhood cancer. Medical Pediatric Oncology 14: 202.

Miller M, Dyson M (1996) Principles of wound care. London: Macmillan Magazines Ltd.

Mills W, Chopra R, Linch DC, Goldstone (1994) Liposomal amphotericin B in the treatment of fungal infections in neutropenic patients: a single centre experience of 133 episodes in 116 patients. British Journal of Haematology 86: 754–60.

MIMS (1994) Handbook of Haematology. Schering Plough Ltd. London: Medical Imprint, Haymarket.

Morgan D (1993) Is there still a role for antiseptics? Journal of Tissue Viability 3(3): 80–84.

Morgan D (1997) Myiasis: the rise and fall of maggot therapy. Journal of Tissue Viability 5(2): 43–51.

Morrow I (1976) Psychological problems following ileostomy and colostomy. Mount Sinai Journal of Medicine 43(4): 368–70.

Morson BC (1974) The polyp–cancer sequence in the large bowel. Proceedings of the Royal Society of Medicine 67: 451–7.

Morton O (1993) Here comes the sun. Nursing Times 89(29): 52–4.

Mould RF (1993) A Century of X-Rays and Radioactivity in Medicine. Bristol: Institute of Physics.

Mountnay L, Sanderson H, Harris J (1994) Colorectal cancer. In: Stevens A, Raferty J (Eds) (1994) Health Care Needs Assessment Vol. 1, Chapter 7. Oxford: Radcliffe.

Moxham J (1995) Smoking medicine 23(2): 83–6.

Muir C, Weiland L (1995) Upper aerodigestive tract cancers. cancer 75: 147–153.

Murphy P (1997) Specialist nursing care of patients with lung cancer. MacMillan Nurse Supplement. December 6.

National Cancer Guidance Group (1998). Vol. 4, No. 3 (June). ISSN 0965-0288.

Nauseef WM et al. (1981) A study of the value of simple protective isolation in patients with granulocytopenia. New England Journal of Medicine 304(8): 448–53.

Navajas MF-C, Chacon DJ, Solvas JFG, Vargas RG (1992) Bacterial contamination of enteral feeds as a possible risk of nosocomial infection. Journal of Hospital Infection Control 21: 111–120.

Nelson-Jones R (1995) The Theory and Practice of Counselling (2nd edition). London: Cassell.

Newacheck P, Taylor W (1992) Childhood chronic Illness: Prevalence, severity and impact. American Journal of Public Health 82(3): 364–70.

Newman V, Altwood M, Oakes R (1989) The Use of Metronidazole gel to control the smell of malodorous lesions. Palliative Medicine 3(4): 303–5.

NHS Centre (1997) Effective Health Care. The management of colorectal cancer. Vol 3.

Gregory et al (1995) National Diet and Nutrition Survey of UK Adults.

Nightingale JMD, Lennard-Jones JE, Walker ER, Farthing MJG (1990) Jejunal efflux in short bowel syndrome. Lancet 336: 765–8.

Noll R et al. (1995) Comparing parental distress for families with children who have cancer and matched comparison families without children with cancer. Family Systems Medicine 13: 11–28.

Non-small Cell Lung Cancer Collaborative Group (NSCLC) (1995) Chemotherapy in non-small cell lung cancer – a meta-analysis. BMJ 3(11): 899–909.

Northern and Yorkshire Cancer Registry and Information Service data 1997. Unpublished.

Office of National Statistics (ONS) (1997) Monitor. HMSO: London.

O'Mary S (1993) Diagnostic evaluation, classification and staging. In: Groenwald S, Frogge M, Goodman M, Yarbo C (Eds) Cancer Nursing: Principles and Practice. London, Boston: Jones and Bartlett.

OPCS (1994) Cancer Statistic Registration. Series MBI No. 22. London: HMSO.

Ottery FD (1994) Cancer Cachexia: Prevention and diagnosis. Cancer Practice 2: 123–31.

Overgaard J (1986) the role of radiotherapy in recurrent and metastatic malignant melanoma: A clinical radiobiological study. International Journal of Radiation Oncology 12: 867–72.

Palmer D, McFie J (1997) Alternative intake. Nursing Times 93(49): 63–6.

Parker BR (1997) Leukemia and lymphoma in childhood. Radiology Clinics of N. America 35(6): 1495–516.

Paterson R, Parker HM (1938) A dosage system for interstitial radium therapy. British Journal of Radiology 11: 252–340.

Paul S, Tarbell NJ, Korf B, Kretschmer CS, Lavally B, Grier H (1991) Stage IV neuroblastoma in infants: Long term survival. Cancer 67(6): 1493–7.

Payne-James J, Khawaja H (1993) First choice for TPN: the peripheral route. Journal of Parenteral and Enteral Nutrition 17(5): 468–78.

Pennington CR (1991) Parenteral nutrition: the management of complications. Clinical Nutrition 10: 133–7.

Pennington CR (1997) Symposium on 'Assessment of nutritional status in disease and other trauma'. Disease and malnutrition in British hospitals. Proceedings of Nutrition Society 56: 393–407.

Penson J, Fisher R (1991) Palliative Care for People with Cancer. London: Edward Arnold.

Peterson (1956) Spontaneous course of cervical pre-cancerous conditions. American Journal of Obstetrics and Gynecology 72: 1063–71.

Peto et al. (1995) Continuing increase in mesothelioma mortality in Britain. Lancet.

Philpott-Howard J, Casewell M (1994) Hospital Infection Control: Policies and practical procedures London: WB Saunders.

Piccart M (1993) Epithelial ovarian cancer. European Cancer News 6(7).

Pierquin B, Dutreix A, Paine CH, Chassagne D, Marinello G, Ash D (1978) The Paris System in Interstitial Therapy. Acta Radiologica Oncology 17: 33–48.

Pollett WG, Nicholls RJ (1983) The relationship between the extent of distal clearance and the survival and local reoccurrence rates after curative anterior resection for carcinoma of the rectum. Annals of Surgery 70: 159–63.

Porter H (1994) Mouthcare in malignancy. Nursing Times 90(14): 27–9.

Price B (1990) Body Image: Nursing concepts and care. London: Prentice-Hall.

Pritchard A, Mallett J (1995) The Royal Marsden Hospital Manual of Clinical Nursing Procedures (3rd edition). Oxford: Blackwell.

Pryor BD, Bologna SG, Kahl SL (1996) Risk factors for serious infection during treatment with cyclophosphamide and high dose corticosteroids for systemic lupus erythromo. Arthritis and Rheumatism 39 (9): 1475–82

Reeves K (1984) More than sticking on bags. Senior Nurse 1(23): 19.

Reheis CE (1985) Neutropenia: causes, complications, treatment and resulting care. Nursing Clinics of North America 20(1): 219–25.

Reid U (1997) Stigma of hair loss after chemotherapy. Paediatric Nursing 9(3): 16–18.

Reyman P (1993) Chemotherapy: Principles of Administration. In: Groenwald, S Frogge M, Goodman M, Yarbo C (Eds) Cancer Nursing: Principles and Practice. London, Boston: Jones and Bartlett.

Richards M, Smith I, Dixon J (1994) Role of systemic treatment for primary operable breast cancer. BMJ 309: 1363–6.

Richardson A (1987) A process standard for oral care. Nursing Times 83(32): 38–40.

Richardson D, Robinson V (Eds) (1993) Introducing Women's Studies. London: Macmillan.

Richelme H, Bereder JM, Mouroux J et al. (1990) La Chirurgie d'exerese du Cancer Bronchique apres 70 ans. Chirurgie 116: 385–94.

Ringden O, Meurier, Tollemar J, Ricci P, Tura S, Kuse E, Viviani MA, Gorin NC, Klastersky J, Fenaux P, Prentice HG, Ksioniski G (1991) Efficacy of amphotericin B encapsulated in liposomes (AmBisone) in the treatment of fungal infection in the immunocompromised patient. Supplement B: 73–82.

Robertson CM, Hawkins MM, Kingston JE (1994) Late deaths and survival after childhood cancer: implications for cure. BMJ 309: 162–6.

Rodgers A (1990) The UK Breast Cancer Screening Programme; an expensive mistake. Journal of Public Health Medicine 12(3/4): 197–204.

Rollins H (1997) A nose for trouble. Nursing Times 93(49): 66–69.

Rous N (1996). Urology: a core textbook (2nd edition) Chapters 9 and 10. Oxford: Blackwell Science.

Royal College of Nursing (RCN) (1995) Breast palpation and breast awareness: guidelines for practice. London: Royal College of Nursing.

Royal College of Pathologists (1996) Standards of Care for Children with Leukaemia: Recommendations of a Working Party. London: Royal College of Pathologists.

Sacks N, Meek R (1997) Nutritional support. In: Ablin AR (Ed) Supportive Care of

Children with Leukaemia: Recommendations of a Working Party. London: Royal College of Pathologists.

Sainsbury J, Anderson T, Morgan D, Dixon J (1994) Breast cancer. BMJ 6962(309): 1150–53.

Salter M (1995) Altered Body Image and the Nurse's Role. Guildford: Wiley & Sons Ltd.

Sawyer M, Antonious G, Nguyen A (1995) A prospective study of the psychological adjustment of children with cancer. American Journal of Pediatric Hematological Oncology 17: 39–45.

Schofield PJD, Jones J (1993) Colorectal Neoplasm II Large Bowel Cancer. ABC of Colorectal Disease. London: British Medical Journal.

Schon D (1987) Educating the Reflective Practitioner. San Francisco: Jossey-Bass.

Shaffer J (1998) Body building. Nursing Times Nutrition Suppl. 94: 63–6.

Shankardass K, Chuchmach S, Chelswick K, Stefanovich C, Spurr S, Brooks J, Tsai M, Saibil FG, Cohen LB, Edington JD (1990) Bowel function of long term tube fed patients consuming formulae with or without dietary fibre. Journal of Parenteral and Enteral Nutrition 14: 508–12.

Sheppard C, Markby R (1995) The partner's experience of breast cancer: a phenomenological approach. International Journal of Palliative Nursing 3: 134–40.

Shills ME (1979) Principles of nutritional support. Cancer 43: 2093–2102.

Shukla VK, Hughes LE (1990) Naevi and melanomas. Surgery pp.1888–95. The Medicine Group UK Ltd.

Silk D (1994) Organisation of Nutritional Support in Hospitals. British Association for Parenteral and Enteral Nutrition (BAPEN).

Sinclair C, Webb B (1993) Aids to Undergraduate Obstetrics and Gynaecology (2nd edition). Edinburgh, London: Churchill Livingstone.

Slade RJ, Laird E, Beynon G, Pickersgill A (1998) Key Topics in Obstetrics and Gynaecology (2nd edition). Oxford: Bios Scientific Publishers.

Snyder-Halpern R, Buczkowski E (1990) Performance based staff development: A baseline for clinical competence. Journal of Nursing Staff Development (Jan/Feb): 7–11.

Sorahan T, Hamilton L, Wallace DMA, Bathers S, Gardiner A, Harrington JM (1998) British Journal of Urology 82: 25–32.

Souhami RL, Norritu L, Ash CM et al. (1998) Identification of patients at high risk of chemotherapy- induced toxicity in small cell lung cancer. Treatment Modalities in Lung Cancer, Antibiotic Chemotherapy. Basel: Karger.

Soutter P (1993) A Practical Guide to Colposcopy. Oxford: Oxford Medical Publications.

Spiro SG (1991) Lung cancer presentation and treatment. Medicine International 91: 3798–807.

Stadva KV, Sandella JA, Bell I (1983) Cited in Testicular Self Examination. Nursing Times 29 (February 1990) 86(9): 39.

Stanford JR (1988) Cited in Laker C Urological Nursing p.270. Oxford: Blackwell Science.

Stanway A (1986) Natural medicine: a guide to natural therapies. London: Penguin Books Ltd.

Stegman S (1986) Basal cell carcinoma and squamous cell carcinoma: Recognition and treatment. Medical Clinics of North America 70(95): 107.

Stiller CA (1994) Population based survival rates for childhood cancer in Britain

1980–1991. BMJ 309: 1612–16.

Stiller CA, Draper GJ (1998) The epidemiology of cancer in children. In: Voute PA, Kalifa C, Barrett A (Eds) Cancer in Children: Clinical Management. Oxford: Oxford University Press.

Stryker JA (1992) Clinical Oncology for Students of Radiation Therapy Technology. Missouri: Warren H Green.

Stutchfield B (1996) In: C Myers (Ed) Stoma Care Nursing. London: Arnold Hodder Headline.

Svoboda V, Kovari J, Morris F (1995) High Dose-Rate Microselectron Moulds in the Treatment of Skin Tumours. International Journal of Radiation Biology Physics 31(4): 967–72.

Sweetenham JW, Macbeth FR, Mead GM, Williams CJH, Whitehouse JMA (1989) Pocket Consultant – Clinical Oncology. Oxford: Blackwell Scientific.

Tanagho EA, McAnich JW (1992) Smith's General Urology (12th edition). Prentice Hall.

Tanaka T (1995) Chemoprevention of oral carcinogenesis. European Journal of Cancer, Part B, Oral Oncology 316: 3–15.

Thomas S (1992) Alginates. Journal of Wound Care 1(1).

Thomas S, Jones M, Shutler S, Jones S (1996) Using larvae in modern wound management. Journal of Wound Care 5(2): 60.

Thomas S, Loveless P (1992) Observations on the fluid handling properties of alginate Dressings. The Pharmaceutical Journal 248: 850–51.

Thompson DG, Cohen DG (1996) Nursing management of the infant with congenital malignancy. Journal of Obstetric Gynecologic and Neonatal Nursing 25(1): 32–8.

Tiffany R (1979) Cancer Nursing – Radiotherapy. London: Faber.

Tiffany R (1988) Oncology for Nurses and Health Care Professionals Vol. 2. London: Harper and Row.

Todd J (1998) Peripherally inserted central catheters. Professional Nurse 13(5): 297–302.

Topham J (1996) Sugar paste and povidone-iodine in the treatment of wounds. Journal of Wound Care 5(8): 364–5.

Toren A, Rechavie G, Ramot B (1996) Pediatric cancer: Environmental and genetic aspects. Pediatric Hematology and Oncology 13(5): 319–31.

Torrance C (1983) Pressure Sores: Aetiology, treatment and prevention. London: Croome Helm.

Trelevan J, Barrett J (1994) Bone Marrow Transplantation in Practice. Edinburgh: Churchill Livingstone.

Trevelyan J, Booth B (1994) Complementary Medicine for Nurses, Midwives and Health Visitors. London: Macmillan.

Trock B, Lanza E, Greenwold P (1990) Dietary fibre, vegetables, and colon cancer: Critical review and meta-analyses of the epidemiologic evidence. Journal National Cancer Institute 82: 650–51.

Tschudin V (1988) Nursing the Patient with Cancer. London: Prentice Hall.

Tschudin V (1995) The emotional cost of caring in caring: the compassion and wisdom of nursing. London: Arnold.

Tulikoura I, Huikuri K (1982) Morphological fatty changes and function of the liver, serum free fatty acids and triglycerides during parenteral feeding. Scandinavian Journal of Gastroenterology 17: 177–85.

Twycross RG, Lack SG (1990) Therapeutics in Terminal Care (2nd edition). Edinburgh: Churchill Livingstone.

UICC (Union Internationale Centre le Cancer) (1978). TNM Classification of Malignant Tumours. Geneva: UICC.

UICC (1997) International Union Against Cancer. TNM Classification of Malignant Tumours (5th edition). New York: Wiley-Liss.

US Preventative Services Task Force (1996) Guide to Preventative Services (2nd edition) Baltimore: Williams and Wilkie.

Valanis (1996) Epidemiology of lung cancer: A worldwide epidemic – Seminars in Oncology Nursing 12(4): 251–9.

Velasco E, Thuler LC, Martins CA, Dias LM, Goncalves VM (1997) Nosocomial infections in an oncology intensive care unit. American Journal of Infection Control 25(6): 458 –62.

Venitt S (1978) The aetiology of human cancers. In: Pritchard P (Ed) Oncology for Nurses and Health Care Professionals Vol. 1 (Pathology, Diagnosis and Treatment). London: Harper and Row.

Ventafridda V et al. (1990) Symptom prevalence and control during cancer patients' last days of life. Journal of Palliative Care 6(3): 7, 11.

Veronesi U, Paganelli G, Galimberti V, Viale G, Zurrida S, Bedoni M, Costa A, Cicco C, Geraghty JG, Luini A, Sacchini V, Veronesi P (1997) Sentinel-node biopsy to avoid axillary dissection in breast cancer with clinically negative lymph nodes. Lancet 349: 1864–7.

Vickery C (1997) Exudate: What is it and what is its function in acute and chronic wounds? In: Cherry C, Harding K (Eds) Management of Wound Exudate. Proceedings of Joint meeting of EWMA and ETRS. London: Churchill Communications.

Vokes EE, Wekselbaum RR, Lippman SM, Hong WK (1993) Head and Neck Cancer. New England Journal of Medicine 328(3): 184–94.

Vost J (1997) Infection control and related issues to intravenous therapy. British Journal of Nursing 6(13): 846–57.

Voute PA, Kalifa C, Barrett A (Eds) (1998) Cancer in Children: Clinical Management. Oxford: Oxford University Press.

Waber DP, Tarbell NJ, Fairclough D, Atmore K (1995) Cognitive sequelae of treatment in childhood acute lymphoblastic leukaemia: cranial radiation requires an accomplice. Journal of Clinical Oncology 10: 2490–96.

Wade B (1998) A Stoma is for Life. London: Scutari.

Wade JC et al. (1982) Staphylococcus Epidermidis: an increasing but frequently recognised cause of infection in granulocytopenia. Annals of International Medicine 97: 503–8.

Walsh M, Ford P (Eds) (1989) Nursing Rituals: Research and rational action. Oxford: Butterworth-Heinemann.

Walter J (1977) Radiation hazards and protection; cytotoxic chemotherapy. In: Walter J (Ed) Cancer and Radiotherapy: A Short Guide for Nurses and Medical Students (2nd edition). London: Churchill Livingstone.

Ward V, Wilson J, Taylor L, Cookson B, Glynn A (1997) Preventing Hospital Acquired Infection – Clinical Guidelines. London: Public Health Laboratory Service.

Watson J, Sainsbury J, Dixon J (1995) Breast reconstruction after surgery. BMJ 6972(310): 117–21.

Watson PG (1985) Meeting the needs of patients undergoing ostomy surgery. Journal of Enterstomal Therapy 12: 121–6.

Wax MK, Yun J, Wetmore SJ, Lu X, Kaufman HH (1995) Adenocarcinoma of the ethmoid sinuses. Head and Neck 17: 303–11.

Weaver (1976) The black cancer – malignant melanoma. Nursing Times 2(15): 582–4.

Wehr M, Richards J, Adair T (1984) Physics of the Atom. Massachusetts: Addison-Wesley.

Weiss RF (1998) Herbal medicine. Beaconsfield Publishers Ltd.

Whale Z (1998) Head and neck cancer: an overview of literature. European Journal of Oncology Nursing 2(2): 99–105.

Whedon MB (1991) Bone Marrow Transplantation: Principles, practice and nursing insights. Boston: Jones and Bartlett.

White C (1997) Living with a Stoma. London: Sheldon Press.

White E, Mackay J, (1997) Genetic screening: risk factors for breast cancer. Nursing Times 93: 41.

Wilkinson S (1991) Facts which influence how nurses communicate with cancer patients. Journal of Advanced Nursing 16(6): 677–89.

Williams C (1994) Kaltostat. British Journal of Nursing 3: 18.

Williams WJ (1996) Haematology Companion Handbook (5th edition). New York: McGraw-Hill.

Wilson J (1995) Infection Control in Clinical Practice. London: Baillière Tindall.

Wingard JR (1995) Importance of Candida species other than C. albicans as pathogens in oncology patients. Clinical Infectious Diseases 20(1): 115–25.

Winter GD (1962) Formation of the scab and rate of epithelialisation of superficial wounds in the skin of a young domestic pig. Nature 193: 293–4.

Wise J (1997) Hormone replacement therapy increases risk of breast cancer. BMJ 315: 969.

World Cancer Research Fund (1997) Food Nutrition and the Prevention of Cancer: a global perspective. Washington DC: American Institute for Cancer Research.

Yamada N et al. (1983) Effect of postoperative total parenteral nutrition as an adjunct to gastrectomy for advanced gastric carcinoma. British Journal of Surgery 70: 267–74.

Websites of interest:

http://www.ncl.ac.uk
http://cancernet.nci.nih.gov
http://oncolink.upenn.edu
http://www.noah.cunny.edu

Useful addresses/support groups

Aromatherapy Organizations Council
3 Latimer Close
Braybrooke
Market Harborough
Leicester
LE16 8LN

BPH and Prostate Cancer – Better Prostate Health
PO Box 2846
London W6 0ZG
British Chiropractic Association
29 Whitley Street
Reading
Berks
RG2 0EG

British Association of Cancer United Patients (BACUP)
(Leaflets and telephone support available)
3 Bath Place
Rivington Street
London EC2A 3JR
Telephone (020) 7608 1661
Freephone 0800 181199

British Colostomy Association
15 Station Road
Reading
Berkshire
RG1 1LI

British Complementary Medicine Association
Exmoor Street
London
W10 6DZ

British Homeopathic Association
27A Devonshire Street
London W1N 1RJ

British Medical Acupuncture Society
Newton House
Newton Lane
Whitely Warrington
Cheshire
WA4 4JA

Cancer Help Centre
Grove House
Cornwallis Grove
Clifton
Bristol
BS8 4PG

Changing Faces
1&2 Junction Mews
Paddington
London
W2 1PN

Children with Leukaemia Trust
London House
100 New Kings Road
London
SW6 1RU

Colon Cancer Concern
4 Rickett Street
London SW6 1 RU
Information line 020 7381 5752

Complementary Therapies in Nursing Forum
Royal College of Nursing
20 Cavendish Square
London
W1M 0AB

Crocus Trust
PO Box 360
Twickenham
TW1 1UN

General Council & Register of Osteopaths
56 London Street
Reading
Berks
RG1 4BQ

Hodgkin's Disease & Lymphoma
PO Box 275
Haddenham
Aylesbury
Bucks
HP17 2UW

Ileostomy Association and the internal pouch support group
Amblehurst House
PO Box 23
Mansfield
Notts
NG18 4TT

Institute of Pure Chiropractic
14 Park End Street
Oxford
OX1 1HH

International Institute of Reflexology
28 Hollyfield Avenue
London
N11 3BY

Let's Face It
(London office)
62 Fortescue Road
Edgware
Middlesex
HAB OHN

or
14 Fallowfield
Yately
Hants
GU46 6LW

Leukaemia Busters
Southampton General Hospital
Tremona Road
Southampton
SO16 6YD

Leukaemia Research Trust
43 Great Ormond Street
London
WC1N 3JJ

Macmillan Cancer Relief
15–19 Britten Street
London
SW3 3TZ

Malcolm Sargent Cancer Fund for Children
14 Abingdon Road
London
W8 6DF

National Association of Laryngectomee Clubs (NALC)
Ground Floor
6 Rickett Street
Fulham
London
SW6 1RU

National Institute of Medical Herbalists
9 Palace Gate
Exeter
Devon
EX1 1JA

National Register of Hypnotherapists & Psychotherapists
12 Cross Street
Nelson
Lancs
BB9 7EN

OVACOME (Ovarian cancer support)
St Bartholomew's Hospital
West Smithfield
London
EC1A 7BE

Tenovous Cancer Information Centre
Telephone 0800 526527

Traditional Acupuncture Society
1 The Ridgeway
Stratford-upon-Avon
Warwickshire
CV37 9JL

Urostomy Association
Central Office
Buckland
Beaumont Park
Danbury
Essex CM3 4 DE

Women's National Cancer Control Campaign
Suna House
128–130 Curtan Road
London
EC2 3AR

Index

acinic cell cancer 193
acral lentiginous melanoma 130
Actisorb 233, 235
acupuncture 308, 315–16, 325
acute lymphoblastic leukaemia (ALL)
    138, 139, 141, 145
  BMT 158
  children 212, 213, 214, 228
acute myeloid leukaemia (AML)
    138–9, 145, 164
  children 214
acyclovir 279
adenocarcinoma 113, 332
  bladder cancer 174
  cervical cancer 103
  colorectal cancer 74, 89
  Fallopian tube cancer 115
  head and neck cancer 193, 194
  lung cancer 93
  prostate cancer 189
  renal cancer 178
adenoid cystic carcinomas 193
adjuvant chemotherapy 35
  breast cancer 63
  colorectal cancer 85
adrenal glands 95
adriamycin 150, 153, 166
Africa and Africans 72, 124, 169, 184
afterloading 17, 21, 22–3, 126
age 1, 6, 7–8, 42, 187
  bladder cancer 174
  body image and sexuality 296, 302
  breast cancer 52, 54–5, 56, 63

cervical cancer 103
childhood cancers 211–29
colorectal cancer 72, 73, 74, 76, 78,
  83, 86
endometrial cancer 110
Fallopian tube cancer 115
haematological cancers 139, 145–7,
  149–50, 152, 167
infection control 278
leukaemia 139, 145, 146–7,
  212–14, 221, 227–8
lung cancer 100, 101
nutritional support 248, 250, 251
ovarian cancer 107, 109, 110
penile cancer 184
prostate cancer 168–9, 173
renal cancer 178
skin cancer 130, 131
smoking 100
testicular cancer 181
vaginal cancer 112, 113, 114
vulva cancer 114
AIDS 154, 271
alcohol 2–3, 10, 152
  breast cancer 56
  colorectal cancer 73
  head and neck cancer 193–4, 207,
   208–10
  lung cancer 93
alginate dressings 238, 242, 243–4
alkylating agents 32, 33, 36–7, 42
allopurinol 144, 165, 166
alopecia 40–1, 222–3, 300

chemotherapy 30, 36–7, 39, 40–1,
    49
  breast cancer 63–4, 69–70
  children 222–3
  colorectal cancer 86
  haematological cancer 153, 164
  radiotherapy 19
alpha interferon 146
alpha particles 12, 14
alprostadil 89
amphotericin 251
anaemia 158, 161–2, 224
  BMT 160
  body image and sexuality 300
  colorectal cancer 74, 77
  Hodgkin's disease 152
  leukaemia 138, 140, 142, 146, 147,
    163–4, 214
  lung cancer 94
  multiple myeloma 194
  non-Hodgkin's lymphoma 155
  prostate cancer 169
  renal cancer 178
anal cancer 76, 841
analgesia 149, 252, 313, 321, 324–5
  children 224
  lung cancer 99, 101
anastomosis 73, 77, 80, 82–3, 87–8,
  200
animal fats 2, 56, 72–3, 112, 169
  nutritional support 252, 263
Ann Arbor classification 10
anorexia 222, 245–7
  colorectal cancer 74
  haematological cancer 146
  Hodgkin's disease 215
  lung cancer 95, 99, 100
  renal cancer 178
anterior resection 81–2, 88
anti-androgens 171
antibiotics 159–60, 233, 256, 262, 280
  cytotoxic 32, 33–4, 36
  herbalism 311
  infection control 264, 276, 278–9,
    280, 281, 293
  leukaemia 142–3, 147, 213, 228
  penile cancer 185
  prostate cancer 170

anti-emetics 40, 49, 166, 252
  breast cancer 63
  children 224
antimetabolites 32–3, 37
antithymocyte globulin 162
anus 21, 81
  see also anal cancer
aplastic anaemia 158, 161–2
Arimidex 61
aromatherapy 307, 310, 312–13, 324
asbestos 5, 93, 94, 194
ascites 109, 115, 118
Asia and Asians 72, 116, 124, 169,
  194, 215
Aspergillus spp 271, 275
astrocytomas 214
atelectasis 94
Australia 72, 132
axillary surgery 29, 59, 62

Babesia spp 271
Bacillus Calmeette-Guerin (BCG) 177
bacteria 275–9
  fungating tumours 232–5, 238, 240,
    242–4
  gram-negative 143, 233, 275
  gram-positive 143
  infection control 266, 269, 271,
    273–4, 275–9
  parenteral feeding 260
  tube feeding 256–7
balanitis 185
barium enema 77, 81, 88
basal cell carcinomas (BCC) 43,
  124–8, 231
  skin cancer 121, 122–3, 124–8,
    129, 135
  vulva cancer 115
basophils 138, 139
Beckwith-Wiedmann syndrome 217
benzene 138, 161
beta particles 12, 14
betel 4, 194
biopsies
  bladder cancer 177, 187, 189
  breast cancer 52, 59
  cervical cancer 28, 104
  childhood cancers 215, 221

colorectal cancer 81
cone 104–5, 117
head and neck cancer 196
leukaemia 141
lung cancer 95
ovarian cancer 118
penile cancer 185
prostate cancer 28, 170, 171, 174,
    189
skin cancer 135
vulva cancer 114
bladder 43
cervical cancer 106
infection control 288
radiotherapy 19, 28, 113
vaginal cancer 113
bladder cancer 3–4, 5, 168, 174–7,
    187–8
body image 177, 296, 302
chemotherapy 43, 176–7, 189
children 218
endometrial cancer 111
radiotherapy 20, 177
bleeding 243–4
chemotherapy 41
children 224
colorectal cancer 74, 81, 88
fungating tumours 230, 231–2, 235,
    238, 243–4
gums 140–1
gynaecological cancer 106, 111,
    113, 115, 119, 120
radiotherapy 20, 28
bleomycin 33, 43, 153
side effects 36, 40
blood 1, 34, 38, 39
metastases 129, 133
with stools 74, 76, 80
see also haematuria
blood/brain barrier 34, 157, 165
body image 294–305
bladder cancer 177, 296, 302
childhood cancers 222
colorectal cancer 81–2, 90
gynaecological cancer 119, 120
haematological cancer 146
head and neck cancer 202, 205–7,
    208–9

penile cancer 186
body mass index (BMI) 249–50
bone marrow
aplastic anaemia 161
chemotherapy 30–1, 38, 39, 150,
    273, 300
children 212, 214, 218, 220–1, 224,
    228
haematological cancer 148, 150,
    153–7, 158–60, 165–6
leukaemia 137, 140–7, 163, 212,
    214, 228
infection control 268–9, 272, 273
radiotherapy 19, 24
suppression 19, 24, 31, 39, 150,
    154, 224
see also myelosuppression
bone marrow transplant (BMT)
    145–6, 150, 154, 157, 158–60
aplastic anaemia 158, 161–2
autologous 150, 154, 158, 164, 219
infection control 271, 292
leukaemia 145–6, 164
parenteral nutrition 262
bone metastases 20, 24, 28, 29, 325
breast cancer 57, 62
childhood cancers 217, 221
colorectal cancer 85
head and neck cancer 197
lung cancer 95, 98
bone tumours in children 219–20
bones
childhood rhabdomyosarcoma 218
haematological cancer 140, 147–8,
    150
pathological fractures 62, 147, 150,
    179
prostate cancer 169, 171
renal cancer 180
bowel 19
habit changes 74, 77–81, 89,
    108–9, 118
obstruction 79, 86, 109
bowel cancer 2, 35, 71–90, 302–4
brachial plexopathy 63
brachytherapy 20, 21–3, 26–8
breast cancer 21–2, 28–9
cervical cancer 22–3, 28

endometrial cancer 111
   lung cancer 98
   prostate cancer 171
brain 19
brain metastases
   breast cancer 57, 62
   childhood Wilm's tumour 217
   lung cancer 95, 97
   renal cancer 179
   skin cancer 133
   vulva cancer 115
brain tumours 214–15
   children 214–15, 221, 227, 229
breast cancer 2, 7, 9, 51–70, 299
   BMT 158
   body image and sexuality 298, 299,
     301–2
   brachytherapy 21–2, 28–9
   chemotherapy 35, 49, 58, 61, 63–4,
     67–70
   compared with lung cancer 92
   fungating tumours 231
   mortality rate 51–2, 53–5, 57, 70,
     71
   nurses 58, 60–1, 67, 69
   radiotherapy 21–2, 28–9, 58, 60,
     62–3, 69–70
   reconstruction 59–61, 67, 68, 301
   screening 7, 51, 52–5, 68, 70
   tamoxifen 52, 56, 61, 68–70, 110
breathlessness *see* dyspnoea
bronchoscopy 95, 100
bronchus cancer 22
bruising 140, 146, 148, 213
Burkitt's lymphoma 4, 156, 213

cachexia 109, 245–6
cadexomers 232, 233–4, 238, 242
cadmium 178
caesium 14, 17, 21, 22–3, 26
   gynaecological cancer 28, 119
Candida 274–5
   infection control 271, 274–5, 284
carbon 235
cardiac problems 146, 227
   chemotherapy 34, 36, 164
   radiotherapy 63
cataracts 19, 162, 204
cell cycle 17–18, 31–3, 35, 38

cell-mediated immunity 269–70
central access 44, 142
   vascular devices 264, 271, 287–8
central nervous system (CNS) 162,
    214–15
   chemotherapy 34
   hypnotherapy 316
   leukaemia 141, 145, 214, 228
   non-Hodgkin's lymphoma 157, 165
cerebrospinal fluid (CSF) 34, 43, 214,
    221
cervical cancer 3, 4, 102–7, 117,
    119–20
   brachytherapy 22–3, 28
   endometrial cancer 111
   mortality rate 105
   pregnancy 116–17
cervical intra-epithelial neoplasia
    (CIN) 103, 104, 112
cervical smears 103–4, 106, 117, 119
chemical exposure as cause of cancer
    2, 5
chemotherapy 30–50, 63–4, 85–6, 97,
    144–5, 204–5, 247
   bladder cancer 43, 177, 189
   breast cancer 35, 49, 58, 61, 63–4,
    67–70
   cervical cancer 105, 106
   children 215, 220, 222–4, 226–7,
    229
     bone tumours 219
     leukaemia 214, 228
     neuroblastoma 218
     non-Hodgkin's lymphoma 216
     rhabdomyosarcoma 219
     Wilm's tumour 217
   colorectal cancer 49–50, 75, 77, 84,
    85–6, 87–9
   curative 34
   Fallopian tube cancer 115
   fungating tumours 231
   haematological cancer 30, 34, 41,
    43, 150, 153–4, 157,
    165–6
   BMT 158–60
   leukaemia 30, 142, 144–5, 146–7,
    164, 214, 228
   head and nick cancer 34, 192, 198,
    204–5
   hydatidiform moles 116

infection control 270–3, 278–9,
   281, 284–5, 287, 292
lung cancer 97
methods of administration 43–4, 45
mouth care 284–5
nurses 48–9
nutritional support 246, 247, 248,
   260
ovarian cancer 109, 110, 118
pain control in palliative care 324
pregnancy 42, 48, 116–17
side effects 30, 36–7, 39–42, 43,
   49–50, 222–4
body image and sexuality 300
infection control 273
skin cancer 127, 133
testicular cancer 184
vaginal cancer 114
children 211–29, 250
leukaemia 31, 138–40, 145,
   212–14, 221, 227–8
renal cancer 178
China 194–5
complementary therapies 309–12,
   315
chiropractic 307, 308–9
chlorambucil 33, 157
side effects 37, 39, 40
choriocarcinomas 110, 116
chromosomes 146, 213, 217, 228
chronic lymphocytic leukaemia (CLL)
   10, 138, 146–7
infection control 271
chronic myeloid leukaemia (CML)
   138, 146, 158
chronic radiation enteritis 247
ciliary escalator system 265, 266
circumcision 184, 185
cisplatin 42
Clark's classification 9, 132
clear cell adenocarcinomas 113
co-analgesics 324–5
cold coagulation 104, 105
colectomy 73, 74, 77–80
colon cancer 2, 3, 71, 73, 75–6, 77–80,
   86
chemotherapy 49–50
colonoscopy 74, 77, 81, 88
colorectal cancer 2, 3, 6, 71–90

chemotherapy 49–50, 75, 77, 84,
   85–6, 87–9
Duke's staging system 9, 75–6,
   87–9
mortality rate 71, 75–7, 85–6
colostomy 80, 81, 83–4, 89
body image and sexuality 304
colposcopy 104, 105, 113, 117
complement system 267, 270, 271
complementary therapies 234,
   306–18, 324
cone biopsy 104–5, 117
constipation 99, 222, 224, 247
contraceptive pill 56, 61, 68, 107
corticosteroids 147, 272
cough 19, 20, 216, 217
lung cancer 94, 97, 98, 100
cryotherapy 126–8
cryptosporidium parvum 271
CT scans 25, 28, 95
bladder cancer 187
children 220, 221, 229
haematological cancer 153, 156,
   165
head and neck cancer 196
lung cancer 95
penile cancer 185
prostate cancer 28, 171
renal cancer 180, 190
currettage 127, 128
cyanosis wheeze 94
cyclophosphamide 33, 38, 97, 150, 157
side effects 36–7
cyclosporin 160, 161–2, 272
cyproterone acetate 171
cystectomy 177, 296
cystitis 36–7, 174
cystodiathermy 177
cystoprostatectomy 188
cysts in the breasts 53
cytology 53, 54, 67, 69
cytomegalovirus (CMV) 280
cytotoxic antibiotics 32, 33–4, 36
cytotoxic drugs *see* chemotherapy

daunorubicin 33, 36, 40
debridement 232, 234–5, 237
deoxyribonucleic acid (DNA) 2, 17,
   31–3

skin cancer 123, 124
depression
  body image and sexuality 297
  breast cancer 62, 64–5, 69
  chemotherapy 49
  complementary therapies 306, 313
  head and neck cancer 206, 208,
    210
  leukaemia 163
dexamethasone 40, 166
diabetes 31, 110, 119, 185, 252, 317
diagnosis 1, 7, 8–10, 245–6, 248,
    328–32
  body image and sexuality 297–9
  breast cancer 51, 53–5, 63, 64–6
  childhood cancers 211–12, 214–17,
    224–5, 228
  colorectal cancer 73, 74, 76, 77, 79,
    81, 87, 89
  complementary therapies 309, 310
  gynaecological cancer 105, 108,
    114–15, 116, 117, 120
  haematological cancer 147–8, 153,
    156, 165–7
  aplastic anaemia 161, 162
  leukaemia 139, 141, 145, 163–4
  head and neck cancer 196, 205–7,
    209–10
  infection control 272, 289
  lung cancer 91–2, 95, 99
  skin cancer 133, 135–6
  urological cancers 186
  bladder 174, 176, 188
  penile 185
  prostate 170, 191
  renal 179–80
  testicular 182–3
  X-rays 16, 24
diarrhoea 224, 246–7, 252, 255–6
  cervical cancer 107
  chemotherapy 41
  colorectal cancer 79, 80
  infection control 275, 276
  parenteral nutrition 262
  radiotherapy 19, 247
  tube feeding 255–6
diazepam 98
diet 2, 10, 245–63

breast cancer 56
  childhood cancers 222–3, 224, 226
  colorectal cancer 72–3
  endometrial cancer 112
  head and neck cancer 194–5,
    203–4
  lung cancer 93
  prostate cancer 169
  renal cancer 178
differentiated teratoma (DT) 182
domperidone 40
doses
  chemotherapy 38
  radiotherapy 11, 15–26, 28–9
dosimetry 26, 28–9
Down's syndrome 138
doxorubicin 33, 34, 38, 227
  breast cancer 49
  lung cancer 97
  side effects 36, 39, 49
dressings 230–1, 233–44, 301
  infection control 282, 287, 288
dry desquamation 19, 203
duanomycin 227
ductal carcinoma in situ (DCIS) 56
Duke's staging system 9, 75–6, 87–9
dyskeratosis congenita 161
dysphagia 247, 261
  head and neck cancer 195, 203
  lung cancer 98
dyspnoea 19, 98–9
  childhood cancers 216, 217
  haematological cancer 140, 146
  head and neck cancer 195
  leukaemia 163–4
  lung cancer 94, 97, 98–9, 209
dysuria 19

ear cancer 23, 192, 196
Egypt 174
  complementary therapies 310, 311,
    312
electromagnetic radiation 12, 15
electrons 12, 14, 17, 20, 23, 24
embryonal carcinomas 110
endocrine disorders 162, 227
endocrine therapy 61–2, 300
  prostate cancer 171, 172–3

renal cancer 178
see also hormone replacement
    therapy
endodermal sinus tumours 110
endometrial cancer 102, 107, 110–12
enteral tube feeding 252, 256–7, 263
enterobacter 271, 275–6
Enterococcus spp 271
enucleation 131
eosinophils 138, 139, 152
epirubicin 33, 36, 39
epithelial ovarian cancer 107, 109
Epstein-Barr virus 4, 195, 215, 280
erythema 19, 44, 62, 203
erythrocyte sedimentation rate (ESR)
    139, 153
erythroplasia of queyrat 184
Escherichia coli 143, 275–6
Eskimos 72
etoposide 33, 37
Ewing's sarcoma 219–20, 221
external beam therapy 20–1, 24–5,
    27–9
    bladder cancer 177
    breast cancer 29
    cervical cancer 28, 105
    endometrial cancer 111
    head and neck cancer 203
    prostate cancer 28
extravasation 44, 46, 273
exudate 238–42
    fungating tumours 230–1, 233–44
    green 233, 242
    red/brown 233, 242
eyes 131
    radiotherapy damage 19, 204

Fallopian tube cancer 102, 115–16
familial adenomatous polyposis (FAP)
    6, 73
family history 55–6, 110, 136
    see also genes and genetics
fanconi anaemia 161
fatigue, malaise, lethargy and tiredness
    aplastic anaemia 161
    body image and sexuality 300
    chemotherapy 30
    childhood leukaemia 213, 227

haematological cancer 140, 146,
    147, 152, 163–4
Hodgkin's disease 215
lung cancer 95, 98–9, 100
radiotherapy 62, 70
renal cancer 178
Wilm's tumour 217
fertility *see* infertility
fever and pyrexia
    childhood leukaemia 213, 227
    haematological cancer 152–3, 155
    Hodgkin's disease 215
    infection control 280
    non-Hodgkin's lymphoma 216
    Wilm's tumour 217
fibre in diet 2, 72–3, 112, 252, 256,
    263
fibroadenomas 53
fibrosis 19, 36
FIGO staging 105–6, 108, 111, 116
flamazine 233
flexible cystoscopy 175, 177, 187,
    188–9, 190
flexible nasoendoscopy 196
flexible sigmoidoscopy 74, 77, 79, 81,
    88
fludarabine 33, 37, 157
5-fluorouracil (5-FU) 33, 43
    side effects 37, 39, 42
5-fluorouracil and folinic acid
    (5FU-FA) 85–6
flutamide 171
foam dressings 235, 238, 242
folic acid 31
French-American-British classification
    10, 163
full blood count 118, 119, 166
    leukaemia 163, 214, 221
fungal infections 269, 273, 274–5, 284,
    313
fungation 20, 62, 185, 230–44, 301

gammaglobulin 270, 271
gamma-rays 12, 13
gangrene 234
gastrectomy 248, 253
gastritis 254
gastrointestinal cancer 3, 245

see also colorectal cancer; stomach
    cancer
gastrointestinal tract 246–8, 252,
    253–5, 266
    chemotherapy 37, 40, 41
    infection control 265, 266, 276,
        279, 283
    melanocytes 129
    radiotherapy 19
gastroscopy 332
gemcitabine 33, 37
genes and genetics 1–2, 6
    aplastic anaemia 161
    bone marrow disease 158
    breast cancer 55–6
    childhood cancers 212, 213, 216
    colorectal cancer 73
    leukaemia 138, 212, 213
    lung cancer 93
    ovarian cancer 108
    prostate cancer 169
    renal cancer 178
genitourinary tract infection control
    265, 275–6, 288
gentamicin 170
germ cell tumours 107, 110, 182
Giardia intestinalis 271
Gleason score 171, 172
gold 22
gonadoblastomas 110
goserelin 173
graft versus host disease (GVHD) 160,
    162, 262
granisetron 40
granulosa cell tumours 110
Grawitz tumour 178
Greeks 308, 310, 311, 312
green bottle fly 235
grief and grieving 327–9, 331
growth hormone 227
gum hypertrophy and bleeding 140–1
gynaecological cancer 102–20
    brachytherapy 22–3, 26, 28
    mortality rates 103

haematological cancer 5, 9–10,
    137–67
    aplastic anaemia 158, 161–2

BMT 158–60
    chemotherapy 30, 34, 41, 43, 150,
        153–4, 157–60, 165–6
    infection control 270, 272
    malignant lymphomas 152–7
    multiple myeloma 147–52
    see also leukaemia
haematuria 20
    cervical cancer 106
    urological cancer 186, 191
    bladder 174–7, 187, 188
    renal 178–9, 190
    Wilm's tumour 217
haemoglobin 160, 119, 138, 166, 139
    chemotherapy 38, 109
    leukaemia 163–4
Haemophilus influenzae 271
haemopoiesis 137–8
haemoptysis 94, 97, 98, 209
hair loss *see* alopecia
half-life 12, 14
hands 23
    hygiene 281–2, 283, 288, 291–3
head and neck cancer 9, 192–210, 218
    chemotherapy 34, 192, 198, 204–5
    nutritional support 247, 255
hepatitis 4
herbalism 307, 310–12
hereditary non-polyposis colon cancer
    (HNPCC) 73
herpes virus 194, 271
histamine 267
histocompatible locus antigens (HLA)
    158, 162
Histoplasma spp 271
hoarseness 94, 195, 208
Hodgkin's disease 10, 152–4, 157,
    215–16
    BMT 158
    chemotherapy 48–9
    children 212, 215–16, 221, 226
homeopathy 234, 307, 313–14
hormone replacement therapy (HRT)
    55, 56, 61, 68, 120
hormones *see* endocrine therapy
Horner's syndrome 218
hospital-acquired infection (HAI) 264,
    271–2, 276–7, 280, 288

human immunodeficiency virus (HIV) 4
human papilloma virus 4, 102, 114, 194
human T-lymphotropic virus (HTLV) 4
humoral immunity 268–9
hydatidiform moles 116
hydroceles 182
hydrocolloids 232, 235, 236, 242, 243
hydrogels 232, 235, 237, 240–1, 242
hydroxydaunorubacin 157
hypercalcaemia 148–9
hyperglycaemia 260–1
hyperkalaemia 144
hypernephroma 178, 190
hypersensitivity reactions 36
hypertension 110, 112, 119
hyperuricaemia 144, 148, 165
hyperviscosity syndrome 148, 149–50
hypnosis and hypnotherapy 308, 316–17
hypoalbuminaemia 250
hypogammaglobulinaemia 270
hypoglycaemia 258
hypothermia caps and scalp cooling 41, 49, 63
hypothyroidism 204
hysterectomy 119, 120
    body image and sexuality 297
    cervical cancer 105, 117
    endometrial cancer 111
    ovarian cancer 109, 118

ifosfamide 33, 37
ileo-anal reservoir 73
ileostomy 73, 80, 83, 88
immune system 264, 265–80, 314
    nutritional support 246, 247
immunosuppression
    childhood cancers 215, 216
    infection control 264, 270–1, 273–80, 282–3, 288, 290
    skin cancer 124, 128
imodium 304
impotence see sexuality and sexual problems
incontinence 186

bladder cancer 177
body image and sexuality 302, 303–4
colorectal cancer 81, 83
infection control 288
ovarian cancer 108
prostate cancer 169, 173, 189–90
India 4
    complementary therapies 309, 310, 311
indigestion 41, 108, 146
infection and infection risk 264–93
    airbone spread precautions 290, 291
    chemotherapy 39, 41, 63
    children 213, 224
    contact spread precautions 290–1
    fungating tumours 233, 238, 241, 242
    haematological cancer 150, 155
    aplastic anaemia 161, 162
    BMT 159–60, 162
    leukaemia 140, 142–3, 147, 213
    head and neck cancer 204
    nutritional support 246, 260, 263
    prostate cancer 170
infertility 42, 119–20, 162, 300
    cervical cancer 117
    chemotherapy 42, 154, 165
    childhood cancers 227
    ovarian cancer 107, 109, 110
    testicular cancer 181
inflammatory response to infection 266–7
inguinal nodes 114–15, 136
interferon 146, 167
International Prostate Symptom Score (IPSS) 170
interstitial brachytherapy 21–2, 26
    breast cancer 22, 29
intracavity brachytherapy 21, 22, 23, 26, 111
intraluminal brachytherapy 22
inverse square law 12, 14–15, 21, 27
iodine 13–14, 22, 24, 26
    fungating tumours 233–4, 238
ionizing radiation 2, 4–5, 13, 17–18
    breast cancer 56

haematological cancer 138
  radiotherapy 11, 13, 15, 17–18, 26
  skin cancer 124, 128
iridium 14, 17, 21–2, 26, 29
  head and neck cancer 203, 209
isolation precautions 283, 290–2, 293
isotopes 13–14

Kaposi's sarcoma 4
kidneys
  cervical cancer 106
  chemotherapy damage 36–7, 142,
    273
  childhood cancers 214, 216–17,
    221
  haematological cancer 147–8, 152,
    165, 166
  aplastic anaemia 162
  leukaemia 142, 144, 214, 221
  infection control 273, 275, 278
  radiotherapy damage 19
  see also renal cancer
Kiel classification 154, 156
Klebsiella 276

lactate dehydrogenase (LDH) 153, 155
laparotomy 115–16, 118
large cell carcinoma 93
larvae therapy 234–5
laryngeal nerve 94, 98
laryngectomy 9, 201–2, 204, 206–7,
    208
  nutritional support 255
laryngoscopy 195, 196
larynx and hypopharynx 3, 9, 192–4,
    195, 197–9, 201, 204,
    209
laser treatment 104, 177, 199, 231
  loop excision 104, 105
latisimus dorsi flap 60
Leishmania spp 271
lentigo melanoma (Hutchinson's
    freckle) 130, 131
lesion infection risk 287
lethargy see fatigue, malaise, lethargy
    and tiredness
leucocytes 139, 162, 213
  fungating tumours 232, 233

leucocytosis 146
leukaemia 4, 10, 137–47, 158, 163–4,
    271, 272
  chemotherapy 30, 142, 144–5,
    146–7, 164, 214, 228
  children 31, 138–40, 145, 212–14,
    221, 227–8
leukoplakia 195
lichen sclerosus 114
limb perfusion 43, 133
linear accelerators (linacs) 16, 20–1,
    24, 27
lip cancer 3, 23, 192
Listeria 271, 278
liver 19, 261, 273
  haematological cancer 152–3, 155
  BMT 160
  leukaemia 141, 147, 213, 221
  infection control 272, 273, 278, 280
  secondaries 100
liver cancer 3, 4, 5
liver metastases
  breast cancer 9, 57, 62
  colorectal cancer 75, 77, 87, 89
  head and neck cancer 197
  lung cancer 95
  prostate cancer 171
  Wilm's tumour 217
lobectomy 96
loop colostomy 80, 83
loop diathermy 104
loop ileostomy 80, 83, 88
lower socio-economic groups 4, 102,
    279
lung cancer 3, 5, 71, 91–101
  head and neck tumours 209–10
  mortality rate 92, 96–7, 101
  nutritional support 245
  radiotherapy 20, 96, 97, 98
lung metastases
  head and neck cancer 197
  prostate cancer 171
  renal cancer 180
  testicular cancer 184
  vulva cancer 115
  Wilm's tumour 217
lungs 19, 196, 275, 278
lymphadectomy 171

lymphadenopathy 147, 169, 185, 280
lymphatic system and lymph nodes 1,
    8–9
  breast cancer 52, 57, 59, 62–3, 68,
    69
  childhood cancers 215–16, 218–19,
    221
  colorectal cancer 75
  endometrial cancer 111
  haematological cancer 141, 147,
    152–3, 155–6
  head and neck cancer 193, 196,
    197–8
  infection control 272, 273, 278
  lung cancer 94
  melanocytes 129
  metastases 128–9, 133, 183, 196,
    197–8
  penile cancer 185
  prostate cancer 169, 173
  radiotherapy 19
  renal cancer 180
  skin cancer 128, 129, 133, 136
  testicular cancer 183
  vaginal cancer 113
  vulva cancer 114–15
  see also TNM classification
lymphoblastic lymphoma 165–6, 213
lymphocytes 139, 160, 218
  B-cells 268, 270
  haematological cancer 138–9, 147,
    152–6
  infection control 268–72
  natural killer cells 270, 272
  T-cells 269, 270, 271, 272
lymphoedema 59, 62, 114, 169, 300
Lyofoam 235, 238
lysozyme 265, 266
lytic lesions 147–9

maceration 240
Macmillan nurses 48–9, 118, 136, 209
macrophages 272
malabsorption of nutrition 247–8,
    262–3
malignant lymphomas 152–7, 165
malignant melanomas (MM) 9, 43,
    129–33, 231

head and neck cancer 193
  skin cancer 121, 129–33, 135–6
  vaginal cancer 114
  vulva cancer 115
malignant teratoma 110
malignant teratoma intermediate
    (MTI) 182
malignant teratoma undifferentiated
    (MTU) 182
malignant transitional cell carcinoma
    174, 189
malignant trophoblastic teratoma
    (MTT) 182
mammography 52–5, 67, 69
Manchester system 26, 28
massage 307, 309–10, 312–13
mastectomy 9, 56, 58, 59, 62–3, 67
  body image and sexuality 297, 299,
    301, 302
mean corpuscular haemoglobin
    (MCH) 139
mean corpuscular volume (MCV) 139
mediastinoscopy 95
medulloblastoma 214
megestrol 61
melanin in skin 121–2, 124
melanocytes 129
melphalan 33, 37, 150
men
  bladder cancer 175
  body image and sexuality 296–7
  chemotherapy side effects 42
  childhood cancers 212, 213, 216,
    217, 219, 227
  colorectal cancer 72, 83
  haematological cancer 147, 152,
    154
  head and neck cancer 193
  lung cancer 3, 92, 99
  penile cancer 184–6
  prostate cancer 168–74
  renal cancer 178
  skin cancer 132
  sperm banking 42, 154, 165
  testicular cancer 181–4
menarche 56
meninges 129, 275
meningitis 275, 277, 278

meningococcal septicaemia 267
menorrhagia 140
mesothelioma 5, 93
metastases 1, 8–9, 20, 24, 28–9, 325
  breast cancer 9, 52, 57, 59, 62, 63
  childhood cancers 217, 218, 221
  colorectal cancer 75, 77, 85, 87, 89
  fungating tumours 231
  gynaecological cancer 106, 108,
    111, 115–16
  head and neck cancer 193, 196,
    197–9
  lung cancer 95–6, 97, 98, 101
  lymph nodes 128–9, 133, 183, 196,
    197–8
  skin cancer 124, 128, 133, 135–6
  urological cancer 186
  bladder cancer 176, 177, 188
  penile cancer 185
  prostate cancer 170, 171, 172
  renal cancer 178–80
  testicular cancer 182–4
  see also TNM classification
methicillin-resistant staphylococcus
    aureus (MRSA) 280
methotrexate 30, 33, 37, 43
  BMT 160
  children 227
  haematological cancer 157, 165
metoclopramide 40
metronidazole 234
mitomycin 33, 36
  bladder cancer 177, 189
mitosis 17, 32, 56
mitozantrone 33, 36
moist desquamation 19, 126
moles and birthmarks 123–4, 135–6
monocytes 138, 139
morphine 98, 209
Mostofi staging 171, 172
mouth care and oral hygiene 41,
    284–6
  children 222
  head and neck cancer 204
  infection control 275, 284–6
  leukaemia 140–1, 143–4, 163
  nutritional support 250, 261
mucoepidermoid carcinomas 193

mucositis 41
  chemotherapy 36–7, 41, 164
  leukaemia 143
  nutritional support 247, 252, 262–3
  radiotherapy 19, 203, 247
multiple myeloma 147–52, 166–7, 271
  BMT 158
mumps 181
mustard gas 30, 194
mustine 33, 37, 39
mycobacterium tuberculosis 271, 278
myeloblastic leukaemia 10
myelodysplastic syndromes 158
myeloid leukaemia 212
myelosuppression 36–7, 164
  see also bone marrow
myometrium 111

nails 41–2
nasal and postnasal cancers 192–4,
    195–6, 199, 204
  possible causes 5
nasojejunal tubes 255
nasopharynx cancer 196, 204, 208
National Breast Screening Programme
    51, 52
nausea and vomiting 39–40
  cancer during pregnancy 116
  chemotherapy 30, 36–7, 39–40,
    49–50, 247, 273
  body image and sexuality 300
  colorectal cancer 86
  lung cancer 97
  haematological cancer 153–4, 164,
    166
  childhood cancers 216, 222, 223–4,
    229
  colorectal cancer 74, 86
  haematological cancer 148, 153–4,
    164, 166
  Listeria 278
  nutritional support 246–7, 252,
    256–7, 262–3
  ovarian cancer 109, 118
  radiotherapy 19, 247
  stomach cancer 332
  tube feeding 256–7
necrosis 273

chemotherapy 31, 44
cryotherapy 127
fungating tumours 230–4
radiotherapy 19, 125, 201, 204
Neisserie spp 271
neoadjuvant chemotherapy 35, 63,
    205
neoplasms 215
nephrectomy 180–1, 191
nephritis 19
nephroblastoma 178, 216
neuroblastoma 158, 217–18, 221
neuroendocrine neoplasms 193
neutrons 12–13
neutropenia 270
    aplastic anaemia 162
    leukaemia 137, 140, 143, 147, 164
neutrophils 38, 109, 138, 143, 214
    aplastic anaemia 161
    infection control 270, 271
    normal haematological values 139
night sweats 146, 152–3, 155
nipple reconstruction 60–1, 68
nitrogen mustard 31, 227
nocturia 169, 189
nodular melanoma 130, 131
non-epithelial (ovarian) cancer 107
non-Hodgkin's lymphoma 10, 152,
    154–7
    children 216, 221
non-small cell lung cancer (NSCLC)
    92, 93, 96
nuclear medicine scans 28, 29, 220–1

oat cell tumours 93
obesity 110, 112, 119
obstruction of bowel 79, 86, 109
occupational causes of cancer 5, 10, 93
    head and neck cancer 194
    urological cancers 174, 187
odour 232–5
    fungating tumours 230–1, 232–5,
        236, 244, 301
odynophagia 195
oesophagitis 254
oesophagus cancer 3, 22, 192, 193,
    196

nutritional support 252, 262
oestrogen 61–2, 110
omentum removal 109
oncovin 157
ondansetron 40
oophorectomy 62, 109, 111, 118
opiates 99
oral cavity cancer 192–4, 195, 197–9,
    209–10
    possible causes 3, 4
orchidectomy 171, 183
oropharyngeal cancer 3, 192, 195,
    197–8, 201
osteoarthritis 325–6
osteogenic carcinoma 219
osteolytic lesions 148, 149
osteopathy 307, 308–9
osteoporosis 214
osteosarcoma 219, 221
ovarian cancer 102, 107–10, 115, 118
    genetics 56
ovaries 62
ozone layer 5, 123

paclitaxel 31
pain 235–6
    bone metastases 95
    breast cancer 53, 62
    cervical cancer 106
    childhood cancers 213, 216,
        217–18, 219
    colorectal cancer 74, 86–7
    complementary therapies 306–8,
        311, 313, 316, 318
    control inventory 321–2
    Fallopian tube cancer 115
    fungating tumours 230–1, 233–4,
        235–6, 237–8, 241–2
    haematological cancer 146–7, 149,
        152, 166, 213
    head and neck cancer 195, 203–4,
        209–10
    infection control 264, 267, 273, 293
    lung cancer 94, 97, 98, 99, 100
    ovarian cancer 108, 118
    palliative care 319–26
    penile cancer 185
    prostate cancer 169, 171, 325

radiotherapy 20, 24, 62
testicular cancer 182
tube feeding 256
urological cancer 186, 188, 190
vaginal cancer 113
palliative treatment 35, 97, 261
    cervical cancer 105
    chemotherapy 345, 49, 50
    breast cancer 63
    colorectal cancer 85–6
    complementary therapies 306, 318
    fungating tumours 230, 235
    head and neck cancer 199, 205,
        207, 209–10
    lung cancer 91–2, 96, 97, 99–100
    pain control 319–26
    radiotherapy 11, 18, 20, 24
        bladder cancer 177
        breast cancer 62
        childhood bone tumours 220
        colorectal cancer 85
        lung cancer 100
        penile cancer 186
    skin cancer 133
    surgery 77
    vulva cancer 114
pallor 140, 146, 163, 213
pamidronate 149
Pancoast's tumour 95
pancreatic cancer 248, 253
pancytopenia 161, 163–4
    BMT 159–60
panendoscopy 196
papilloma 174
paraproteins 147–9, 166–7
parenteral feeding 252, 257–61, 262–3
Paris system 26
particulate radiation 12–13
Paterson-Brown Kelly syndrome 194
penile cancer 168, 184–6
peripheral neuropathy 37
peripherally inserted central catheter
        (PICC) 44, 45, 142
    parenteral feeding 258–60
phagocytes 266, 267, 268, 269
pharyngitis 254
Philadelphia chromosome 146
phlebitis 44

phosphorus 24
pilocarpine 204
piriform fossa tumours 195, 199
plasma 147–9, 166, 250
    infection control 267, 269
plasmapheresis 149
Plasmodium spp 271
platelets 38, 39
    aplastic anaemia 161
    BMT 160
    haematological cancer 138–9, 142,
        147, 163, 166
    childhood leukaemia 214, 221
pneumocystis carinii 271
pneumonectomy 96
pneumonitis 19, 63, 160, 280
pneumothorax 254, 259, 260
pollutants 2, 5–6
polycythaemia rubra vera 24
polyps 73, 74–5
polyuria 148
predisposing factors 1, 2–6
    breast cancer 51, 55–6
    childhood cancers 211–12, 215,
        219
    gynaecological cancer 102, 107,
        109, 110, 112, 120
    head and neck cancer 193–5
    infection control 275–9
    leukaemia 138
    lung cancer 92–3
    skin cancer 121, 128, 132
    urological cancer 169, 174, 178,
        181, 185
prednisolone 99, 227
    haematological cancer 150, 153,
        157, 165
pregnancy 116–17
    breast cancer 56, 61, 68
    chemotherapy 42, 48, 116–17
    infection control 275, 278
    ovarian cancer 107, 109
    stilboestrol and vaginal cancer 113
primary tumours 8–9, 19
    see also TNM classification
procarbazine 42, 227
prochlorperazine 40
proctocolectomy 73

progestogens 111
prognosis 8, 92, 245
  breast cancer 52, 56–7, 66
  childhood cancers
    bone tumours 220
    Hodgkin's disease 215–16
    leukaemia 213, 214, 228
    neuroblastoma 218
    rhabdomyosarcoma 218–19
    Wilm's tumour 217
  colorectal cancer 80, 81
  gynaecological cancers 120
    cervical 117
    endometrial 110
    Fallopian tube 115
    hydatidiform moles 116
    ovarian 109
    vaginal 113, 114
    vulva 115
  haematological cancer 145, 152
    Hodgkin's disease 153–4,
    215–16
    leukaemia 145, 163, 213, 214,
    228
    multiple myeloma 152
    non-Hodgkin's lymphoma 155,
    157
  head and neck cancer 193, 197,
    206
  lung cancer 91, 92, 97, 101
  skin cancer 130, 131, 132, 136
  urological cancers 186
    bladder 174, 177
    prostate 172, 173, 191
    renal 178
    testicular 182
promiscuity 102, 107, 117, 119–20
prostaglandins 267
prostate 22
prostate cancer 168–74, 189–90, 191,
  325
  radiotherapy 25, 28, 171, 189
prostatectomy 171, 173, 189–90, 325
prostatic specific antigen (PSA) 170,
  173, 189–90
prostheses
  body image and sexuality 301, 302
  breast cancer 60–1

head and neck cancer 199–200,
  208, 209
protection from chemotherapy drugs
  47–8
protection from radiation 11, 26–7
protective clothing 283
protons 12–13
pruritus 114, 152
pseudomonas 143, 271, 277–8
pseudomons 233, 242
psychological effects 10, 64–6, 330
  alopecia 40, 49
  bladder cancer 177
  body image and sexuality 294–7,
    299, 301, 305
  breast cancer 51, 58–9, 63, 64–6, 70
  chemotherapy 40, 48, 49–50
  childhood cancers 224–6
  colorectal cancer 90
  complementary therapies 307, 316
  head and neck cancer 202, 205–7
  isolation 291–2, 293
  pain control in palliative care 319,
    324
  parenteral feeding 259
  skin cancer 136
purpura 140, 141, 163

QUASAR study 86

radiation 12–15, 29
  exposure as possible cause of cancer
    2, 4–5, 213
  intensity 14–15
  penetration 14, 16, 20, 25
  safety 11, 26–7
  see also radiotherapy
radioactivity 13–14
  decay 12, 14
  radiotherapy 12, 13–14, 16–17,
    21–4, 26–7
radiosensitivity 17–18, 24
radiotherapy 9, 11–29, 35
  breaking bad news 330
  breast cancer 21–2, 28–9, 58, 60,
    62–3, 69–70
  childhood cancers 215, 220, 222–4,
    226–7, 228–9

bone tumours 219–20
  leukaemia 214
  neuroblastoma 218
  rhabdomyosarcoma 219
  Wilm's tumour 217
colorectal cancer 75, 77, 84–5,
  88–9
fractionated 17–20
fungating tumours 231–2
gynaelogical cancers 119, 120
  cervical 105–6, 117
  endometrial 111–12
  ovarian 110
  vaginal 112, 113
  vulva 114
haematological cancer 149, 153–4,
  156–7, 166
  BMT 158–60
  leukaemia 145, 147, 214
head and neck cancer 9, 192,
  198–9, 201, 203–5, 209–10
lung cancer 20, 96, 97, 98
mouth care 284
nutritional support 246, 247, 248,
  257, 260
pain control in palliative care 324,
  326
pregnancy 117
radical 18–27, 29
side effects 19, 28, 222–4
  body image and sexuality 300
skin cancer 125–6, 128, 133, 135
urological cancer
  bladder 20, 177
  penile 186
  prostate 25, 28, 171, 189
  renal 181
  testicular 184
radium 13, 14, 16–17, 26
radon 93
Rai classification 10
ranitidine 258
5HT receptor antagonists 40, 224
rectal cancer 3, 71–2, 75–6, 80–3, 84,
  111
  body image and sexuality 296
rectum 28, 113
rectus abdominis myocutaneous flap
  60

recurrence
  bladder cancer 177, 189
  breast cancer 58–9, 70
  childhood cancers 219
  colorectal cancer 85, 88–9
  head and neck cancer 199, 205,
    209
  penile cancer 186
  renal cancer 191
  skin cancer 125, 127, 128
  vaginal cancer 113
  see also relapse
red blood cells 139, 266
  leukaemia 138–9, 163
  multiple myeloma 149
redistribution 18
Reed-Sternberg cells 152
referred otalgia 195
reflexology 307, 309–10
relapse 35
  BMT 162
  endometrial cancer 111
  Hodgkin's disease 154
  leukaemia 145, 214
  myeloma 167
  non-Hodgkin's lymphoma 157
  ovarian cancer 109
  see also recurrence
remission
  childhood cancers 218, 228
  haematological cancer 150, 154,
    157, 159, 166–7
  BMT 159
  leukaemia 144, 145, 228
renal cancer 168, 178–81
renal cell carcinoma (RCC) 178
reoxygenation 18
repair of cells 17–18
repopulation/replication of cells 18
  chemotherapy 31–3, 39, 41
reticulocytes 139
  index 161
retinitis 280
retinoblastoma 6
rhabdomyosarcoma 218–19, 221
rhodococcus 271
ribonucleic acid (RNA) 2, 31–2
rodent ulcers 124
Romans 310, 311, 312

rye classification 216

salivary glands 222
    cancer 192, 193, 199
salmonellae 271, 276
salvage chemotherapy 35
sarcoma 4, 113, 174, 219–20, 221
sarcoma botryoids 113
scalp tourniquets 41
schistosomiasis 174
Schofield equations 251
Schwachman diamond syndrome 161
screening 7–8
    breast cancer 7, 51, 52–5, 68, 70
    cervical cancer 103–4, 106–7, 117,
        119, 120
    childhood cancers 221
    colorectal cancer 71, 73, 76–7
    endometrial cancer 110
    lung cancer 91, 99
    ovarian cancer 107–8, 109
    prostate cancer 173–4, 191
    renal cancer 178
scrotum cancer 5
sebum 265, 266
self concept *see* body image
self-esteem
    body image and sexuality 297–8,
        304
    breast cancer 64
    colorectal cancer 82, 90
    head and neck cancer 205
    urological cancer 177, 186
seminomas 182
sentinel node biopsy 59
septicaemia 143
    infection control 267, 274–5,
        277–8, 288
serotonin 246
serum CA125 levels 108, 109, 118
sex cord tumours 107, 110
sexuality and sexual problems 28, 296,
        300
    bladder cancer 188
    BMT 162
    body image 294–305
    breast cancer 64–5
    colorectal cancer 83, 89–90
    gynaecological cancers 119

penile cancer 186
prostate cancer 173, 189–90
shigellae 276
siblings of children with cancer 225
sickle cell anaemia 271
side effects
    body image and sexuality 299–300
    chemotherapy 30, 36–7, 39–42, 43,
        49–50, 222–4, 273
    body image and sexuality 300
    breast cancer 63–4, 69–70
    colorectal cancer 86
    haematological cancer 153–4
    head and neck cancer 205
    children 221–4
    complementary therapies 306, 311,
        314
    endocrine therapy 61, 300
    node dissection 114
    opiates 99
    pain control in palliative care 319
    radiotherapy 19, 28, 222–4
    bladder cancer 177
    body image and sexuality 300
    breast cancer 62–3, 70
    head and neck cancer 204
    prostate cancer 189
    skin cancer 125
sigmoid colon 76, 79–80
silver 233, 235
sinus cancer 5
skin
    damage by radiotherapy 19
    infection control 265, 266, 278
skin cancer 5–7, 121–36, 245
    body image and sexuality 297
    fungating tumours 231
    mortality rate 130
    ultraviolet radiation 5–7, 122–3,
        128, 131–5
skin-tunnelled lines 44, 45, 142
sloughing tissues 232, 234, 237,
        239
small cell carcinomas 3, 193, 93, 97
smoking and tobacco 2, 3–4, 6, 10, 92,
        99–100
    cervical cancer 102, 117
    childhood cancers 212, 219
    colorectal cancer 73

head and neck cancer 193–4, 207,
  208–10
lung cancer 91, 92, 99–100, 101
urological cancer 174, 178, 187
specific immune response 268–73
spinal compression 149, 151, 218
spinal cord 19, 149, 151
spiritual dimension of treatment 330
  complementary therapies 307, 309
  pain control in palliative care 319,
    326
spleen 141, 146, 147, 152, 155
  childhood leukaemia 213
  infection control 270, 271, 272
splenectomy 270
squamous cell carcinoma (SCC) 28,
  128–9
  fungating tumours 231
  gynaecological cancer 28, 112, 114
  head and neck cancer 193, 194,
    208, 209
  lung cancer 93
  skin cancer 5, 121, 128–9, 135
  urological cancer 174, 185
staging 1, 8–10
  bladder cancer 175, 176
  childhood cancers 215–16, 217,
    218–19
  colorectal cancer 75
  gynaecological cancer 104, 105–6,
    108, 111, 115, 116
  head and neck cancer 192, 193,
    196–8, 206
  Hodgkin's disease 153, 215–16
  lung cancer 92, 95–6
  penile cancer 185
  prostate cancer 170, 171, 172
  renal cancer 180
  skin cancer 132
  testicular cancer 183, 184
staphylococcus 143, 277, 280
  fungating tumours 233, 242
steroids 100, 150, 160, 209
  nutritional support 255, 259
stilboestrol 113
stomach cancer 3, 77, 332
stomas
  body image and sexuality 302–4

colorectal cancer 80–1, 83, 85,
  87–8, 89–90
head and neck cancer 201–2, 208
nutritional support 259, 261
stomatitis 222
streptococcus 143, 271, 276–7
  fungating tumours 233
stricture of bowel 19
stridor 195, 209
strontium 24
sugar paste 232, 234
suicide 206
sunburn 122, 128, 132, 133–4, 135,
  136
  alopecia 223
superficial spreading melanoma 130
superficial treatment machines 20
surface applicator (mould) radiotherapy 21, 23, 26
  skin cancer 126
surgery 29
  bladder cancer 177, 188
  body image and sexuality 294,
    296–7, 299–301
  breast cancer 54, 58–9, 60, 62
  chemotherapy 35
  childhood cancers 215, 217, 227,
    229
  bone tumours 219
  neuroblastoma 218
  colorectal cancer 73–5, 77–85,
    87–8
  fungating tumours 231
  gynaecological cancers 119, 120
    cervical 105, 117
    endometrial 111–12
    Fallopian tube 115
    ovarian 108–9, 110, 118
    vaginal 113
    vulva 114–15
  head and neck cancer 192–3, 198,
    199–202, 205–7, 209–10
  infection control 271, 282
  lung cancer 96
  nutritional support 246, 247–8,
    251, 253, 255, 262
  pain control in palliative care 324
  penile cancer 186

prostate cancer 171, 189–90
renal cancer 180–1, 191
skin cancer 125, 128, 133, 135–6
spinal cord compression 149
testicular cancer 183

tachycardia 146
tamoxifen 52, 56, 61, 68–70, 110
taste alteration
   chemotherapy 247
   nutritional support 246, 247, 261
   radiotherapy 203, 222, 247
technetium 221
teletherapy see external beam therapy
tenesmus 74, 81, 107
TENS machine 325
teratoma 110, 158, 182
teratoma with seminoma (MTU + S)
   182
testicles 173
   leukaemia 141, 145, 214
testicular cancer 168, 181–4, 191
   teratoma 158
testosterone 173
thioguanine 33
thoracoscopy 95
thrombocytopenia 138, 140–2, 155,
   163–4
thrombophlebitis 164
thyroid 24
   cancer 5, 24
thyrotoxicosis 24, 26
tissue expanders 60
TNM (tumour, nodes, metastases)
   classification 8–9
   bladder cancer 176
   Fallopian tube cancer 116
   head and neck cancer 196–7
   lung cancer 95
   penile cancer 185
   prostate cancer 171
   renal cancer 180
tobacco see smoking and tobacco
tongue cancer 21, 192, 200
total body irradiation (TBI) 162
toxohormones 178
toxoplasma gondi 271
tracheostomy 201–2, 204, 209

transitional cell carcinoma 174,
   178–9, 181, 189
transurethral resection of prostate
   (TURP) 170, 171
transurethral resection of tumour 177
trophoblastic disease 116
tropisetron 40
tryptophan 246
tuberculosis 271, 278–9
tumour lysis syndrome 144, 165, 166
tube feeding 254–7, 262, 263

ulceration 20, 41, 62, 185, 195
   fungating tumours 231, 232
   nutritional support 246, 247
   skin cancer 124–5, 128, 135
ultrasound
   bladder cancer 175
   breast cancer 29, 53, 67
   cancer during pregnancy 116
   colorectal cancer 77, 89
   ovarian cancer 108, 118
   prostate cancer 28, 170, 171
   renal cancer 180, 190
ultraviolet radiation 133–4
   skin cancer 5–7, 122–3, 128,
      131–2, 133–4, 135
United States of America 3–4, 116,
   271
   colorectal cancer 72–3
   complementary therapies 308
   endometrial cancer 110
   prostate cancer 169
   skin cancer 123
   vaginal cancer 113
unsealed source therapy 20, 23–4, 26,
   27
uraemia 148–9
ureter cancer 168
ureterectomy 181
urinary catheters and infection control
   264, 271, 288–9
urinary frequency 19, 108, 169, 175
urinary retention 28, 269, 171, 186
urinary urgency 169, 188, 189
urological cancers 168–91
urothelial tumours 174
uterine cancer 22, 61, 102, 107

uterus 22, 28
uveal melanoma 131

vagina 22, 28, 41, 106
    body image and sexuality 297, 300
    infection control 265, 275, 277, 283
vaginal cancer 22, 102, 112–14, 218
    mortality rate 113
varicella (chickenpox) 279
vascular access devices 43–6, 264, 271,
    287–8
vesicants 36–7, 43–4, 142, 166
vinblastine 31, 33, 37, 42
vinca alkaloids 32, 33, 37
vincristine 31, 33
    childhood cancer 224, 227
    haematological cancer 150, 153,
        157, 166
    lung cancer 97
    side effects 37, 39, 42
vindesine 33, 37
vinorelbine 33
viruses 2, 4, 279–80
    cervical cancer 102
    childhood cancers 213, 215
    complementary therapies 313
    gynaecological cancer 114
    head and neck cancer 194, 195
    infection control 269, 271, 279–80
    renal cancer 178
    testicular cancer 181
Von Hippel-Lindau disease 178
vulva 21
vulva cancer 102, 114–15
vulval intra-epithelial neoplasia (VIN)
    114
vulvectomy 114–15

washing and bathing patients 284
wedge dissection for breast cancer 29
weight loss
    body image and sexuality 300
    colorectal cancer 74, 77, 80, 88
    haematological cancer 146, 152–3,
        155
    Hodgkin's disease 215
    lung cancer 95, 98–9, 100

nutritional support 245, 249–50,
    259
urological cancer 169, 178, 187
Wertheim's hysterectomy 111, 117
white blood cells 139
    chemotherapy 38, 39, 109
    childhood leukaemia 212
    haematological cancer 137–9, 146,
        152, 163, 166
    infection control 266, 267, 272
wide local excision 58–9, 61, 62, 69,
    301
Wilm's tumour 178, 216–17
wind 74, 90
Wiskott-Aldrich syndrome 216
women 3–4
    bladder cancer 175
    body image and sexuality 297, 299,
        301–2
    breast cancer 7, 51–70
    chemotherapy 42, 154
    childhood cancers 212, 216
    colorectal cancer 72, 83
    gynaecological cancer 102–20
    head and neck cancer 193
    lung cancer 3, 92, 100
    renal cancer 178
    skin cancer 132
wounds
    complementary therapies 313
    dressings 230–1, 233–44, 301
    infection control 275, 277–8, 282,
        286–7, 288

xerostomia 203, 204
X-rays 12, 13, 14, 16–17
    bladder cancer 188
    brachytherapy 26
    breast cancer 29
    childhood cancers 213–14, 219,
        221
    colorectal cancer 77, 83, 87
    diagnosis 16, 24
    external beam therapy 20, 24–5
    head and neck cancer 196
    Hodgkin's diseae 153
    lung cancer 100

malignant lymphomas 153, 156, 165
myeloma 166
penile cancer 185
prostate cancer 171

renal cancer 190
tube feeding 254, 256, 260

zoladex 62, 173
zoster (shingles) 279